HEALTH EQUITY, SOCIAL JUSTICE, AND HUMAN RIGHTS

Important links between health and human rights are increasingly recognised, and human rights can be viewed as one of the social determinants of health. A human rights framework provides an excellent foundation for advocacy on health inequalities, a value-based alternative to views of health as a commodity, and an opportunity to move away from public health action being based on charity. This text demystifies systems set up for the protection and promotion of human rights globally, regionally, and nationally. It explores the use and usefulness of rights-based approaches as an important part of the toolbox available to health and welfare professionals and community members working in a variety of settings to improve health and reduce health inequities.

Global in its scope, *Health Equity, Social Justice, and Human Rights* presents examples from all over the world to illustrate the successful use of human rights approaches in fields such as HIV/AIDS, improving access to essential drugs, reproductive health, women's health, and improving the health of marginalised and disadvantaged groups.

Understanding human rights and their interrelationships with health and health equity is essential for public health and health promotion practitioners, as well as being important for a wide range of other health and social welfare professionals. This text is valuable reading for students, practitioners, and researchers concerned with combating health inequalities and promoting social justice.

Fiona H. McKay is Senior Lecturer in the School of Health and Social Development, Deakin University, Australia.

Ann Taket was Professor of Health and Social Exclusion in the School of Health and Social Development, Deakin University, Australia, and Director of the Centre for Health through Action on Social Exclusion (CHASE) until her retirement at the end of 2019.

HEALTH EQUITY, SOCIAL JUSTICE, AND HUMAN RIGHTS

Second Edition

Fiona H. McKay and Ann Taket

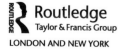

LONDON AND NEW YORK

Second edition published 2020
by Routledge
2 Park Square, Milton Park, Abingdon, Oxon, OX14 4RN

and by Routledge
52 Vanderbilt Avenue, New York, NY 10017

Routledge is an imprint of the Taylor & Francis Group, an informa business

First edition published by Routledge 2012

British Library Cataloguing-in-Publication Data
A catalogue record for this book is available from the British Library

Library of Congress Cataloging-in-Publication Data
Names: McKay, Fiona H., author. | Taket, A. R. (Ann R.), author.
Title: Health equity, social justice and human rights / Fiona H. McKay, Ann Taket.
Description: 2nd edition. | New York, NY : Routledge, 2020. | Includes
    bibliographical references and index.
Identifiers: LCCN 2019056714 (print) | LCCN 2019056715 (ebook) |
    ISBN 9780367281373 (hardback) | ISBN 9780367281380 (paperback) |
    ISBN 9780429299841 (ebook)
Subjects: LCSH: Health services accessibility. | Equality—Health aspects. | Medical
    policy—Social aspects.
Classification: LCC RA418 .T354 2020 (print) | LCC RA418 (ebook) |
    DDC 362.1—dc23
LC record available at https://lccn.loc.gov/2019056714
LC ebook record available at https://lccn.loc.gov/2019056715

ISBN: 978-0-367-28137-3 (hbk)
ISBN: 978-0-367-28138-0 (pbk)
ISBN: 978-0-429-29984-1 (ebk)

Typeset in Bembo
by Apex CoVantage, LLC

CONTENTS

ILLUSTRATIONS

Figures

Tables

CASE STUDIES

CONTRIBUTORS

Kate Anderson is Senior Lecturer in Disability and Inclusion in the School of Health and Social Development, Deakin University, Australia.

Susan Balandin was the Inaugural Chair in Disability and Inclusion in the School of Health and Social Development, Deakin University, Australia until her retirement at the beginning of 2020.

Patsie Frawley is Associate Professor in Disability and Inclusion in the School of Health and Social Development, Deakin University, Australia.

Fiona H. McKay is Senior Lecturer in the School of Health and Social Development, Deakin University, Australia.

Ann Taket was Professor of Health and Social Exclusion in the School of Health and Social Development, Deakin University, Australia, and Director of the Centre for Health through Action on Social Exclusion (CHASE) until her retirement at the end of 2019.

Joanne Watson is Senior Lecturer in Disability and Inclusion in the School of Health and Social Development, Deakin University, Australia.

ACKNOWLEDGEMENTS

We'd like to acknowledge with enormous thanks the interest and enthusiasm of the different cohorts of students who have taken the unit in health equity and human rights while undertaking masters degrees in public health, health promotion, social work, and health and human services management at Deakin University, Australia. Their interest in the topic prompted the research necessary to explore the workings of different human rights systems at global, regional, and national levels, with the aim of offering some demystification of a highly complex and interconnected web of systems.

ACRONYMS

ABS	Australian Bureau of Statistics
ACHPR	African Commission on Human and Peoples' Rights
ACT	Australian Capital Territory
AHRC	Asian Human Rights Commission (an NGO) OR Australian Human Rights Commission (an NHRI)
AHRD	ASEAN Human Rights Declaration
AICHR	ASEAN Intergovernmental Commission on Human Rights
AIDA	Australian Indigenous Doctors' Association
AIDS	Acquired Immunodeficiency Syndrome
ALAC	Active Learning for Active Citizenship, UK programme 2004–2006
ANNI	Asian NGO network of NHRIs
ANC	African National Congress
APF	Asia Pacific Forum: one of the four regional NHRI networks
ARV	Antiretroviral therapy or antiretrovirals
ASEAN	Association of Southeast Asian Nations
AU	African Union
CEDAW	Convention on Elimination of All Forms of Discrimination Against Women OR Committee on the Elimination of Discrimination against Women
CERD	Committee on the Elimination of Racial Discrimination
CESCR	Committee on Economic, Social and Cultural Rights
CHRAJ	Commission on Human Rights and Administrative Justice, NHRI of Ghana
CIHRS	Cairo Institute for Human Rights Studies
CRC	Convention on the Rights of the Child OR Committee on the Rights of the Child
CRPD	Convention on the Rights of Persons with Disabilities
CSDH	Commission on the Social Determinants of Health
DO	Equality Ombudsman, Sweden

ECHR	European Convention on Human Rights
ECOSOC	Economic and Social Council, UN
ESCR–Net	International Network for Economic, Social and Cultural Rights
EU	European Union
FRA	European Union Agency for Fundamental Rights
GANHRI	Global Alliance of NHRIs
HIV	Human Immunodeficiency Virus
HRC	Human Rights Council, intergovernmental body within the UN system (since 2006, Commission on Human Rights before then)
HRU	Human Rights Unit
HRW	Human Rights Watch
IACHR	Inter-American Commission on Human Rights
ICC	International Criminal Court
ICCPR	International Covenant on Civil and Political Rights
ICD	International Classification of Diseases
ICERD	International Convention on the Elimination of All Forms of Racial Discrimination
ICESCR	International Covenant on Economic, Social and Cultural Rights
ICFDH	International Classification of Functioning, Disability and Health
ICRMW	International Convention on the Protection of the Rights of All Migrant Workers and Members of Their Families
ICTR	International Criminal Tribunal for Rwanda
ICTY	International Criminal Tribunal for the former Yugoslavia
ILO	International Labour Organization
IMT	International Military Tribunal
IRO	International Refugee Organization
IPHRC	Independent Permanent Human Rights Commission
LGBTIQ	Lesbian, gay, bisexual, trans, intersex, and queer
MSF	Médicins Sans Frontières, international NGO
NANHRI	Network of African National Human Rights Institutions, one of the four regional NHRI networks
NATO	North Atlantic Treaty Organization
NGO	Non-governmental organisation
NHRC	National Human Rights Commission, India's national human rights institution
NHRI	National Human Rights Institution
NHS	National Health Service
NTER	Northern Territory Emergency Response
OAS	Organization of American States
OAU	Organization of African Unity
OHCHR	Office of the United Nations High Commissioner for Human Rights
OIC	Organisation of Islamic Cooperation, formerly Organisation of the Islamic Conference
OPCAT	Optional Protocol to the Convention Against Torture
PAC	Pan-Africanist Congress
PACHR	Permanent Arab Commission on Human Rights

PAHO	Pan American Health Organization, Regional Office of WHO for the Americas
PHM	People's Health Movement
RINDHCA	Red de Instituciones Nacionales para la Promoción y Protección de los Derechos Humanos del Continente Americano, one of the four regional NHRI networks
RBA	Rights-based approach
SAPATAFHR	Solidarity for Asian People's Advocacy Task Force on ASEAN and Human Rights
SARS	Severe acute respiratory syndrome
SDGs	Sustainable Development Goals
SEARO	WHO, Regional Office for South-East Asia
SHRC	Scottish Human Rights Commission
TRIPS	Trade-Related Aspects of Intellectual Property Rights
UDHR	Universal Declaration of Human Rights
UN	United Nations
UNAIDS	UNAIDS, the Joint United Nations Programme on HIV/AIDS
UNFPA	United Nations Population Fund
UNEP	United Nations Environment Programme
UNHCR	United Nations High Commissioner for Refugees, the UN agency for Refugees
UNICEF	United Nations Children's Fund
UNRWA	United Nations Relief and Works Agency
UPR	Universal Periodic Review
VEOHRC	Victorian Equal Opportunity and Human Rights Commission, state level human rights body in the state of Victoria, Australia
WGNRR	Women's Global Network for Reproductive Rights
WHO	World Health Organization
WTO	World Trade Organization

1

INTRODUCTION

Ann Taket and Fiona H. McKay

Introduction

Since the late twentieth century, a growing body of work has demonstrated the importance of a human rights approach within disciplines concerned with seeking reductions in health inequities. This work has a number of identified, interrelated issues. First is the growing recognition of the important links between health and human rights, both direct and indirect, and across the short, medium, and long term, as well as the considerable overlaps between human rights, the social determinants of health, and the Sustainable Development Goals (SDGs). Second, human rights argumentation provides an excellent foundation for advocacy on health inequities, providing a value-based alternative to views of health as a commodity to be bought and sold in the marketplace, and a move away from argumentation for public health action based on paternalistic concepts of charity. Finally, human rights-based approaches are highly congruent with empowerment-based approaches, now regarded as the foundation of effective health promotion, and with current thinking about the appropriate base for interactions between health professionals and their clients in many fields of practice.

Successful examples of the use of human rights approaches can be seen in the response to HIV/AIDS, improved access to essential drugs, greater reach of reproductive health, and improved health of marginalised and disadvantaged groups. Knowledge of human rights is important at all levels in the health and social welfare arena – from the interactions between a professional and their client, through various levels of planning and policy making, to global health policy and health-related policies in other sectors. Human rights analysis provides us with an important tool to help identify the human rights effects (intended or otherwise) of different policies, programs, and interventions, while rights-based approaches can be used to design policies and programs that will support and promote human rights, rather than hinder them through neglect or ignorance.

Despite a growing body of work on human rights, there remain low levels of awareness of human rights in the public health workforce, by public health students, and in the general public. As an illustration, in a class of forty students commencing a course on Health Equity and Human Rights in March 2010 (with students from all continents across the globe, all with at least two years public health practice), only one was aware of the Universal Declaration of Human Rights (UDHR), highlighting the need for a book such as this.

This book is distinctive in a number of ways. First, it introduces readers to the human rights systems that exist at global, regional, and national levels. Second, it examines how rights-based approaches can be useful at all levels in the health and social welfare arenas. Third, it provides a global view of the range of monitoring approaches to human rights. Finally, it details the role of advocacy for human rights in the design of health-related policies and programs and in interventions to better support reductions in health inequities. The book is global in its scope, discussing examples from all regions of the world. It aims to encourage the reader to appreciate the value of a critical approach to health and human rights by presenting a critical appraisal of successful right-based approaches and a discussion of their limitations.

Social justice, health equity, and human rights

> *Public health should be a way of doing justice, a way of asserting the value and priority of all human life . . . public health is ultimately and essentially an ethical enterprise committed to the notion that all persons are entitled to protection against the hazards of this world and to the minimisation of death and disability in society.*
>
> (*Beauchamp 1976: 13*)

The Ottawa Charter lists social justice and equity among the prerequisites for health, alongside peace, shelter, education, food, income, a stable ecosystem, and sustainable resources (WHO 1986). The report of the Commission on the Social Determinants of Health emphasises the importance of social justice and broad political and economic determinants in the world's health agenda (Muntaner et al. 2009). The work of the Commission involved direct engagement with human rights experts and discussion of the close links between human rights and the social determinants of health (Venkatapuram et al. 2010). However, there remains some contention surrounding the extent to which the Commission's final report granted a sufficiently central role to human rights (see Hunt (2009) and Chapman (2010) for further discussion).

Justice can be understood as fairness, while social justice is defined as 'redistributing goods and resources to improve the situations of the disadvantaged' (Bankston 2010: 165). These ideas are most closely associated with the theory of justice expounded by liberal philosopher John Rawls (1971) and consistent with Amartya Sen's (2009) important contribution on the idea of justice. Sen's work is particularly valuable in terms of its focus on the issue of comparative judgments (comparing social arrangements to identify which is more or less just), rather than focusing on the question of the nature of just institutions and the behavioural norms implicated in these, as Rawls's work did. Sen's work is also fascinating in exploring a much wider ranges of sources, both Western and non-Western, in support of his argument.

Equity means social justice or fairness: 'the term inequity has a moral and ethical dimension. It refers to differences which are unnecessary and avoidable but, in addition, are also considered unfair and unjust' (Whitehead 1990: 5). The concept of equity is inherently normative, that is, value based, while the concept of equality, understood as 'a lack of difference' is not. Unfortunately, the term 'health inequality' is sometimes used as a synonym for 'health inequity', perhaps because inequity is seen as having an accusatory, judgmental, or morally charged tone. However, it is important to recognise that, strictly speaking, these terms are not synonymous. Social justice and fairness can also be interpreted differently by different people in different settings, meaning that Whitehead's definition does not provide a universal standard of measurement. Braveman and Gruskin (2003: 254) attempt to get around this problem by offering the following:

> Equity in health is the absence of systematic disparities in health (or in the major social determinants of health) between groups with different levels of underlying social advantage/disadvantage – that is, wealth, power, or prestige. Inequities in health systematically put groups of people who are already socially disadvantaged (for example, by virtue of being poor, female, and/or members of a disenfranchised racial, ethnic, or religious group) at further disadvantage with respect to their health; health is essential to wellbeing and to overcoming other effects of social disadvantage.

This concept of health inequity, Braveman and Gruskin argue, focuses attention on the distribution of resources and other processes that drive a kind of health inequality – that is, a systematic inequality in health (or in its social determinants) between more and less advantaged social groups, or in other words, a health inequality that is unjust or unfair. As Chapter 2 will demonstrate, equity is closely related to human rights principles. The problem is that while Braveman and Gruskin's definition appears more operationalisable, it still does not remove the element of judgment entirely, although it clarifies it by referring to social disadvantage, understood in terms of wealth, power, and/or prestige. Braveman and Gruskin conclude (2003: 257):

> Equity in health means equal opportunity to be healthy, for all population groups. Equity in health thus implies that resources are distributed and processes are designed in ways most likely to move toward equalising the health outcomes of disadvantaged social groups with the outcomes of their more advantaged counterparts. This refers to the distribution and design not only of health care resources and programmes, but of all resources, policies, and programmes that play an important part in shaping health, many of which are outside the immediate control of the health sector.

Historical background: from the League of Nations to the United Nations

Within Western 'civilisation' the development of the concept of human rights included centuries during which the 'rights of man' covered only restricted subgroups of humans, usually tax-paying male citizens (De Baets 2015). Individuals and groups campaigned for the rights of some groups, such as women and slaves; other 'vulnerable' groups received attention through a variety of treaties, but these did not formally recognise any entitlements included as human rights.

The League of Nations, established in 1920 in the aftermath of the First World War, and grounded in the broad, international revulsion against the unprecedented destruction of that war, was envisaged as a standing international organisation dedicated to fostering international cooperation, providing security for its members, and ensuring a lasting peace (Pedersen 2015). While the League of Nations did formulate pioneering treaties for minorities, refugees, and Mandate Territories (see Chapter 7 for one example) (De Baets 2015), it did not formally recognise human rights (Moyn 2012; De Baets 2015). This recognition of human rights was left for the succeeding organisation, the United Nations (UN), created in 1945 in the aftermath of the Second World War. The UN identifies the importance of human rights in its founding charter (United Nations 1945). Human rights are one of what has become known as the three pillars of UN operations: human rights, peace and security, and development.

Human rights systems: global, regional, national, and subnational

Since 1945, the world has seen the progressive development of a complex set of interacting human rights systems: the UN global system, various regional systems, and a variety of national or subnational systems. These systems are considered in Chapters 2 to 4.

Chapter 2 focuses on the UN global human rights system. It begins by considering the UDHR and the key treaties and covenants within the UN human rights system before giving a short overview of the ongoing development of the system. Next it covers the right to health, provides guidance on how this right is to be interpreted, and examines the considerable overlap between the social determinants of health, human rights, and the SDGs. Chapter 2 then discusses government responsibilities to respect, protect, and fulfil rights, and considers how global monitoring and reporting systems assist in holding governments to account for progress in realising human rights. The chapter concludes by examining some of the key debates surrounding the global system.

Regional human rights systems are considered in Chapter 3. Beginning with an overview, this chapter then considers a number of different regions and their systems in turn: Africa, the Americas, Asia-Pacific, Europe, the Middle East, and the Organisation of the Islamic Conference. An overview is given of the regional charters or statements of rights, as well as the operation of any relevant monitoring system(s). Short case studies illustrate the operations of the different systems, particularly in relation to achievements on the right to health and the social determinants of health.

Chapter 4 considers examples of different national systems. The concept of the National Human Rights Institution (NHRI) is introduced first. The selection of different countries serves to illustrate some contrasts in national systems as well as some challenges in particular types of systems and NHRIs. Sweden, Ghana, Australia, India, and Japan are considered in turn. The chapter then turns to examine NHRIs and their increasing development and integration within the global system, before concluding with an examination of the limited research that exists into the effectiveness of different aspects of national human rights systems.

As subsequent chapters in this book move through the different levels of human rights systems, the intersections with questions of global health governance will be considered in a number of different ways: through the operation of law and the legislature, through policy formulation and implementation, and in practice and service provision. From the 1990s onwards, the increasing pace of globalisation under neoliberal capitalism, accompanied by increasing economic interdependence, as exemplified by the global financial crisis of 2008–2009, together with increasing international movements of people and products, means that consideration of global health governance is increasingly pertinent.

Tools for public health advocacy and action: rights-based approaches to seeking social justice and health equity

A major concern of this book is to examine the many ways that human rights approaches can be used to support health and social welfare advocacy and action in order to achieve social justice and health equity and thus provide an important toolbox for public health practice. Figure 1.1 depicts the different paths that may come into play, through the UN systems, through regional or national legislative routes, and through policy and programming processes. In each

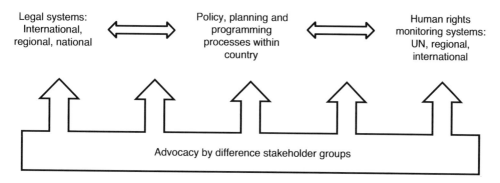

FIGURE 1.1 Multiple paths for rights–based accountability and action

of these different paths, advocacy by relevant stakeholders may be highly significant in affect–ing the outcome.

The different pathways for accountability and action are considered in multiple places throughout this book. In Chapter 2 the use of the UN system is considered, and the links between the social determinants of health and rights are explored; the use of legislative sys–tems at the regional level are considered in Chapter 3 and at the national level in Chapter 4. In Chapter 5 the use of rights-based advocacy and human rights approaches to support policy or program planning is examined. Here the concern is with different rights-based approaches that can be used in real-world processes of policy development and/or program planning and delivery.

In Chapters 6 to 9, four individual human rights instruments are used as a way to discuss issues relating to a range of different groups. Chapter 6 considers the Convention on the Rights of the Child, exploring the role of this Convention in protecting children and the mechanisms within which this Convention works. Specific case studies of child labour and the right to an education are included. Chapter 7 focuses on the Refugee Convention, link–ing its provisions to earlier international efforts to assist refugees. The chapter includes cover–age of Palestinian refugees, stateless people, LGBTIQ+ refugees, and people seeking asylum in Germany. Chapter 8 concentrates on the Convention on the Rights of Persons with Dis–abilities. This chapter captures some of the emerging discussion relating to the rights of people with disabilities in a range or countries and settings. Chapter 9 explores the International Convention on the Elimination of All Forms of Racial Discrimination, including consider–ation of hate speech, the criminalisation of membership in racist organisations, implicit bias, and the negative health impacts of racism. It concludes with a discussion of colonialism and segregation, and the Rights of Indigenous Peoples.

Chapters 10 and 11 then consider the question of human rights monitoring and respond–ing to human rights breaches in more depth. This allows for the inclusion of a detailed discus–sion of different mechanisms for the enforcement and monitoring of human rights, including the Universal Periodic Review System, introduced in Chapters 2 to 4, and the intergovern–mental courts that deal with the most severe breaches. These chapters include examples at different levels: global, regional, national and state, and local.

Chapter 12 will present a range of approaches to advocating for human rights. This includes advocacy from a range of organisations for an issue at a point in time, as well as working to advocate for human rights more generally. This chapter includes a discussion of the role of NGOs in human rights advocacy and of human rights defenders. The work of several different NGOs, including Médecins Sans Frontières, Amnesty International, Human Rights Watch, and Care International, is discussed, and common features of and differences between organisations are explored.

Throughout Chapters 2 to 12, the uses of rights-based approaches are subject to a critical appraisal to the extent permitted by the research and evaluation evidence available. These chapters focus on where rights-based approaches have worked well and identify where their use has been limited or less successful.

The final chapter in the book summarises the value of rights-based approaches and explores current challenges and future issues for exploration. It discusses whether the complex multi-level human rights system represents necessary complexity or needless bureaucracy, explores the challenges of transnational corporations and philanthrocapitalism, and considers the rights of non-human agents.

This book invites the reader to consider whether the value of a rights-based approach in public health is rhetoric or reality, or more specifically, under what circumstances have rights-based approaches been useful and for what purpose. In adopting this critical questioning approach, the reader is encouraged to think about a number of different important dimensions in the contexts in which rights-based approaches are applied: in terms of different levels – global, regional, national, local, and various sublevels, right down to including policy and practice in individual care or service provision; in terms of geography – different countries with diverse socio-economic and cultural contexts; in terms of different topics – such as HIV/AIDS, harm reduction, sexual and reproductive health, and poverty; and finally in terms of different population groups – women, children, refugees, asylum seekers, migrants, disabled people, and people with mental illness. As the various chapters in the book will emphasise, achieving progress towards human rights is inextricably linked with achieving better health for all. It depends crucially on critically examining power relations within communities and societies, and on examining how economic and political structures serve to create and recreate power relations that reinforce and reinscribe various positions of disadvantage and advantage (Taket et al. 2009). While it is probably self-evident that rights-based approaches are not a universal panacea for the public health professional, or any other group for that matter, it will be demonstrated that there is considerable untapped potential in their use.

References

Bankston, CL III 2010. Social justice: Cultural origins of a perspective and a theory, *Independent Review*, 15(2): 165–178.

Beauchamp, DE 1976. Public health as social justice, *Inquiry*, 13(1): 3–14.

Braveman, P, & Gruskin, S 2003. Defining equity in health, *Journal of Epidemiology and Community Health*, 57(4): 254–258. doi.org/10.1136/jech.57.4.254

Chapman, AR 2010. The social determinants of health, health equity, and human rights, *Health and Human Rights*, 12(2): 17–30.

De Baets, A 2015. *Human Rights, History of, International Encyclopedia of the Social & Behavioral Sciences*, 2nd edn (pp. 367–374). doi.org/10.1016/B978-0-08-097086-8.62085-8

Hunt, P 2009. Missed opportunities: Human rights and the commission on social determinants of health, *Global Health Promotion*, 1757–1759(Suppl 1): 36–41. doi.org/10.1177/1757975909103747

Moyn, S 2012. Substance, scale, and salience: The recent historiography of human rights, *Annual Review of Law and Social Science*, 8: 123–140. doi.org/10.1146/annurev-lawsocsci-102811-173847

Muntaner, C, Sridharan, S, Solar, O, & Benach, J 2009. Commentary: Against unjust global distribution of power and money: The report of the WHO commission on the social determinants of health: Global inequality and the future of public health policy, *Journal of Public Health Policy*, 30(2): 163–175. doi.org/10.1057/jphp.2009.15

Pedersen, S 2015. *The Guardians: The League of Nations and the Crisis of Empire*, Oxford: Oxford University Press. doi.org/10.1093/acprof:oso/9780199570485.001.0001

Rawls, J 1971. *A Theory of Justice*, Oxford: Oxford University Press.

Sen, A 2009. *The Idea of Justice*, London: Penguin. doi.org/10.2307/j.ctvjnrv7n

Taket, AR, Crisp, BR, Nevill, A, Lamaro, G, Graham, M, & Barter-Godfrey, S 2009. *Theorising Social Exclusion*, London: Routledge. doi.org/10.4324/9780203874646

United Nations 1945. *Charter of the United Nations* [Online], Geneva: UN. Available: www.un.org/en/charter-united-nations/ [Accessed 31/07/2019].

Venkatapuram, S, Bell, R, & Marmot, M 2010. The right to sutures: Social epidemiology, human rights, and social justice, *Health and Human Rights*, 12(2): 3–16.

Whitehead, M 1990. *The Concepts and Principles of Equity in Health, Discussion Paper*, Copenhagen: World Health Organization, Regional Office for Europe.

WHO 1986. *Ottawa Charter for Health Promotion*, First International Conference on Health Promotion, Ottawa, WHO, WHO/HPR/HEP/95.1.

2

THE GLOBAL HUMAN RIGHTS SYSTEM

Ann Taket and Fiona H. McKay

Introduction

> *Our contemporary human rights system is heir to demands for human dignity throughout history and across cultures. It expresses the enduring elements of the world's great philosophies, religions and cultures.*
>
> Boutros Boutros Ghali (AHRC 2009: 1)

As the quote from Boutros Boutros Ghali, former United Nations (UN) Secretary General, emphasises, it is important to acknowledge the lengthy history of human struggles that have resulted in the creation of our contemporary human rights system. Work investigating the chronology of human rights finds that the notion that all human beings have rights by virtue of being human, back through history and in terms of different major religions, including Buddhism, Christianity, and Islam, from the earliest entry of 3000 BCE (before the common era) until 2002 (Levinson 2003; for a further exploration of this history see Ishay (2008) and Moyn (2010)). Despite this long history, human rights were only recognised on a global scale after the Second World War. Agreement between nation-states that all people are 'born free and equal in dignity and rights' was reached in 1945 when the promotion of human rights was identified as one of the principal purposes of the newly created UN (UN 1945).

The global human rights system provides one important mechanism for holding the performance of governments to account and stimulating changes to protect, promote, or fulfil human rights. This chapter focuses on the basic components of the global human rights system. It begins by looking at the Universal Declaration of Human Rights (UDHR) and then moves on to describe the key treaties and covenants in the UN human rights system, as well as the ongoing development of the system. It looks briefly at the right to health and guidance on how this is to be interpreted. The chapter then turns to examine government responsibilities to respect, protect, and fulfil rights, and discusses how global monitoring and reporting systems assist in holding governments to account for their achievements, or lack thereof. The chapter concludes by reviewing briefly some of the key debates surrounding the global system.

The Universal Declaration of Human Rights

The UN charter established general obligations that apply to all its member states, including respect for human rights and dignity. In 1948, the UDHR (provided in full in Appendix 1), containing 30 Articles, was adopted as a common standard of achievement for all people and all nations (UN General Assembly 1948). Article 1 begins with the basic statement that 'All human beings are born free and equal in dignity and rights'. The key principle of non-discrimination, found in Article 7, states that 'All are equal before the law and are entitled without any discrimination to equal protection of the law'. The UDHR prohibits slavery, torture, and arbitrary detention, while it protects freedom of expression, assembly, and religion, the right to own property, and the right to work and receive an education. Of particular relevance to public health is Article 25, which states in part that 'Everyone has the right to a standard of living adequate for the health and well-being of himself and his family, including food, clothing, housing and medical care and necessary social services'. A universal declaration that specified the rights of individuals was considered necessary to give effect to the UN Charter's provisions on human rights. The Commission on Human Rights, a standing body of the UN, initially chaired by Eleanor Roosevelt, was constituted to undertake the work of preparing the UDHR. For an analysis of the drafting process, particularly in relation to Article 25, see Claude and Issel (1998).

The rights contained in the UDHR are often described in terms of different groups or generations of rights. The so-called first generation are the civil and political rights, including the right to life, the right to liberty, the right to freedom from torture and slavery, and the rights to freedom of opinion, expression, and religion. Second generation rights cover economic and social rights, including rights to education, work, food, shelter, a reasonable standard of living, medical care, and social services. Later in the development of the system, third and fourth generations rights were distinguished; they include the rights to self-determination, natural resources, and cultural heritage, as well as group or collective rights.

The UDHR is a declaration; as such, it does not have the legal standing of a treaty. However, it was intended to provide clarification on the meaning of the terms 'fundamental freedoms' and 'human rights' appearing in the binding UN Charter. The declaration has served as the foundation for two binding UN human rights covenants, the International Covenant on Civil and Political Rights (ICCPR) and the International Covenant on Economic, Social, and Cultural Rights (ICESCR), and the principles of the Declaration are further elaborated in other international treaties considered later in this chapter.

Key features of human rights

As the UDHR makes clear, human rights are founded on respect for the dignity and worth of each person. They are universal, meaning applied equally to all people, without discrimination. They are also inalienable, meaning that no one can have their human rights taken away. Human rights, however, can be limited in specific situations (for example, the right to liberty can be limited if a person is found guilty of a crime by a court of law); this is considered further in the next section.

Perhaps the most important feature of human rights is the notion of universality; human rights are the rights of all human beings. In other words, the most important right of all is everyone's right to human rights. The universality of human rights implies that human rights are fundamental to every type of society. In this way, everyone has the same basic human rights. Individuals may exercise different rights, or exercise the same rights differently, depending on which group they belong to within society. Relevant different groups include women and children, as well as groups defined by culture, ethnicity, or religion. Even if the form or content of human rights changes over time, the principle of their universality remains constant.

Human rights as a set are indivisible, interrelated, and interdependent; individual human rights do not exist in isolation from each other. Consequently, it is insufficient to respect some human rights and not others; if one right is violated, this will often affect respect for several other rights. This, however, does not mean that rights always reinforce one another positively. Sometimes they complement one another; at other times, there is tension or conflict between them. Sometimes they are in direct contradiction; for example, the right to cultural or religious practice for one group may clash with the right not to be discriminated against on certain grounds for other groups. Tensions between rights may also occur when they are effectively in competition with each other for limited resources, for example, the rights to a healthy environment, to an education, to health care, or to welfare benefits. A fourth feature of human rights is that they are inabrogable, meaning that they cannot voluntarily be given up or traded for other privileges.

When considering human rights, it is also important to consider the role of intersectionality. Intersectionality emerged from several theories, including black feminist, Indigenous feminist, third-world feminist, queer, and post-colonial theory. The term was first coined by American sociologist Kimberlé Crenshaw (1989). Intersectionality allows for an examination of rights beyond individual factors such as biology, socioeconomic status, sex, gender, and race, to focus on relationships and interactions between factors and across multiple levels of society. By investigating human rights through the lens of intersectionality, the factors that mean some groups have poorer access to human rights can be examined within the context within which they exist. Such an examination can also allow for the investigation of the role of power and influence from governments, policy makers, families, and communities, among others, in an investigation of the structural influence of discrimination and the prevention of some groups achieving their human rights (Kapilashrami and Hankivsky 2018).

Two different types of rights can be distinguished: absolute and relative. Absolute rights are those where no restrictions or limitations may be placed on them, even if argued as necessary for some public good. Absolute rights include the right to be free from torture, slavery, or servitude; the right to a fair trial; and the right to freedom of thought. The right to life is not absolute; what is forbidden is arbitrary deprivation of life. Note also that the right to freedom of thought or opinion and the right to hold any opinion does not include unlimited right to free expression of opinion. It is qualified by certain restrictions or limitations that are provided by law and that are necessary for (a) respecting the rights or reputations of others, or (b) the protection of national security or of public order, or of public health or morals. This illustrates the complex interdependence that exists between the achievement of rights of different groups within the same community. Some articles in the conventions provide guidance on when rights can justifiably be restricted; this is discussed further when these other human rights instruments are considered.

The ongoing development of the system

Once the UDHR had been put into place, work began on developing more explicit human rights standards and to set in place specific monitoring and reporting mechanisms. This ushered in an extended period of development that resulted in the two International Covenants, of Civil and Political Rights, and of Economic, Cultural and Social Rights, that were adopted in 1966; the UDHR together with the ICCPR and ICESCR are referred to as the 'International Bill of Human Rights'. Building on these, other instruments have developed and expanded the rights for particular population groups and issues. The key features of the process can be illuminated by considering the creation of the Convention on the Rights of Persons with Disabilities (CRPD), one of the latest conventions to be adopted. This began with the passing of resolution 56/168 on 19 December 2001, by UN General Assembly which established an Ad Hoc Committee to negotiate for a comprehensive and integral international convention to promote and protect the rights and dignity of persons with disabilities. The first meeting of this committee was held from 29 July to 9 August 2002. Drafting of the text began in May 2004, and the final text was agreed in the eighth and final session of the Ad Hoc Committee held from 14 to 25 August 2006. Delegates to the Committee represented non-government organisations (NGOs), Governments, National Human Rights Institutes (NHRI), and international organisations. This was the first time that NGOs had actively participated in the formulation of a human rights instrument.

This continuing development of human rights emphasises their discursive and evolving nature. Although the UDHR can be seen as an impressive and inspirational achievement, with significant social justice implications, it is important to recognise that the language used would be rather different if the text were being authored today, in that a more gender-neutral formulation would be highly likely.

CASE STUDY: PROTECTING THE RIGHTS OF INTERSEX PEOPLE

In July 2013, the Office of the United Nations High Commissioner for Human Rights (OHCHR) launched UN Free & Equal – an unprecedented global UN public information campaign aimed at promoting equal rights and fair treatment of LGBTI people. In 2017, UN Free & Equal reached 2.4 billion social media feeds around the world and generated a stream of widely shared materials – including videos, graphics, and plain-language fact sheets. National UN Free & Equal campaigns and events have been organised in almost thirty countries, with visible support from UN, political, community and religious leaders and from celebrities in all regions of the world.

UN Free & Equal has a whole series of subsidiary campaigns, including one on intersex awareness. The intersex awareness campaign runs under the title 'Perfect just the way they are'. Intersex people are born with sex characteristics that do not fit typical definitions of male and female. In many countries, intersex children are subjected to repeated surgery and treatment to try to change their sex characteristics and appearance, causing physical, psychological, and emotional pain – and violating their rights. The UN is calling on governments and parents to protect intersex children from harm.

Carpenter (2018) documents the continuing struggle by human rights defenders and NGOs to modify the International Classification of Diseases, ICD-11 codes for intersex people by introducing neutral terminology and by ensuring that all relevant codes do not specify practices that violate human rights.

See www.unfe.org/intersex-awareness/ for the UN campaign.

A convention (sometimes called a covenant) is a binding treaty, coming into force upon ratification by a certain number of states. Once an instrument is adopted by the General Assembly of the UN or other relevant committee or grouping, it is then opened for signature. Countries sign the treaty to indicate their willingness to proceed through necessary steps to be bound by the treaty. Where the signature is subject to ratification, acceptance or approval, the signature does not establish the consent to be bound, it signals intention, not commitment. However, it is a means of authentication and expresses the willingness of the signatory state to continue the treaty-making process. The signature qualifies the signatory state to proceed to ratification, acceptance, or approval. It also creates an obligation to refrain, in good faith, from acts that would defeat the object and the purpose of the treaty. Ratification or accession are the terms used when a country indicates its agreement to be bound by a treaty. If one were cynical, one might suspect that this allows some countries to maintain a façade of compliance by remaining signatories for a long period or even indefinitely. For example, the ICESCR has been signed but not ratified (as at 11 March 2019) by Comoros, Cuba, Palau, and the United States. In the case of the United States, the signature was dated 5 October 1977, but ratification has still not taken place, while Cuba has indicated the challenges of making progress while the subject of an economic blockade. Once an instrument has come into force, the term accession is used for further countries who agree to be bound by the instrument, this is equivalent to ratification. Table 2.1 shows the nine core human rights instruments, and for each, the date of adoption, and the date the instrument came into force.

Key treaties and covenants in the UN human rights systems

Each of the nine core international human rights instruments create legally binding obligations on those countries that have ratified them and have a committee of experts to monitor implementation of their provisions by states. As well as the core instruments, there are a variety of other universal instruments relating to human rights, a selection is shown in the lower half of Table 2.1, together with the date of adoption.

Particularly important treaties are the ICCPR and the ICESCR; both were adopted by the UN General Assembly on 16 December, 1966. The creation of two covenants, with much overlap (and even more interrelationship) but distinct focuses, deserves some comment. Part of the reason for their division flows from the history of the Cold War, but there is also the distinct form and nature of the two sets of rights they contain (Gruskin et al. 2005). Civil and political rights can be seen as 'negative' rights or freedoms, generally requiring states not to interfere in the affairs of their citizens (for example, privacy, freedom of expression, thought, and religion, freedom of movement and assembly, and freedom from torture, arbitrary arrest, and discrimination); these rights are often referred to as 'first generation' rights. In contrast, economic, social, and cultural rights can be considered 'positive' rights, requiring states to actively implement measures to secure these rights (for example, the right to a clean environment, rights to education, health, and welfare assistance); these are the 'second generation' rights. The Convention of the Rights of the Child (CRC), the first human rights treaty to be opened for signature after the end of the Cold War includes civil, political, economic, and social rights considerations not only within the same treaty, but within the same right; see Chapter 6 for a discussion of the CRC.

TABLE 2.1 Core international human rights treaties and selected universal human rights instruments

Acronym	Full name	Date of adoption	Date of coming into force
Core international human rights treaties			
ICERD	International Convention on the Elimination of All Forms of Racial Discrimination	21 December 1965	4 January 1969
ICCPR	International Covenant on Civil and Political Rights (*)	16 December 1966	23 March 1976
ICESCR	International Covenant on Economic, Social and Cultural Rights (*)	16 December 1966	3 January 1976
CEDAW	Convention on the Elimination of All Forms of Discrimination against Women (*)	18 December 1979	3 September 1981
CAT	Convention against Torture and Other Cruel, Inhuman or Degrading Treatment or Punishment (*)	10 December 1984	26 June 1987
CRC	Convention on the Rights of the Child (*)	20 November 1989	2 September 1990
ICRMW	International Convention on the Protection of the Rights of All Migrant Workers and Members of Their Families	18 December 1990	1 July 2003
CRPD	Convention on the Rights of Persons with Disabilities (*)	13 December 2006	3 May 2008
CPPED	International Convention for the Protection of All Persons from Enforced Disappearance	20 December 2006	23 December 2010
Selected universal human rights instruments (#)			
	Convention Relating to the Status of Refugees	28 July 1951	
	Convention Relating to the Status of Stateless Persons	28 September 1954	
	Protocol Relating to the Status of Refugees	16 December 1966	
	Convention on the Reduction of Statelessness	30 August 1961	
	Declaration on the Human Rights of Individuals Who are not Nationals of the Country in which They Live	13 December 1985	
	Indigenous and Tribal Peoples Convention	27 June 1989	
	United Nations Principles for Older Persons	16 December 1991	
	Declaration on the Rights of Persons Belonging to National or Ethnic, Religious and Linguistic Minorities	18 December 1992	
	Declaration on the Rights of Indigenous Peoples	2 October 2007	

(*) Indicates that the covenant or convention concerned has one or more optional protocols that were adopted and came into force at later dates.

(#) Only a very limited selection has been given here; a full list can be found on www.ohchr.org, by selecting universal human rights instruments.

Source: compiled from information given on www.ohchr.org and treaties.un.org

More recently, during the closing decades of the twentieth century, a third generation of collective rights has been identified, to some extent this arises out of Asian critiques of the first- and second-generation rights as not responding adequately to cultures with more collective than individual norms. These rights include the right to economic development, the right to benefit from world trade and economic growth, and environmental rights. This set of rights is less well represented in treaties and conventions, and remain an important area for future development, this issue is returned to in the last section of this chapter. Sometimes a fourth generation of rights is distinguished to cover the collective rights of Indigenous peoples (for example, Messer 1993; Brinton Lykes 2001; Broderstad 2010). At other times the term 'fourth generation' is used to refer to information or communication rights (Neshat 2004; Shade 2004), and at still other times to refer to intergenerational justice or the rights of future generations (Grech 2009).

When can rights be restricted or limited?

The interdependence of rights has been noted earlier. This subsection looks at the question of what constitutes 'valid' or justifiable limitations on human rights. The UDHR and the two covenants both discuss the issue, setting out the circumstances in which limitation of rights can be justified. They do this in two different ways, first in general articles and second specifically in relation to particular rights. Relevant articles from the UDHR, ICCPR, and ICESCR are shown in Table 2.2. The form of the limitation varies as shown in the table; of particular interest are those rights that may be limited on public health grounds, including freedom of movement and association, but also freedom of expression, and freedom to manifest one's religion or beliefs.

ICCPR Article 4 contains an important exclusion, that of any limitation that involves discrimination on specific grounds. The corresponding article in the ICESCR is perhaps less precise (and thus less useful) in its formulation. Recognising the difficulty of the judgments that need to be exercised in deciding whether a specific limitation of rights is justified or not, work was carried out to formulate a series of principles to help decide whether limitations are just or not. This resulted in the five Siracusa Principles (ECOSOC 1984). These principles state that, when a government limits the exercise or enjoyment of a right, this action must be taken as a last resort and will only be considered legitimate if the following five criteria are met: the restriction is provided for and carried out in accordance with the law; the restriction is in the interest of a legitimate objective of general interest; the restriction is strictly necessary in a democratic society to achieve this objective; there are no less intrusive and restrictive means available to reach the same goal, and; the restriction is not imposed arbitrarily, that is, in an unreasonable or otherwise discriminatory manner. In the case of restriction on the grounds of protection of public health, Gostin, quoted in Coker (2001), suggests the following specific criteria for use: risk posed should be demonstrable and significant; proposed interventions should be demonstrably effective; approach should be cost-effective; sanctions should be least restrictive necessary; policy should be fair and non-discriminatory.

Within public health, infectious diseases present one of the clearest examples where restrictions of human rights need to be considered. The HIV/AIDS pandemic, SARS (Lam et al. 2003), swine flu (Pada and Tambyah 2011), and Ebola (Barbisch et al. 2015), have provided many instances where restrictions have been introduced affecting rights to freedom of movement. Some websites (for example, www.hivtravel.org) give information about restrictions

TABLE 2.2 Articles relating to limitation or restriction of rights

Treaty and article	Text
UDHR, Article 29	1. Everyone has duties to the community in which alone the free and full development of his personality is possible. 2. In the exercise of his rights and freedoms, everyone shall be subject only to such limitations as are determined by law solely for the purpose of securing due recognition and respect for the rights and freedoms of others and of meeting the just requirements of morality, public order and the general welfare in a democratic society. 3. These rights and freedoms may in no case be exercised contrary to the purposes and principles of the United Nations.
ICCPR, Article 4	i. [I]n time of public emergency which threatens the life of the nation and the existence of which is officially proclaimed, the States Parties to the present Covenant may take measures derogating from their obligations under the present Covenant to the extent strictly required by the exigencies of the situation, provided that such measures are not inconsistent with their other obligations under international law and do not involve discrimination solely on the grounds of race, colour, sex, language, religion or social origin.'
ICESCR, Article 4	The States Parties to the present Covenant recognize that, in the enjoyment of those rights provided by the State in conformity with the present Covenant, the State may subject such rights only to such limitations as are determined by law only in so far as this may be compatible with the nature of these rights and solely for the purpose of promoting the general welfare in a democratic society.
ICCPR, Article 12, freedom of movement	. . . . not be subject to any restrictions except those which are provided by law, are necessary to protect national security, public order (ordre public), public health or morals or the rights and freedoms of others
ICCPR, Article 18, para 3. freedom to manifest one's religion or beliefs	Freedom to manifest one's religion or beliefs may be subject only to such limitations as are prescribed by law and are necessary to protect public safety, order, health, or morals or the fundamental rights and freedoms of others.
ICCPR, Article 19, para 2. freedom of expression	The exercise of the rights provided for in paragraph 2 of this article carries with it special duties and responsibilities. It may therefore be subject to certain restrictions, but these shall only be such as are provided by law and are necessary: (a) For respect of the rights or reputations of others; (b) For the protection of national security or of public order (ordre public), or of public health or morals.
ICCPR, Article 21, peaceful assembly and ICCPR, Article 22, freedom of association with others, including the right to form and join trade unions	No restrictions may be placed on the exercise of this right other than those imposed in conformity with the law and which are necessary in a democratic society in the interests of national security or public safety, public order (ordre public), the protection of public health or morals or the protection of the rights and freedoms of others.
ICESCR, Article 8, trade unions	. . . . subject to no limitations other than those prescribed by law and which are necessary in a democratic society in the interests of national security or public order or for the protection of the rights and freedoms of others;

Source: compiled from www.ohchr.org

on the freedom of movement for people who are HIV positive, including requirements for HIV testing prior to entry for different countries. Application of the public health version of the Siracusa Principles suggests that none of these restrictions can be justified on public health grounds. In applying the public health version of the Siracusa Principles given above, Gostin and Lazzarini on HIV (1997: 66) stress the importance of careful determination of significant risk:

> *Significant risk must be determined on a case by case basis through fact specific individual inquiries. Blanket rules or generalizations about a class of persons with HIV infection do not suffice. The risk must be 'significant', not merely speculative or remote. For example, theoretically, a person could transmit HIV by biting, spitting, or splattering blood, but the actual risk is extremely low (approaching zero). Likewise, an HIV positive health professional who does not perform deeply invasive procedures is highly unlikely to transmit HIV to a patient. Present knowledge does not support screening or excluding that person from the health care profession because, lacking a real and substantial possibility of HIV transmission, such policies do not meet the significant risk test.*

Human rights, the social and cultural determinants of health, and the sustainable development goals

> *There is a powerful synergy between health and rights. By design, neglect or ignorance, health policies and programs can promote and protect or conversely restrict and violate human rights. Similarly, the promotion, protection, restriction or violation of human rights can have direct impacts on health.*
>
> *Brundtland (2005: 61)*

In this quote Gro Harlem Brundtland, the Director General of WHO in 2005, refers to the understanding that the major determinants of better health often lie outside the health system and include the fulfilment of an array of rights that are relevant to promoting and protecting health. Health policies, programs, and practices, in and of themselves, can promote and protect, or restrict and violate, human rights, by design, neglect, or ignorance. Throughout the rest of the book, many examples are given of the rights implications of policies and programs. There are many areas where human rights have an impact on health. Firstly, human rights violations can directly affect health, for example, harmful traditional practices, torture, slavery, and violence against women and children; these effects on health can be in the short, medium, or long term. Secondly, vulnerability to ill health can be reduced through the promotion of human rights, for example, the rights to health, to education, to food and nutrition, and to freedom from discrimination. Promotion, protection, and restriction or violations of human rights all have both direct and indirect impacts on health and wellbeing; these can be proximal or distal. Since the 1980s, the HIV/AIDS pandemic and reproductive and sexual health concerns in particular have been instrumental in clarifying the interrelationships between health and human rights (Gruskin et al. 2007). This is considered further in Chapter 5.

The year 2015 saw the formulation of the seventeen Sustainable Development Goals (SDGs), which

> *seek to build on the Millennium Development Goals and complete what they did not achieve. They seek to realize the human rights of all and to achieve gender equality and the empowerment*

of all women and girls. They are integrated and indivisible and balance the three dimensions of sustainable development: the economic, social and environmental.

(UN 2015: 5)

The links between human rights, the social and cultural determinants of health and the SDGs are many and direct; see Table 2.3. Rights to education, employment and occupation, food, shelter, water, sanitation, safety, and freedom of movement and expression include many of the factors understood as social determinants of health (CSDH 2008). Thus, action taken to support a broad range of human rights can be understood as supporting health, and similarly action on many social determinants of health, with attention to moving towards health equity, is also action to support human rights. Similarly, achievements in different SDGs will support the achievement of human rights and vice versa. The SDGs can be regarded as giving a useful analytic framework for considering the social, economic, and environmental determinants of health.

The 'right to health'

The enjoyment of the highest attainable standard of health is one of the fundamental rights of every human being.

(Preamble to the WHO Constitution)

One particularly important human right for public health practitioners is the 'right to health'. This is stated directly in the preamble to the WHO constitution; Article 25 of the UDHR mentions 'health and wellbeing', and Article 12 of the ICESCR is more explicit (see Table 2.3). This explicit recognition of the highest attainable standard of health as a 'human right' as opposed to a good or commodity with a charitable construct provides a very powerful basis for public health and health promotion advocacy. It is important to note that the ICESCR mentions explicitly both mental health and physical health but does not include social health (as the WHO Constitution did); many have seen this as unfortunate. Other international human rights instruments also address the right to health, both generally and in relation to specific groups, for example: ICERD Article 5(e)(iv); CEDAW Articles 11(1)(f), 12, and 14(2)(b); CRC Article 24; ICRMW Articles 28, 43(e), and 45(c); and CRPD Article 25. In thinking about the implications of the right to health, Mary Robinson, a previous UN High Commissioner for Human Rights, expresses some important key features:

The right to health does not mean the right to be healthy, nor does it mean that poor governments must put in place expensive health services for which they have no resources. But it does require governments and public authorities to put in place policies and action plans which will lead to available and accessible health care for all in the shortest possible time. To ensure that this happens is the challenge facing both the human rights community and public health professionals.

WHO (2002: 9)

The monitoring committee responsible for the ICESCR formulated General Comment 14, issued by the UN Committee on Economic, Social, and Cultural Rights in 2000 (CESCR 2000), and the UN Office of the High Commissioner for Human Rights and WHO have

TABLE 2.3 Human rights, the social and cultural determinants of health, and the sustainable development goals

Social and cultural determinants of health	References in UDHR and key conventions	Social development goals: 'No-one left behind'
Income and poverty Living conditions, including food, water, sanitation Housing	**UDHR, Article 25.** (1) Everyone has the right to a standard of living adequate for the health and well-being of himself and of his family, including food, clothing, housing and medical care and necessary social services, and the right to security in the event of unemployment, sickness, disability, widowhood, old age or other lack of livelihood in circumstances beyond his control. (2) Motherhood and childhood are entitled to special care and assistance. All children, whether born in or out of wedlock, shall enjoy the same social protection.	1: No Poverty 2: Zero Hunger 3: Good Health and Wellbeing 5: Gender Equality 6: Clean Water and Sanitation 7: Affordable and Clean Energy 11: Sustainable Cities and Communities 16: Peace, Justice and Strong Institutions
Employment and occupation	**UDHR, Article 23.** (1) Everyone has the right to work, to free choice of employment, to just and favourable conditions of work and to protection against unemployment. (2) Everyone, without any discrimination, has the right to equal pay for equal work. (3) Everyone who works has the right to just and favourable remuneration ensuring for himself and his family an existence worthy of human dignity, and supplemented, if necessary, by other means of social protection. (4) Everyone has the right to form and to join trade unions for the protection of his interests. **Article 24.** Everyone has the right to rest and leisure, including reasonable limitation of working hours and periodic holidays with pay.	8: Decent Work and Economic Growth 10: Reduced Inequality
Education	**UDHR, Article 26.** (1) Everyone has the right to education. Education shall be free, at least in the elementary and fundamental stages. Elementary education shall be compulsory. Technical and professional education shall be made generally available and higher education shall be equally accessible to all on the basis of merit. (2) Education shall be directed to the full development of the human personality and to the strengthening of respect for human rights and fundamental freedoms. It shall promote understanding, tolerance, and friendship among all nations, racial or religious groups, and shall further the activities of the United Nations for the maintenance of peace. (3) Parents have a prior right to choose the kind of education that shall be given to their children. See also ICESCR, Article 13	4: Quality Education

Transport | None explicitly | 11: Sustainable Cities and Communities

Culture and ethnicity
Gender and age

5: Gender Equality
8: Decent Work and Economic Growth
10: Reduced Inequality
11: Sustainable Cities and Communities
12: Sustainable Consumption and Production

UDHR, Article 1

All human beings are born free and equal in dignity and rights. They are endowed with reason and conscience and should act towards one another in a spirit of brotherhood.

UDRH, Article 2

Everyone is entitled to all the rights and freedoms set forth in this Declaration, without distinction of any kind, such as race, colour, sex, language, religion, political or other opinion, national or social origin, property, birth or other status.

Furthermore, no distinction shall be made on the basis of the political, jurisdictional, or international status of the country or territory to which a person belongs, whether it be independent, trust, non-self-governing or under any other limitation of sovereignty.

ICCPR, Article 18

1. Everyone shall have the right to freedom of thought, conscience, and religion. This right shall include freedom to have or to adopt a religion or belief of his choice, and freedom, either individually or in community with others and in public or private, to manifest his religion or belief in worship, observance, practice, and teaching.

2. No one shall be subject to coercion which would impair his freedom to have or to adopt a religion or belief of his choice.

3. Freedom to manifest one's religion or beliefs may be subject only to such limitations as are prescribed by law and are necessary to protect public safety, order, health, or morals or the fundamental rights and freedoms of others.

4. The States Parties to the present Covenant undertake to have respect for the liberty of parents and, when applicable, legal guardians to ensure the religious and moral education of their children in conformity with their own convictions.

ICCPR, Article 26

All persons are equal before the law and are entitled without any discrimination to the equal protection of the law. In this respect, the law shall prohibit any discrimination and guarantee to all persons equal and effective protection against discrimination on any ground such as race, colour, sex, language, religion, political or other opinion, national or social origin, property, birth or other status.

See also Conventions on: Elimination of Racial Discrimination; Elimination of All Forms of Discrimination against Women; Rights of the Child; Rights of Migrant Workers and their Families; Rights of Persons with Disabilities; Protection of All Persons from Enforced Disappearances.

(Continued)

TABLE 2.3 (Continued)

Social and cultural determinants of health	References in UDHR and key conventions	Social development goals: 'No-one left behind'

Population-based services and facilities	**ICESCR, Article 12**
	
	 1. The States Parties to the present Covenant recognize the right of everyone to the enjoyment of the highest attainable standard of physical and mental health.
	 2. The steps to be taken by the States Parties to the present Covenant to achieve the full realization of this right shall include those necessary for:
	   (a) The provision for the reduction of the stillbirth-rate and of infant mortality and for the healthy development of the child;
	   (b) The improvement of all aspects of environmental and industrial hygiene;
	   (c) The prevention, treatment and control of epidemic, endemic, occupational, and other diseases;
	   (d) The creation of conditions which would assure to all medical service and medical attention in the event of sickness.
		3: Good Health and Wellbeing

Social cohesion and social support	**UDHR, Article 22** Everyone, as a member of society, has the right to social security and is entitled to realization, through national effort and international cooperation and in accordance with the organization and resources of each State, of the economic, social, and cultural rights indispensable for his dignity and the free development of his personality. **UDHR, Article 29.** (1) Everyone has duties to the community in which alone the free and full development of his personality is possible. (2) In the exercise of his rights and freedoms, everyone shall be subject only to such limitations as are determined by law solely for the purpose of securing due recognition and respect for the rights and freedoms of others and of meeting the just requirements of morality, public order, and the general welfare in a democratic society. (3) These rights and freedoms may in no case be exercised contrary to the purposes and principles of the United Nations.	10: Reduced Inequality 11: Sustainable Cities and Communities 16: Peace, Justice and Strong Institutions

produced a fact sheet on the right to health to assist countries move towards the right to health (WHO 2008). One of the key normative points about the right to health is that it extends to the underlying determinants of health (CESCR 2000, paragraph 4, 10 and 11); this specifically includes many of the other rights that have considerable overlaps with the social and cultural determinants of health and the SDGs. Also important is the participation of the population in all health-related decision-making at community, national, and international levels (CESCR 2000, paragraph 11, 17, 34 and 54).

General Comment 14 (CESCR 2000) makes clear that the right to health is not to be understood as the 'right to be healthy', this being impossible to achieve or guarantee. The notion of 'the highest attainable standard of health' in ICESCR Article 12.1 takes into account both the individual's biological and socio-economic preconditions and a state's available resources. Genetic factors, individual susceptibility to ill health, and the adoption of unhealthy or risky lifestyles all influence an individual's health. The right to health contains both freedoms and entitlements. The freedoms include the right to control one's health and body, including sexual and reproductive freedom, and the right to be free from interference, such as the right to be free from torture, non-consensual medical treatment, and experimentation. Entitlements include the right to a system of health protection which provides equality of opportunity for people to enjoy the highest attainable level of health and the participation of the population in all health-related decision-making at the community, national, and international levels.

The right to health includes the right of access to a variety of facilities, goods, services, and conditions necessary for the realisation of the highest attainable standard of health. According to General Comment 14 (CESCR 2000), the right to health contains four interrelated and essential elements: availability, accessibility, acceptability, and quality. Within some of the elements, there is the potential for tensions or outright conflicts, for example potential conflicts may occur in the item on acceptability through differences between medical ethics and the notions of cultural appropriateness held by particular groups. The notion of core obligations is also important. These were introduced in General Comment 3 on 'The nature of states parties' obligations' (CESCR 1990) which confirms that states parties have a core obligation to ensure the satisfaction of, at the very least, minimum essential levels of each of the rights in the Covenant. General Comment 14 (CESCR 2000) expands this by stating that the core obligations of the right to health include those given as the essential components of primary health care enshrined in the Alma Ata Declaration (CESCR 2000, paragraphs 43 and 44). In the case of HIV/AIDS, more specific elaborations have been given by WHO and the UN Human Rights Commission (World Health Assembly 2000; Commission on Human Rights 2001) ensuring the provision and affordability of drugs.

The appearance of the content of the Alma Ata Declaration within General Comment 14 was a direct result of WHO's re-engagement with the developing global human rights system from 1973 onwards (Meier 2010). Meier (2010) distinguishes three separate periods of WHO's involvement in global human rights. During the first (1948–1952), WHO was closely involved with the initial stages of discussion and drafting for what was to become the ICESCR, arguing for the broad understanding of health given in WHO's Constitution, and for explicit consideration of health promotion. During the second period (1953–1973), as the drafting process was completed, WHO remained on the side lines, concentrating on a biomedical approach with vertical disease specific approaches to international public health, and the resulting Article 12 in the ICESCR, reflects a much narrower conception of health.

By the 1973 election of Halfdan Mahler as Director General of WHO, the epidemiological transition and the recognition of the challenges of non-communicable diseases, coupled with the failure of vertical disease-based programs in cases such as malaria, had created a different climate, and WHO re-engaged with human rights, initially through espousing a needs-based approach to health development through primary health care, and resulting, in 1978, in Article 1 of the Alma Ata Declaration:

> *The Conference strongly reaffirms that health, which is a state of complete physical, mental and social wellbeing, and not merely the absence of disease or infirmity, is a fundamental human right and that the attainment of the highest possible level of health is a most important world-wide social goal whose realization requires the action of many other social and economic sectors in addition to the health sector.*

Throughout the foregoing and specifically in discussion of accessibility, the right to freedom from discrimination has been argued as particularly important. According to Jonathan Mann, Director of the Global Programme on HIV/AIDS from 1986 to 1990 and founding Director of the Francois-Xavier Bagnoud Center for Health and Human Rights at Harvard University:

> *Public health practice is heavily burdened by the problem of inadvertent discrimination. For example, outreach activities may 'assume' that all populations are reached equally by a single, dominant-language message on television; or analysis 'forgets' to include health problems uniquely relevant to certain groups, like breast cancer or sickle cell disease; or a problem 'ignores' the actual response capability of different population groups, as when lead poisoning warnings are given without concern for financial ability to ensure lead abatement. Indeed, inadvertent discrimination is so prevalent that all public health policies and programmes should be considered discriminatory until proven otherwise, placing the burden on public health to affirm and ensure its respect for human rights.*
>
> *(Mann 1997: 9)*

As of 2019, 170 of 197 countries have ratified the ICESCR (UN 2019), while more than 100 countries have included the right to health in their national constitutions (Dittrich et al. 2016). In earlier work, Backman et al. (2008) examine achievement in relation to the right to health in terms of a variety of different indicators for 194 countries; they find a very mixed picture of achievement; for example, only 56 of the 160 countries that have ratified ICESCR have legally recognised the right to health.

Global monitoring and reporting systems

Governments are responsible not only for not directly violating rights but also for ensuring the conditions which enable individuals to realise their rights as fully as possible. This is understood as an obligation to respect, protect, and fulfil rights. The UN system relies, to a great extent, on powers of persuasion, or as some have put it 'naming and shaming', to encourage governments to change laws, policy, or practice in the direction necessary to promote, protect, or fulfil rights. By ratifying the different human rights instruments, governments also acquire reporting requirements which enable the monitoring of progress within the UN human rights system. There are nine core human rights treaties, corresponding to these are nine bodies/committees that monitor the performance of those countries who have ratified or acceded to the treaty in their efforts to comply with the treaty's provisions.

A central feature of the monitoring process is that all committees have reporting requirements. Each country is required to first lodge a report with the committee (usually referred to as 'country reports') detailing the status of its compliance with the treaty in question at the time of the country becoming a party to the treaty. Subsequently, countries are required to lodge supplementary reports at four- or five-year intervals. In addition, the committees conduct hearings with government representatives during which aspects of country reports are examined in detail. NGOs may submit 'Alternative' reports to the relevant committees; these may also be referred to during the committee hearings.

All committees have the capacity to issue 'General Comments'. The object of these General Comments is to provide countries with guidance in their efforts to meet their treaty obligations. This guidance is gleaned from the committees' experiences in reviewing the country reports submitted to them. The General Comments are intended to assist countries in this regard by providing greater detail about what the requirements are and how best they can be met. Where appropriate, the General Comments also draw upon the committees' own published opinions in respect of individual communications or cases. They cover such matters as: expanded definitions of key terms; the use of reservations and derogations; and reporting requirements and standards.

There are two levels at which all seven committees may receive complaints (usually called 'communications') that human rights violations have occurred. First, they may receive communications from governments, that is, where one government alleges that another has violated rights protected by a treaty to which it is a party. It is not surprising that this mechanism is rarely used given diplomatic reluctance between governments to accuse each other of breaches in their human rights obligations. Second, a committee may be empowered to receive and consider individual communications, that is, complaints from individuals that their rights have been infringed upon by the government. As of March 2019, eight of the human rights treaty bodies (CCPR, CERD, CAT, CEDAW, CRPD, CED, CESCR and CRC) may, under particular circumstances, consider individual complaints or communications from individuals. The Convention on Migrant Workers also contains provision allowing individual communications to be considered by the Committee on Migrant Workers; these provisions will become operative when ten state parties have made the necessary declaration under Article 77.

The Committee's opinions or 'views' in relation to individual complaints are not the same as the judgments of international or domestic courts. Although they may pronounce on the compatibility of government actions with treaty obligations, their opinions are not enforceable in any legal sense. However, their persuasive force is often such that the government concerned may be inclined to adjust its laws or policies accordingly as can be seen in the examples considered later in this chapter.

The OHCHR also has a regional structure and in some cases also a country presence. Regional offices and centres are established on the basis of a standard agreement between OHCHR and the host country, following consultations with countries within the same region (OHCHR 2009). Regional offices and centres focus on cross-cutting regional human rights concerns and support, at national level, follow-up to treaty bodies and special procedures as well as matters relating to the Universal Periodic Review (UPR) – discussed in detail in Chapter 10. Regional offices and centres work closely with regional and subregional intergovernmental organisations, including to provide support on institutional and thematic issues. The activities, analyses, conclusions, and recommendations of regional bodies are reported to the High Commissioner, including through their annual report to the Human Rights Council.

Human Rights Council

The Human Rights Council was established by the UN General Assembly in March 2006, as a successor to the Commission on Human Rights. The Human Rights Council is an inter-governmental body within the UN system. It is made up of representatives from forty-seven countries and is responsible for strengthening the promotion and protection of human rights around the globe. One year after holding its first meeting, on 18 June 2007, the Council adopted its 'Institution-building package' providing direction for its future work. As a result of this, a UPR mechanism was created. Other features included a new Advisory Committee which serves as the Council's 'think tank', providing it with expertise and advice on the-matic human rights issues, and the revised 'Complaints Procedure' mechanism which allows individuals and organisations to bring complaints about human rights violations to the atten-tion of the Council. The Human Rights Council also continues to work closely with the UN Special Procedures established by the former Commission on Human Rights and now assumed by the Council.

Universal Periodic Review

The Universal Periodic Review (UPR) is a process that involves a review of the human rights records of all UN member states once every four years. The UPR is a state-driven process, under the auspices of the Human Rights Council, which provides the opportunity for each state to declare what actions they have taken to improve the human rights situations in their countries and to fulfil their human rights obligations. The UPR is designed to ensure equal treatment for every country when their human rights situations are assessed. The UPR was created through the UN General Assembly on 15 March 2006 by resolution 60/251, which established the Human Rights Council itself. It is a cooperative process which, on 13 October 2011, com-pleted its first cycle, having reviewed the human rights records of every country. Currently, no other universal mechanism of this kind exists. The aim of this new mechanism is to improve the human rights situation in all countries and address human rights violations wherever they occur.

Special procedures and special rapporteurs

'Special procedures' is the general name given to the mechanisms established by the Human Rights Council to address either specific country situations or thematic issues in all parts of the world. At the beginning of August 2017, there were forty-four thematic and twelve country mandates (HRC 2018). The OHCHR provides these mechanisms with personnel, policy, research, and logistical support for the discharge of their mandates. The mandate hold-ers report and advise on human rights from a thematic or country-specific perspective. The aim is that their independence, impartiality, and flexibility enable the Special Procedures to play a critical role in promoting and protecting human rights. The experts deal with situations wherever they may occur in the world, including in the context of crises and emergencies.

With the support of the OHCHR, mandate holders discharge their responsibilities in several different ways. Firstly, they undertake country visits (fact-finding missions). Secondly, they act on individual cases and concerns of a broader, structural nature by sending communications to states in which they bring alleged violations to their attention. Thirdly, they can conduct thematic studies and convene expert consultations, develop international human rights standards, engage in advocacy, raise public awareness, and provide advice and support for technical cooperation. Special Procedures report annually to the Human Rights Council; the majority of the mandates also report to the General Assembly.

Mandate holders are referred to as Independent Experts or Special Rapporteurs; they serve in a personal capacity, are not UN staff members, and do not receive financial remuneration. Thematic mandates include Special Rapporteurs on: the right of everyone to the enjoyment of the highest attainable standard of physical and mental health (since 2002); the sale of children, child prostitution, and child pornography (since 1990), violence against women (since 1994); the situation of human rights and fundamental freedoms of Indigenous peoples (since 2001); and trafficking in persons, especially women and children (since 2004).

Ongoing debates, ongoing development

While it is often argued that rights are culturally independent, as highlighted by the quote from Boutros Boutros Ghali that begun this chapter, not all agree. Some argue that the concept of universality is culturally constructed. Human rights are viewed as representing the belief systems of some cultures and societies rather than those of all cultures and societies. This is the 'cultural relativist' argument, the very rationale of which is to deny claims of universality. Accordingly, in their modern form, human rights are considered a Western construct of limited application to non-Western nations. Some Asian political leaders have adopted this cultural relativist argument. This argument can be seen in the work of Kausikan (1996), who suggests that within Asian countries (discussed more in Chapter 3), the adoption of the norm of human rights has occurred through the recognition of the compatibility of human rights with Asian cultures and values. However, this is countered by the significant role played by India during the creation of the UDHR (Bhagavan 2010).

A further example of both the influence of culture and the need for ongoing development of our understanding of human rights is provided by Goldingay (2007, 2009) in her research on young female prisoners in New Zealand. Goldingay (2007, 2009) problematises the notion of 'best interests' as it is written in the Convention on the Rights of the Child, which is often taken as supporting separate facilities for young prisoners. Young Maori prisoners in New Zealand in a non-age-separated prison for women reported that for a number of reasons, ongoing close relationships with adults were essential for their wellbeing (Goldingay 2007). Her larger study Goldingay (2009) illustrated how in Maori and Pacific Islander cultures, the notion of 'best interests' of the child may not align well with separation into age-specific facilities, which may deny young people access to their culture with negative consequences for health and wellbeing. Her findings certainly point to the need to consider cultural factors carefully in interpreting 'best interests'.

Another area of debate is the notion of intergenerational rights, in two senses, firstly in terms of the responsibility for action by present generations to provide redress for past human rights violations, and secondly in terms of consideration of the rights of future generations. As relevant examples of the first of these, the Canadian government has provided significant funds for the Canadian Aboriginal Healing Foundation in reparation for the human rights violations of Canadian Indigenous peoples in the residential school system, as well as compensation payments to individual survivors (Castellano et al. 2008). In Australia, although there was an important symbolic apology on 13 February 2008 delivered by the then Prime Minister Kevin Rudd to the stolen generations of Indigenous children who were forcibly removed from their families (Corntassel and Holder 2008), debate continues about whether monetary compensation should also be provided, as the original report of the national inquiry recommended (Bringing Them Home 1997). When considering the rights of future generations, environmental movements argue that there is a moral obligation to respect and protect the rights of future generations exists in the context not only of environmental pollution, but by the increasing evidence of the likely adverse effects of climate change, for example see Knox and Pejan (2018).

Fulfilling human rights is a necessary prerequisite for health of individuals and populations. In the wake of globalisation and privatisation, increasing attention must be paid to the role of non-state actors who influence the health and wellbeing of people to an unprecedented extent – comparable to (or even greater than) the influence of governments (OHCHR 2000). Among other things, this calls for a need to reinforce the commitment and capacity of governments to ensure that actions taken by the private sector, as well as other actors, are informed by and comply with human rights principles. Current structures are generally insufficient for NGOs or governments to monitor effectively and hold corporations operating on a national scale accountable; the problem is compounded for multinationals, who may escape accountability within states, and for whom there is no international human rights law that applies directly to them or their actions.

References

Throughout this chapter, in discussing the basic history and structures of human rights systems use has been made of websites and a few key references. The following list provides both sources that have been directly cited in text and key sources that are not directly referred to.

AHRC 2009. *Human Rights Explained: Facts Sheet 2: Human Rights Origins*, Canberra, Australia: Australian Human Rights Commission.

Backman, G, Hunt, P, Khosla, R, Jaramillo-Strouss, C, Fikre, BM, Rumble, C, Pevalin, D, Páez, DA, Pineda, MA, Frisancho, A, Tarco, D, Motlagh, M, Farcasanu, D, & Vladescu, C 2008. Health systems and the right to health: An assessment of 194 countries, *The Lancet*, 372(9655): 2047–2085. doi. org/10.1016/S0140-6736(08)61781-X

Barbisch, D, Koenig, KL, & Shih, FY 2015. Is there a case for quarantine? Perspectives from SARS to Ebola, *Disaster Medicine and Public Health Preparedness*, 9(5): 547–553. doi.org/10.1017/dmp.2015.38

Bhagavan, M 2010. A new hope: India, the United Nations and the making of the universal declaration of human rights, *Modern Asian Studies*, 44(2): 311–347. doi.org/10.1017/S0026749X08003600

Bickenbach, JE 2009. Disability, culture and the UN convention, *Disability and Rehabilitation*, 31(14): 1111–1124. doi.org/10.1080/09638280902773729

Bisaillon, LM 2010. Human rights consequences of mandatory HIV screening policy of newcomers to Canada, *Health and Human Rights*, 12(2): 119–134.

Bringing Them Home 1997. *Bringing Them Home: Report of the National Inquiry into the Separation of Aboriginal and Torres Strait Islander Children from Their Families*, Sydney: Commonwealth of Australia.

Brinton Lykes, M 2001. Human rights violations as structural violence, in DJ Christie, RV Wagner, & DA Winter (eds.) *Peace, Conflict, and Violence: Peace Psychology for the 21st Century*, Englewood Cliffs, NJ: Prentice-Hall.

Broderstad, EG 2010. *Indigenous Rights and Citizenship Rights: Contradictory or Coherent?* Presentation at the 11th annual Forum for Development Cooperation with Indigenous Peoples, 24th–26th of October 2010, Norway, The Centre for Sámi Studies, University of Tromsø. Full conference report available in Munin at http://hdl.handle.net/10037/2941 [Accessed 03/08/2019].

Brundtland, GH 2005. The UDHR: Fifty years of synergy between health and human right, in S Gruskin, M Grodin, S Marks, & G Annas (eds.) *Perspectives on Health and Human Rights*, New York: Routledge.

Carpenter, M 2018. Intersex variations, human rights and the International Classification of Diseases, *Health and Human Rights*. Available: www.hhrjournal.org/2018/08/intersex-variations-human-rights-and-the-international-classification-of-diseases/ [Accessed 11/03/2019].

Castellano, MB, Archibald, L, & DeGagné, M 2008. *From Truth to Reconciliation: Transforming the Legacy of Residential Schools*, Ottawa: Aboriginal Healing Foundation.

CESCR 1990. *General Comment No. 3: The Nature of State Parties' Obligations*, Geneva: United Nations.

CESCR 2000. *General Comment No. 14: The Right to the Highest Attainable Standard of Health*, Geneva: United Nations.

Claude, RP, & Issel, BW 1998. Health, medicine and science in the drafting of the Universal Declaration of Human Rights, *Health and Human Rights*, 3(2): 126–142. doi.org/10.2307/4065304

Coker, R 2001. Just coercion? Detention of nonadherent tuberculosis patients, *Annals of the New York Academy of Sciences*, 953: 216–223. doi.org/10.1111/j.1749-6632.2001.tb11380.x

Commission on Human Rights 2001. *Access to Medication in the Context of Pandemics such as HIV/AIDS, Resolution 2001/53*, Geneva: OHCHR.

Corntassel, J, & Holder, C 2008. Who's sorry now? Government apologies, truth commissions, and Indigenous self-determination in Australia, Canada, Guatemala, and Peru, *Human Rights Review*, 9(4): 465–489. doi.org/10.1007/s12142-008-0065-3

Crenshaw, K 1989. Demarginalizing the intersection of race and sex: A black feminist critique of anti-discrimination doctrine, feminist theory and antiracist politics, *University of Chicago Legal Forum*, 139.

CSDH 2008. *Closing the Gap in a Generation: Health Equity through Action on the Social Determinants of Health*, Geneva: World Health Organization.

Dittrich, R, Cubillos, L, Gostin, L, Chalkidou, K, & Li, R 2016. The international right to health: What does it mean in legal practice and how can it affect priority setting for universal health coverage? *Health Systems & Reform*, 2(1): 23–31. doi.org/10.1080/23288604.2016.1124167

Durrant, JE 2008. Physical punishment, culture, and rights: Current issues for professionals, *Journal of Developmental and Behavioral Pediatrics*, 29(1): 55–66. doi.org/10.1097/DBP.0b013e318135448a

ECOSOC 1984. *UN Sub-Commission on Prevention of Discrimination and Protection of Minorities, Siracusa Principles on the Limitation and Derogation of Provisions in the International Covenant on Civil and Political Rights: UN Document E/CN.4/1984/4, Annex*, Geneva: UN.

Goldingay, S 2007. Jail mums: The status of adult female prisoners among young female prisoners in Christchurch Women's Prison, *Social Policy Journal of New Zealand*, 31: 56–73.

Goldingay, S 2009. *Separation or Mixing: Issues for Young Women Prisoners in Aotearoa New Zealand Prisons*, Doctoral thesis, Canterbury: University of Canterbury. Social Work and Human Services. Available: http://hdl.handle.net/10092/3740 [Accessed 03/08/2019].

Gostin, LO, & Lazzarini, Z 1997. *Human Rights and Public Health in the AIDS Pandemic*, New York: Oxford University Press.

Grech, O 2009. Human rights and development, in C Regan, B Borg, & T Meade (eds.) *80:20 Development in an Unequal World*, Birmingham: Tide Global Learning.

Gruskin, S, Grodin, M, Marks, S, & Annas, G (eds.) 2005. *Perspectives on Health and Human Rights*, New York: Routledge.

Gruskin, S, Mills, EJ, & Tarantola, D 2007. History, principles and practice of health and human rights, *Lancet*, 370: 449–455. doi.org/10.1016/S0140-6736(07)61200-8

HRC 2018. *Report on the Twenty-Fourth Annual Meeting of Special Rapporteurs/Representatives, Independent Experts and Chairpersons of Working Groups of the Special Procedures of the Human Rights Council* (Geneva, 27 to 30 June 2017), including updated information on special procedures, A/HRC/37/37.

Ishay, MR 2008. *The History of Human Rights: From Ancient Times to the Globalization Era*, 2nd edn, Berkeley, CA: University of California Press.

Kapilashrami, A, & Hankivsky, O 2018. Intersectionality and why it matters to global health, *The Lancet*, 391(10140): 2589–2591. doi.org/10.1016/S0140-6736(18)31431-4

Katsumata, H 2009. ASEAN and human rights: Resisting Western pressure or emulating the West?, *Pacific Review*, 22(5): 619–637. doi.org/10.1080/09512740903329731

Kausikan, B 1996. Asia's different standard, in HJ Steiner & P Alston (eds.) *International Human Rights in Context*, Oxford: Clarendon Press.

Kinney, ED 2001. The international human right to health: What does this mean for our nation and world?, *Indiana Law Review*, 34(4): 1457–1477. doi.org/10.2139/ssrn.296394

Knox, JH, & Pejan, R (eds.) 2018. *The Human Right to a Healthy Environment*, Cambridge: Cambridge University Press.

Lam, WK, Zhong, NS, & Tan, WC 2003. Overview on SARS in Asia and the world, *Respirology*, 8(Suppl): S2–S5. doi.org/10.1046/j.1440-1843.2003.00516.x

Levinson, D. (ed.) 2003. *The Wilson Chronology of Human Rights*. New York: H.W. Wilson Company.

Manea, MG 2009. How and why interaction matters: ASEAN's regional identity and human rights, *Cooperation and Conflict*, 44(1): 27–49. doi.org/10.1177/0010836708099720

Mann, J 1997. Medicine and public health, ethics and human rights, *The Hastings Center Report*, 27(3): 6–13. doi.org/10.2307/3528660

Meier, BM 2010. Global health governance and the contentious politics of human rights: Mainstreaming the right to health for public health advancement, *Stanford Journal of International Law*, 46(1): 1–50.

Meijknecht, A, & De Vries, BS 2010. Is there a place for minorities' and indigenous peoples' rights within ASEAN? Asian values, ASEAN values and the protection of Southeast Asian minorities and indigenous peoples, *International Journal on Minority and Group Rights*, 17(1): 75–110. doi.org/10.1163/157181110X12595859744204

Mertus, J 2009. *The United Nations and Human Rights: A Guide for a New Era*, London/New York: Routledge. doi.org/10.4324/9780203878019

Messer, E 1993. Anthropology and human rights, *Annual Review Anthropology*, 22: 221–249. doi.org/10.1146/annurev.anthro.22.1.221

Moss, LC 2010. Opportunities for nongovernmental organization advocacy in the universal periodic review process at the UN Human Rights Council, *Journal of Human Rights Practice*, 2(1): 122–150. doi.org/10.1093/jhuman/hup031

Moyn, S 2010. *The Last Utopia: Human Rights in History*, Cambridge, MA: Harvard University Press.

Nagengast, C 1997. Women, minorities, and indigenous peoples: Universalism and cultural relativity, *Journal of Anthropological Research*, 53(3): 349–369. doi.org/10.1086/jar.53.3.3630958

Neshat, NS 2004. *Rights: Fourth Generation Human Rights? Human Rights in Information Society*, Toronto, Canada: Olive Leaf Publishing.

OHCHR 2000. *Business and Human Rights: A Progress Report*, Geneva: OHCHR. Available: www.ohchr.org/Documents/Publications/BusinessHRen.pdf [Accessed 03/08/2019].

OHCHR 2003. *Human Rights: A Compilation of International Instruments*, Vol. 1. United Nations Publications. Available: www.ohchr.org/Documents/Publications/Compilation2en.pdf [Accessed 03/08/2019].

OHCHR 2009. *High Commissioner's Strategic Management Plan 2010–2011*, Geneva: OHCHR. Available: www.ohchr.org/Documents/Press/SMP2010-2011.pdf [Accessed 03/08/2019].

Pada, S, & Tambyah, PA 2011. Overview/reflections on the 2009 H1N1 pandemic, *Microbes and Infection*, 13(5): 470–478. doi.org/10.1016/j.micinf.2011.01.009

SEARO 2011. *The Right to Health in the Constitutions of Member States of the World Health Organization South-East Asia Region*, New Delhi: WHO, Regional Office for South-East Asia.

Shade, LR 2004. Situating communication rights historically, in M Moll & LR Shade (eds.) *Seeking Convergence in Policy and Practice: Communications in the Public Interest*, Vol. 2, Ottawa: Canadian Centre for Policy Alternatives.

Tilley, JJ 2000. Cultural relativism, *Human Rights Quarterly*, 22(2): 501–547. doi.org/10.1353/hrq.2000.0027

UN 1945. *Charter of the United Nations and Statute of the International Court of Justice*, New York: United Nations.

UN 2015. *Transforming Our World: The 2030 Agenda for Sustainable Development, UN Doc. A/RES/70/1*, New York: United Nations.

UN 2019. *Treaty Collection* [Online], Geneva. Available: https://treaties.un.org/ [Accessed 08/04/2019].

UN General Assembly 1948. *Universal Declaration of Human Rights, UN Doc. A/810*, New York: United Nations.

WHO 2002. *25 Questions and Answers on Health and Human Rights*, Geneva: World Health Organization. Available: www.who.int/hhr/activities/publications/en/

WHO 2008. *The Right to Health: Fact Sheet 31*, Geneva: WHO.

World Health Assembly 2000. *HIV/AIDS: Confronting the Epidemic, Resolution WHA53:14*, Geneva: World Health Organization.

3

REGIONAL HUMAN RIGHTS SYSTEMS

Ann Taket and Fiona H. McKay

Introduction

This chapter focuses on the various regional human rights systems. These systems exist in a number of different forms: first in terms of systems that link a group of countries or member states, and second in terms of systems that link different national human rights institutions. Complementing these are non-government organisations (NGOs), both regionally based and global NGOs that have a regional structure to their operations. While the Office of the High Commissioner for Human Rights (OHCHR) also presides over a global, regional system, it does not exactly align with the regional systems discussed in this chapter. There is considerable variation in these systems, both in terms of their operation, and the extent to which they can exert direct influence on the states within their boundaries. Established regional human rights systems, based on a human rights charter, together with some regional enforcement mechanisms exist in Africa, Asia, the Americas, and Europe, each of which is considered here. Also discussed in this chapter is the limited regional developments that have taken place in Asia and the Middle East. Finally, this chapter considers the Organisation of Islamic Cooperation, which brings together Muslim countries across the globe.

It is impossible in a single chapter to include a comprehensive review of the achievements of each regional system, made more difficult as there is only limited research available. Instead the aim of this chapter is to incorporate different examples of the operation and effectiveness of systems. These have been selected to illustrate the potential impact of the systems in tackling health inequity and increasing social justice while also identifying some of the challenges and difficulties that remain. Table 3.1 presents some key features of the regional human rights systems, summarising their origins, membership, and organisation.

Africa

The Organization of African Unity (OAU) was established in 1963. At this time, much of Africa was concerned with increasing economic activity, as well as with decolonialisation and independence from a range of European rulers, and as a result, a serious human rights instrument was not considered important (Umozurike 1983). While there were discussions

TABLE 3.1 Summary features of regional human rights systems

	Origins	Membership	Organization/operation
Africa	1981 – African Charter on Human and Peoples' Rights (Banjul Charter)	Charter applies to the 55 states who are members of the African Union. 30 African states have acknowledged the Court's jurisdiction	Through two bodies: African Commission on Human and Peoples' Rights based in Banjul, Gambia and African Court on Human and Peoples' Rights, Arusha, Tanzania. Individuals may raise complaints.
Americas	1948 – American Declaration of the rights and duties of man 1969 – American Convention on Human Rights Other protocols and conventions	22 American states recognise jurisdiction of the court (a further 3 ratified the Convention only, 2 of those 3 later denounced convention)	Through two bodies: Inter-American Commission on Human Rights (IACHR) based in Washington, D.C., and Inter-American Court of Human Rights, San José, Costa Rica. Individuals may petition the Commission
Asia	1967 – Association of Southeast Asian Nations (ASEAN) established 2012 ASEAN Human Rights Declaration adopted	10 member states	ASEAN Intergovernmental Commission on Human Rights (AICHR) set up in 2009. AICHR cannot receive complaints from individuals.
Europe – 1	1950 – European Convention on Human Rights, entered into force 1953	Council of Europe members, currently 47	Through European Court of Human Rights. Individuals can take cases there. Can direct changes in country law.
Europe – 2	2000 – Charter of Fundamental Rights of the European Union	EU member states	Originally, 'soft' law – rules of conduct that have no legally binding force*, powers strengthened in 2009
Middle East	1968 – Council of the League of Arab States founded the Permanent Arab Commission on Human Rights (PACHR)	22 member states	Modernised version of Arab charter on Human Rights came into force in 2008. PACHR works mainly around rights of Arabs living in Israeli-occupied territories.
Organisation of the Islamic Conference (OIC)	1969 – OIC established, present Charter adopted 2008, 1990 – Cairo Declaration on Human Rights in Islam 2004 – Covenant on the rights of the child in Islam	57 member states across four continents	No reporting or monitoring mechanisms exist.

* Definition from Trubek and Trubek (2005)

regarding a human rights instrument, it took several decades of debate and negotiation between member states and the OAU Secretary General, jurists, the United Nations (UN), and strong support from non-African and NGO observers before a Charter specifically concerning the human rights of African peoples would be adopted (Evans and Murray 2008). The African Charter on Human and Peoples' Rights, also known as the Banjul Charter, after the place where it was drafted, the city of Banjul in The Gambia, was adopted in June 1981 by the Assembly of Heads of State and Government of the OAU (replaced by the African Union, AU in 2000). The Charter came into force in October 1986, and is a reflection of the membership of the OAU seeking to develop a continent-wide human rights instrument, building on the Universal Declaration of Human Rights (UDHR) and in line with those that already existed in Europe and the Americas (Ssenyonjo 2012). As of 2019, fifty-three states who are also member states of the AU have ratified the Charter.

Human and Peoples' Rights are set out in Articles 1 to 26 of the Charter. It is worth noting the particular formulation used in the Charter, as well as the title of the Commission and Court, with reference to 'human and peoples' rights' rather than simply 'human rights'. This can be seen as a move to explicitly include the notion of 'collective rights' held by a group as well as 'individual rights' held by every person. The Charter recognises most of what are regarded as universally accepted civil and political rights, including the rights to: freedom from discrimination; equality; life and personal integrity; dignity; freedom from slavery; and freedom from cruel, inhuman, or degrading treatment or punishment, as well as rights to due process concerning arrest and detention; the right to a fair trial; freedom of religion; freedom of information and expression; freedom of association; freedom to assembly; freedom of movement; freedom of political participation; and the right to property (African Union 1988). Problematic with the civil and political rights is the lack of a right to privacy, a right against forced or compulsory labour, and the right to a fair trial (Heyns 2003). Compared with other international instruments, there is also little consideration of political participation. For example, while the Charter does include the right to participate freely in the government of his (sic) country, it is not stipulate that this should occur through regular, free, and fair elections based on universal suffrage (Evans and Murray 2008).

Health is explicitly and implicitly referred to in several sections of the Charter. Article 16 makes an explicit statement on the right to health:

1 *Every individual shall have the right to enjoy the best attainable state of physical and mental health.*
2 *State Parties to the present Charter shall take the necessary measures to protect the health of their people and to ensure that they receive medical attention when they are sick.*

Health is also referred to in items 1 and 4 of Article 18, which read respectively:

The family shall be the natural unit and basis of society. It shall be protected by the State which shall take care of its physical health and moral needs
and
The aged and the disabled shall also have the right to special measures of protection in keeping with their physical or moral needs.

Other Articles in the Charter relate closely to the social determinants of health, in particular the right to work (Article 15), the right to education (Article 17), and the provision of environment favourable to development (Article 24). Article 21 also recognise the deleterious effects that foreign exploitation, in particular by 'international monopolies' has had, and makes provision for compensation and recovery. The final clauses in this Article, clauses 4 and 5 state:

4   *State Parties to the present Charter shall individually and collectively exercise the right to free disposal of their wealth and natural resources with a view to strengthening African Unity and solidarity.*

5   *State Parties to the present Charter shall undertake to eliminate all forms of foreign exploitation particularly that practised by international monopolies so as to enable their peoples to fully benefit from the advantages derived from their national resources.*

The Charter also recognises certain economic, social, and cultural rights. These rights, however, have said to be slow in being adopted in Africa (Ssenyonjo 2012). Part of this may be related to the minimalist approach that went into drafting these rights, so as to not overburden young states. As a result of this approach, the Charter explicitly recognises only the right to property, a right to work under equitable and satisfactory conditions, a right to enjoy the best state of mental and physical health, the right to education, the protection of the family and cultural rights, and a number of group rights, such as self-determination, free disposal of wealth and natural resources, economic, social and cultural development, national and international peace and security, and a general satisfactory environment (African Union 1988).

Unlike other human rights instruments, the Charter recognises group rights in addition to individual rights. These include harmonious development in family, not to compromise the security of the state, and to strengthen social and national solidarity (African Union 1988).

CASE STUDY: THE RIGHTS OF THE OGONI PEOPLE IN THE NIGER DELTA REGION

In 1996, the Social and Economic Rights Action Center and the Center for Economic and Social Rights in Nigeria lodged a communication in respect of the actions of the government of Nigeria in collaboration with the Shell Petroleum Development Corporation. Their communication alleged that the oil operations in the Niger Delta Region were causing environmental degradation and health problems of the Ogoni people as a result of environmental contamination. There were further charges regarding the direct involvement of the military in attacking, burning and destroying Ogoni villages and homes under false pretext. The Commission found that the government was in violation of multiple articles of the Charter (ACHPR 2001) and appealed to the government to ensure protection of the environment, health, and livelihood of the Ogoni people, supporting this with a number of specific recommendations. Nigeria's periodic country report on the implementation of the African Charter on Human and Peoples' Rights, covering 2005–2008 (Federal Ministry of Justice 2008), describes a variety of measures put in place to address the problems, including the creation of a new ministry of the Niger Delta with a view to ensuring effective implementation of a comprehensive master plan, programs, and direct intervention projects in the region. Research over the period 2000 to 2010 documents the involvement of Shell, through payments to groups linked to violence, in cases of serious violence and human rights abuses in the Delta region (Amunwa 2011). UNEP (2011) provides a comprehensive environmental assessment and summarises the public health impacts of the degradation, in particular arising through water contamination, making comprehensive recommendations for environmental restoration including at the regulatory, operational, and monitoring levels. In Nigeria's latest periodic country report covering 2015–2016 (Federal Ministry of Justice 2017), a number of projects were reported as being set up with representatives of Ogoni local communities for 'immediate implementation', including those that cover the provision of clean drinking water; training; centre of excellence; integrated soil management centre; pilot remediation project; and a health study. The report was submitted in May 2018 and as at March 2019 concluding observations and recommendations from the Commission on this report were not yet available.

African Commission and the African Court on Human and Peoples' Rights

The African Commission on Human and Peoples' Rights was established by Article 30 of the Banjul Charter. The Commission is composed of eleven members elected by secret ballot by the Assembly of Heads of State and Government each for a six-year renewable term. The Commission elects two members as Chairperson and Vice-Chairperson for a two-year renewable period; the Secretary to the Commission is appointed by the Chairperson of the AU Commission. The members serve in their personal and individual capacity and have full independence in the discharge of their duties, and diplomatic privileges and immunities. They are supported by a Secretariat provided by the OAU, later AU.

The African Court on Human and Peoples' Rights was established by a Protocol to the African Charter on Human and Peoples' Rights. This Protocol was adopted by member states of the then OAU in Ouagadougou, Burkina Faso, in June 1998, and entered into force in January 2004. The Court started its operations in Addis Ababa, Ethiopia in November 2006 and moved to its permanent seat in Arusha, Tanzania in August 2007.

In July 2008, the AU made the decision to merge the Court with the African Court of Justice (established through the Constitutive Act of the AU) to create a single African Court of Justice and Human Rights. This will not however come into force until ratification of the relevant Protocol by fifteen African states; as of February 2019, this had still not occurred.

Americas

The regional system in the Americas is operated by the Organisations of American States (OAS). The OAS came into existence in 1948, and currently has thirty-five member states and a number of observer states. The First International Conference of American States was held in Washington, D.C., between October 1889 and April 1890; however, the Charter governing the present-day operation of the OAS did not come in force until 1970.

The main human rights instrument of the Americas is the American Convention on Human Rights. The Convention defines the human rights that ratifying states have agreed to respect and guarantee, and was adopted in 1969, coming into force in 1978. As of March 2019, a total of twenty-three member states were party to the Convention: Argentina, Barbados, Bolivia, Brazil, Chile, Colombia, Costa Rica, Dominica, the Dominican Republic, Ecuador, El Salvador, Grenada, Guatemala, Haiti, Honduras, Jamaica, Mexico, Nicaragua,

Panama, Paraguay, Peru, Suriname, and Uruguay. Two states, Trinidad and Tobago, and Venezuela became parties to the Convention, but later denounced it. Trinidad and Tobago first acceded to the Convention, then denounced it over the issue of the death penalty (OAS 2019). Venezuela first ratified and then denounced the Convention after accusing the Inter-American Court and Commission of undermining its government's stability by interfering with domestic issues (OAS 2019).

The American Convention on Human Rights lists substantive rights within two chapters. The twenty-three Articles of Chapter II cover individual civil and political rights due to all persons, including the rights to life (Article 4) (controversially, this is expanded as 'in general, from the moment of conception'), to humane treatment, to a fair trial, to privacy, to freedom of conscience, to freedom of assembly, and to freedom of movement. Chapter III contains a single Article covering economic, social, and cultural rights; this limited treatment was expanded some ten years later with the Protocol of San Salvador, which covers such areas as the right to work, the right to health (Article 10), the right to a healthy environment (Article 11), the right to food, and the right to education; thus far this Protocol has only been ratified by sixteen states.

There are two bodies responsible for the promotion and protection of human rights, through compliance with the American Convention on Human Rights in the Inter-American System: the Inter-American Commission on Human Rights (IACHR); and the Inter-American Court of Human Rights.

The IACHR is an organ of the OAS, established in 1959, holding its first meeting in 1960, and based in Washington, D.C. (IACHR 2011). The IACHR derives its human rights obligations from three documents; the OAS Charter; OAS Declaration of the Rights and Duties of Man (with content is broadly similar to the UDHR), and the American Convention on Human Rights. The IACHR consists of seven members who carry out their functions independently, without representing any particular country. Members are elected by the General Assembly of the OAS for a period of four years and may be re-elected once. The Executive Secretariat carries out the tasks delegated to it by the IACHR and provides the Commission with legal and administrative support in pursuit of its functions. Since 1961, it has carried out visits to countries to produce country reports and reports on particular topics, and since 1965, it has heard individual petitions regarding alleged human rights violations (IACHR 2011).

Any person, group of persons, or non-governmental entity that is legally recognised in one or more OAS member states may petition the Commission with regard to the violation of any right protected by the American Convention, by the American Declaration, or by any other pertinent instrument. Under the terms of Article 45 of the American Convention, the IACHR may consider communications from a state alleging rights violations by another state. Petitions may be filed in any of the four official languages of the OAS (English, French, Spanish, or Portuguese) by the alleged victim of the rights violation or by a third party or, in the case of interstate petitions, by a government. In addition to examining complaints of violations of the American Convention against countries party to the Convention, the IACHR has competence, in accordance with the OAS Charter and with the Statute of the IACHR, to consider alleged violations of the American Declaration by OAS member states that are not yet parties to the American Convention (IACHR 2011). This means that although the United States is not a party to the Convention, the Commission can hear cases brought by US citizens.

The IACHR publishes reports documenting its activities comprehensively on its website, these include country reports, topic-based reports, and reports on individual cases. Comprehensive annual reports are also produced; these contain a summary of cases and petitions and their follow-up.

CASE STUDY: ADVISORY OPINION ON GENDER IDENTITY

The state of Costa Rica presented a request for an advisory opinion on 18 May 2016, for the Inter-American Court to interpret:

(a) the protection provided by the American Convention on Human Rights to recognition of the change of name in accordance with the gender identity of the individual concerned;

(b) the compatibility with the American Convention of the practice of applying article 54 of the Civil Code of the Republic of Costa Rica to those wishing to change their name based on their gender identity, considering that 'this procedure entails expenses for the applicant and entails a lengthy delay'.

There was also a third part to the opinion requested, not covered here as it did not relate to gender identity.

In the Advisory Opinion, the Court defined gender identity as 'the internal and individual experience of gender as each person feels it, which may or may not correspond to the sex assigned at birth.' The right to gender and sexual identity is related to the concept of freedom and every individual's possibility of self-determination and free choice of the options and circumstances that give a meaning to his or her existence, based on their own options and convictions. The Court asserted that 'State recognition of gender identity is critical to ensuring that transgender persons can fully enjoy all human rights'. These include, among others, the right to protection against all forms of violence, torture, and ill-treatment, as well as the guarantee of the right to health, education, employment, housing, access to social security, and freedom of expression and of association.

Consequently, responding to the questions raised by Costa Rica, the Court considered that the change of name, adaptation of the photograph, and rectification of the mention of sex or gender in public records and on identity documents so that these conform to the self-perceived gender identity was a right protected by the American Convention. Accordingly, states are obliged to recognise, regulate, and establish appropriate procedures to this end.

The Inter-American Court also specified the minimum conditions that these domestic procedures should meet. They should be aimed at reflecting the self-perceived gender identity; be based on free and informed consent; not require medical or psychological certifications that would be unreasonable or pathologising; be confidential, protect personal data, and not reflect changes in gender identity; be prompt and cost-free insofar as possible; and not require providing evidence of surgical and/or hormonal treatments. In addition, the Court concluded that procedures of an administrative nature are those most adapted to these requirements. The Court also clarified that such a procedure need not necessarily be regulated by law.

Regarding the question raised by Costa Rica on the name change procedure established in Article 54 of the Civil Code, the Court considered that this could be compatible with the American Convention in order to change identity data to confirm with the gender identity of applicants, provided that it was either interpreted by a court or regulated administratively to correspond to a materially administrative procedure and to comply with the minimum requirements described above.

Lastly, the Court also indicated that the state of Costa Rica, in order to guarantee the protection of human rights as effectively as possible, could issue regulations incorporating the above-mentioned standards into the materially administrative procedure that it could provide in parallel.

Source: Adapted from Inter-American Court of Human Rights 2018, page 116–117

Activities of the IACHR and the Court with specific relevance to health

To illustrate the scope of the IACHR and the Court in relation to health particularly, this section considers some examples taken from across the range of the functions of the Commission and the Court. There are also two detailed case studies. The first of these (page 36–37) examines the part of the recent advisory opinion handed down by the Court in relation to gender identity. The second case study looks at the rights of people living with HIV/AIDS and shows the important role of the IACHR in improving access to services, in this case antiretrovirals.

The IACHR has been particularly active in women's health, most specifically in tackling gender-based violence, and in reproductive health. Cabal et al. (2003) provide a useful overview of cases brought regarding rape and domestic violence. The cases of rape brought before the Commission have often involved the detention and rape of women by military personnel. Cases concerned with rape by doctors within the health system have resulted in legislative and administrative measures to improve the treatment of rape survivors and the provision of services to them. Cases brought in connection with domestic violence have succeeded in winning compensation for the complainants, but also changes in policy and practice in the countries concerned. Experience from cases regarding reproductive health is also growing, leading IACHR to produce a publication containing specific recommendations in terms of legislation, public policies, and services (IACHR 2010), and setting out the duties of the states in guaranteeing women's human rights without discrimination in terms of access by women to maternal health services.

A recent annual report of the IACHR (2016) focused on a number of different population groups that merit further consideration. In 2016, IACHR identified high levels of extreme violence against women and girls, structural discrimination, and the persistent denial of their sexual and reproductive rights in several countries as being of particular concern.

Indigenous women are the subject of a comprehensive report produced by the IACHR (IACHR 2017) exploring the multiple forms of discrimination based on their gender, ethnicity, and situation of poverty, which heightens their exposure to human rights violations in different contexts. In relation to Indigenous peoples, IACHR (2016: 501) notes:

the most prominent challenges relate to the failure by various States to properly register, demarcate and title the ancestral territories of their Indigenous communities; the failure to respect and guarantee the right to prior consultation in the continent; the impact of extractive and development industries on the rights of Indigenous peoples; as well as the situation of violence, intimidation and threats faced by indigenous communities, including the repression of social protest and the criminalization of Indigenous defenders. IACHR

(2016: 501)

This is despite the IACHR's earlier report on Indigenous and tribal peoples' rights over their ancestral lands and natural resources (IACHR 2009a), which analysed the scope of these rights in the light of the jurisprudence of the Inter-American system and put forward specific guidelines and best practices.

CASE STUDY: RIGHTS OF PEOPLE LIVING WITH HIV/AIDS, IACHR CASE 12.249

Jorge was HIV-positive, living in El Salvador and head of an NGO that works to improve the quality of life and promote the empowerment those living with HIV/AIDS, their family members, and other loved ones. Jorge and his group filed a petition with the IACHR alleging responsibility on the part of his Government for violations of various provisions in binding human rights conventions relating to: the right to life; humane treatment; equal protection before the law; juridical protection; and economic, social, and cultural rights (IACHR 2001). This claimed that by not providing Jorge and twenty-six other HIV-positive individuals with the triple therapy medication needed to prevent them from dying and to improve their quality of life, the state had violated the right to life, health, and wellbeing of the alleged victims. Following recommendations from the IACHR the state reported to the human rights body the decision to authorise the purchase of medication for the provision of therapy and to adopt measures for strengthening and stepping up activities aimed at preventing the transmission of AIDS through education and the promotion of hygiene and preventive health among sectors most at risk for this disease. Additionally, the Government announced its intention to create a fund aimed at purchasing antiretroviral medications for the provision of triple therapy to HIV-infected persons. The national health authorities began administering antiretroviral treatment (IACHR 2009b). According to the most recent annual report of the IACHR (IACHR 2018a), the case still remains under monitoring as only partial compliance has been reported, with the legislative changes recommended still not implemented.

Regarding the situation of the Afro-descendant population in the hemisphere, the IACHR (2016) confirmed that there are still serious problems regarding the persistence of types of structural discrimination and violence (see Chapter 9 for further discussion of racism in the United States). The IACHR (2016) expressed profound concern regarding incidents that reveal a pattern of impunity, or exemption from punishment, with respect to the killings of Afro-Descendants committed by the police in the United States. The IACHR emphasised that the ineffectiveness of the state's response is fostering high levels of impunity, making such killings chronic and leaving victims and their next of kin defenceless (IACHR 2016).

Asia-Pacific

The Association of Southeast Asian Nations (ASEAN) was established in 1967; the current ten member states are Brunei Darussalam, Cambodia, Indonesia, Lao PDR, Malaysia, Myanmar, Philippines, Singapore, Thailand, and Vietnam. Only two conventions have been ratified by all ASEAN member states, the Convention on the Rights of the Child and the Convention on the Elimination of All Forms of Discrimination Against Women. Four of the ten ASEAN countries have entered reservations to these conventions, which have significantly impacted their applicability within the states concerned.

The ASEAN Intergovernmental Commission on Human Rights (AICHR) was set up in 2009 based on Article 14 of the ASEAN Charter, with a remit for promoting and protecting human rights. Item 4 of the AICHR's terms of reference (ASEAN 2009), covering mandate and functions, charges the AICHR with developing an ASEAN Human Rights Declaration, as well as with other functions covering public education on human rights, research, studies, and other functions connected with promoting and protecting human rights. A history of its creation can be found in Yen (2011) and Phan (2019). The ASEAN Human Rights Declaration (AHRD) was adopted in November 2012.

There are wide range of regional NGOs addressing human rights issues. One particularly important body is Forum-Asia, the Asian Forum for Human Rights and Development. This is a regional human rights organisation with forty-seven member-organisations across Asia, in seventeen countries: Bangladesh, Cambodia, India, Indonesia, Japan, Malaysia, Mongolia, Myanmar, Nepal, Pakistan, Philippines, Singapore, South Korea, Sri Lanka, Taiwan, Timor Leste and Thailand. Forum-Asia is a membership-based regional human rights organisation committed to the promotion and protection of all human rights including the right to development. Forum-Asia was founded in 1991 in Manila and its regional Secretariat has been located in Bangkok since 1994. Membership is open to independent, non-profitable, non-partisan, non-violent, and non-governmental civil society organisations working in the field of human rights and human development in Asia. To be included, the organisation must have been in existence for at least two years. Forum-Asia is the co-convenor of Solidarity for Asian People's Advocacy Task Force on ASEAN and Human Rights (SAPATFAHR). Forum Asia and SAPATFAHR have been active in terms of raising thematic issues and specific cases of human rights violations to the AICHR, these include a submission on the removal of mandatory HIV testing for migrant workers presented to the AICHR meeting in September 2010, and submissions on the rights of women, migrant workers, and press freedom (SAPATFAHR 2010). More recently they have prepared a detailed report on a human rights based approach to the SDGs (Forum-Asia 2018) which offer a historical perspective on the concept of development as human right, as well as highlighting critical issues and ways forward in relation to the SDGs; this is of global relevance as well. Their most recent report Baizer and Monk (2018), look across the region at how legislative changes are affecting freedom of expression, peaceful assembly, and association, identifying particular threats and actions against NGOs supporting reproductive health rights and taking action against adverse environmental health effects, such as from mining.

ASEAN Human Rights Declaration

The ASEAN Human Rights Declaration (AHRD) has similarities with the UDHR, since neither has the status of a treaty. However, as Phan (2019) points out, within the context of

ASEAN, declarations are regarded as having the same expectations of implementation as trea-ties, conventions, protocols, and other agreements. It does not include important political and civil rights, or freedom from enforced disappearance, or freedom of association, nor does it explicitly include the rights of people of Indigenous groups and the rights of lesbian, gay, bisexual, and transgender people (Phan 2019). It does however recognise, in Article 4, that the rights of 'vulnerable and marginalised groups are an inalienable, integral and indivisible part of human rights and fundamental freedoms'. It also sets standards that can be interpreted as lower than those provided under major international human rights instruments, in relation to the right to asylum, right to life, and right to form and hold membership of trade unions (Phan 2019). Despite this, Article 40, explicitly confirms that these do not amount to the 'destruc-tion' of any of the rights and freedoms set out in international human rights instruments to which ASEAN countries are party (AHRD 2012).

Another positive point of the AHRD is the explicit inclusion of age and disabilities as grounds for prohibition of discrimination in Article 2, something that is not found in the UDHR, ICCPR, ECHR, the American convention, or the African Charter on Human and People's Rights. It also uses 'gender' as a ground for non-discrimination rather than 'sex'. Article 13 provides for the right not to be subject to human smuggling or trafficking, not something explicit in the UDHR or ICCPR. The AHRD also includes the right to sustain-able development and the right to peace, which are not recognised under many other interna-tional and regional instruments, except the African Charter on Human and Peoples' Rights.

ASEAN Intergovernmental Commission on Human Rights (AICHR)

Forum-Asia reports regularly on the performance of the ASEAN human rights mechanisms. The latest report (Hanung et al. 2018), from 2017, is highly critical of AICHR's perfor-mance, arguing that compared to other regional and international human rights mechanisms, they have the weakest protection record. They note AICHR's complete silence in the face of violations of rights of women and children in 2017, including the rapes, murders, and mass deportation of Rohingya by the Myanmar military. They argue that a limited protec-tion mandate is implied by the terms of reference, but a lack of political will lies behind the failure to operationalise. As a counter to this, Phan (2019) reports an analysis of the first ten years of operation of the AICHR. Phan argues that by design, the AICHR is not a protective mechanism, but that the promotional initiatives undertaken, despite being limited in scope, can provide the initial foundation for the long-term goal of building a protective human rights mechanism for Southeast Asia. In particular the promotion of the rights of women, children and persons with disabilities has been a major area for work by the AICHR in its first ten years (Phan 2019).

Europe

Within Europe there are two separate (though interlinked) systems to consider, one associated with the Council of Europe and the other with the European Union (EU). The Council of Europe's European Convention on Human Rights (ECHR) was signed in 1950 and entered into force in 1953; its original title was the Convention for the Protection of Human Rights and Fundamental Freedoms.

The ECHR was created in response to two concerns (Greer 2006). The first was after-math of the Second World War, with the creation of the Council of Europe and the ECHR coinciding with the creation of the UDHR, and a widespread response to the impacts of violence and violation of human rights at the time. The second was the growth of communism in Central and Eastern Europe and concerns that communist ideology might extend into other parts of Europe. As a result of these concerns, the ECHR has a focus on the rights and responsibilities that are necessary for a democratic society (Council of Europe 1950). The ECHR consists of fifty-nine Articles originally agreed to in 1950, with the main rights and freedoms found in Section I. There are seventeen key Articles relating to rights and freedoms in the ECHR outlined in Section I (Articles 2–18). This includes the right to life, the prohibition of torture, the prohibition of slavery and forced labour, the right to liberty and security, the right to a fair trial, protection against retroactivity of law, the right to private family life, freedom of thought, conscience and religion, and freedom of expression (Council of Europe 1950).

In addition to the fifty-nine Articles agreed to in 1950, there are fifteen Protocols to the ECHR. Protocols can be grouped into two broad categories. The first are those that amend the framework of the ECHR, Protocol 11 (superseding other Protocols, allowing individuals to apply directly to the Court) and Protocol 14 (increasing the efficiency of the Court). The second category include Protocols that increase the number of rights that are protected under the ECHR. These include Protocol 1 that allows for the rights to property, education, and election. During the original drafting these rights could not be agreed on by all states and so were left off the original ECHR. As of 2019, only Monaco and Switzerland have not signed this Protocol. Protocol 4 deals with civil imprisonment, freedom of movement within a country when lawfully there, and the expulsion of foreigners. Greece and Switzerland have not signed this Protocol, and Turkey and the UK have signed but not ratified. Protocol 6 requires states to restrict the death penalty to times of war and has been signed and ratified by all except Russia, while Protocol 13 seeks the complete abolition of the death penalty. Protocol 7 relates to the requirement to conduct fair trials and the right to appeal court decisions and provides for equity between spouses. Finally, Protocol 12 relates to the definition and application of discrimination laws. This protocol has only been ratified by twenty states; those who have not ratified state concerns about the broad nature of the anti-discrimination measures (Council of Europe 2019).

The European Court of Human Rights, set up in 1959, covers forty-seven Council of Europe member states that have ratified the convention. The ECHR is widely regarded as an effective instrument for the protection and promotion of human rights (Helfer 1993).

The European Court of Human Rights has considered persons for whom the state has a particular responsibility, such as detainees, persons with disabilities, the elderly, or children, in support of the positive obligation to protect the right to life and to prevent certain risks. In these cases, the Court has found violations of Article 2 (the right to life) of the ECHR in cases where detainees were not effectively protected against violence by other inmates or did not enjoy sufficient medical support in case of suicidal tendencies (EU Network 2006). While states are bound to uphold the rights in the ECHR, as Keller and Sweet (2008) argue, the Court has no authority to invalidate legal norms and its capacity to control change within states is weak at best.

Bioethics and the case law of the Court is covered in European Court of Human Rights (2016). Bioethics is understood in terms of 'the protection of the human being (his/her human rights and in particular human dignity) in the context of the development of biomedical sciences' (page 3). The report covers reproductive rights (prenatal diagnosis and the right to a legal abortion), medically assisted procreation, assisted suicide, consent to medical examination or treatment, ethical issues concerning HIV, the retention of biological data by the authorities and the right to know one's biological identity. The report anticipates an increase of applications concerning subjects such as gene therapy, stem cell research, and cloning in the future.

The other important human rights structure in Europe is the EU. The Charter of Fundamental Rights of the European Union (EU 2000) was proclaimed in Nice in December 2000 (Peers and Ward 2004). Initially its powers amount to 'soft' law, rules of conduct that have no legally binding force (Trubek and Trubek 2005). The Charter contains fifty-four Articles divided into seven titles. The first six titles deal with substantive rights (under the headings of dignity, freedoms, equality, solidarity, citizens' rights, and justice), while the last title deals with the interpretation and application of the Charter. Much of Charter is based on the ECHR, the case-law of the European Court of Justice and pre-existing provisions of European Union law.

Since coming into force in 2009, the Treaty of Lisbon (December 2007) has changed the status of the EU Charter of Fundamental Rights, so that the charter provisions now become 'general principles' of EU law and this means that both EU and member states, when implementing EU law will need to comply with the EU Charter (FRA 2010). Several EU states, including the UK, Poland, and the Czech Republic, have insisted upon a Protocol governing national application of the Charter in their case, although interpretations differ as to exactly what this protocol will actually mean in practice. While Jirasek (2008) argues that the Protocol will act as an opt-out that excludes the application of the Charter to Poland and the UK. Pernice (2008) argues that the Protocol is an interpretative protocol which will either have limited or no legal consequences. The current situation explained on the website of the European Commission in its Justice section (accessed 20 March 2019) is that the Union institutions (for example, the European Commission, the Council, and the European Parliament) must respect the rights enshrined in the Charter. In particular, all proposals for EU legislation must respect the Charter and guidelines have been produced for taking account of fundamental rights in policy impact assessments. The Charter also applies to member states, but only when they implement Union law. The Charter's provisions do not extend the EU's competences as defined in the Treaties. The EU cannot intervene in fundamental rights issues in areas over which, according to the Treaty, it has no competence. The Lisbon Treaty also provides for the legal basis for the EU to accede to the European Convention on Human Rights which will make the European Court of Human Rights in Strasbourg competent to review acts of the EU institutions. The European Commission also has no general powers to intervene in individual cases of alleged violations of fundamental rights. It can intervene only when EU law comes into play (for example, when EU legislation is adopted or when a national measure applies an EU law in a manner incompatible with the Charter). McHale (2010) suggests that although the Charter potentially has considerable implications for health law and health policy throughout the EU, it is uncertain whether the EU Charter will make any considerable difference over the long term. Article 35 of the Charter contains the right to health care, stating that 'Everyone has the right of access to preventive health care and the right to benefit from medical treatment under the conditions established by national laws and practices. A high level of human health protection shall be ensured in the definition and implementation of all Union policies and activities.'

The European Union Agency for Fundamental Rights (FRA) is an advisory body of the European Union. It was established in 2007 by a legal act of the European Union and is based in Vienna, Austria, and replaced an earlier organisation, the European Monitoring Centre for

Racism and Xenophobia (McHale 2010). The FRA helps to ensure that fundamental rights of people living in the EU are protected. It does this by collecting evidence about the situation of fundamental rights across the European Union and providing advice, based on evidence, about how to improve the situation. The FRA also informs people about their fundamental rights. In doing so, it helps to make fundamental rights a reality for everyone in the European Union. As McHale (2010) points out however, its role does not extend to systematic permanent monitoring of human rights in member states. The annual reports of the FRA provide an insight into the situation in the European Union, although, drawing as they do on the specific projects they have recently completed, the overview they offer is by no means a comprehensive analysis. Their most recent annual report (FRA 2018) suggests that equality bodies and national human rights institutions lack resources, independence, and often have very weak mandates. It remains to be seen how influential the FRA will prove in encouraging EU member states to address the problems identified.

Middle East

Human rights in the Middles East region have been less developed since the 1940s than other regions; reasons for this can be located in its frequently turbulent political history. A Permanent Arab Commission on Human Rights (PACHR) was founded in September 1968 by the Council of the League of Arab States (An-Na'im 2001). The work of the PACHR has been preoccupied primarily with the rights of Arabs living in Israeli-occupied territories. The Arab Charter on Human Rights was adopted by the Council of the League of Arab States in September 1994, but never came into force. The Charter contains a specific article in relation to culture and religion for minorities, stating: 'Minorities shall not be deprived of their right to enjoy their culture or to follow the teachings of their religions'.

The Charter includes no specific mention of health or the right to health but Articles 38 and 39 deal with health matters for the family, and young persons:

Article 38

(a)   *The family is the basic unit of society, whose protection it shall enjoy.*
(b)   *The State undertakes to provide outstanding care and special protection for the family, mothers, children and the aged.*

Article 39

Young persons have the right to be afforded the most ample opportunities for physical and mental development.

The Charter was the subject of considerable criticism by NGOs (Mann 2004). These criticisms pointed out that it does not correspond to many international human rights standards as set forth in previous international declarations and treaties, particularly the UDHR. During the Arab Summit held in Tunis in May 2004, a 'modernised' version of the Arab Charter on Human Rights was adopted. Although this has addressed some of the concerns, some remain, including the possibility of sentencing people under 18 years of age to death, allowing for non-discrimination laws that are applicable only for citizens, and limitations on the freedom of expression and association and gender equality (Mann 2004). The Charter, which entered into force in March 2008 (Rishmawi 2010, 2015), contains a number of traditional human rights as well as provisions of a more political nature. As Rishmawi (2010) identifies, the real test of the Arab Human Rights Committee set up to fulfil monitoring functions will come when it considers the first reports from countries; the committee will also consider parallel reports submitted by NGOs (Rishmawi 2015). No further updated report in English was available as at March 2019.

The Charter and League of Arab States currently lack any enforcement mechanisms and there is no regional court of justice or human rights. The Ministerial Council of the League of Arab States approved a Statute of the Arab Court of Human Rights on 7 September 2014. According to Magliveras (2017) only two states have ratified the Statute. There has been much criticism by NGOs of the Statute, with calls for states not to ratify it until it is comprehensively amended (Rishmawi 2015).

In a report on the state of human rights in the Arab Region in 2008, the Cairo Institute for Human Rights Studies (CIHRS 2008) reported that the status of human rights in the Arab region had increasingly worsened. Their latest report, released in August 2018 (CIHRS 2018), identified a worsening in the situation with increasing militarisation of politics, the failure to find peaceful, radical solutions to the region's internal and international conflicts, and the resurgence of authoritarianism since the Arab Spring revolutions. The report also notes however, increasing public demand for economic and social justice, seeing this as offering hope for a more equitable, just, and democratic future.

Organisation of Islamic Cooperation

The Organisation of Islamic Cooperation (OIC), formerly the Organisation of the Islamic Conference, has a membership of fifty-seven states from four continents. The Organisation aims to be the collective voice of the Muslim world and to safeguard and protect the interests of the Muslim world in the spirit of promoting international peace and harmony. The OIC was established in a summit meeting which took place in Morocco in September 1969 following the arson attack on Al-Aqsa Mosque in Jerusalem. The present Charter of the Organisation was adopted by the Eleventh Islamic Summit held in Dakar in March 2008. The Organisation has consultative and cooperative relations with the UN and other intergovernmental organisations to protect the vital interests of Muslim people, and to work for the settlement of conflict and disputes involving member states.

Under the Charter, the Organisation's aims include: reaffirming support for the rights of peoples as stipulated in the UN Charter and international law; upholding and promoting, at the national and international levels, good governance, democracy, human rights, fundamental freedoms, and the rule of law. The OIC adopted the Cairo Declaration on Human Rights in Islam in 1990, and the Covenant on the Rights of the Child in Islam in 2004. The Independent Permanent Human Rights Commission (IPHRC) is an expert body with advisory capacity established by the 2008 Charter and formally launched in 2011. From March 2017, the IPHRC secretariat has been located in independent headquarters provided by Saudi Arabia.

Regional systems: developments into the future

While the development of regional human rights systems is promising, providing the opportunity for an additional layer of human rights governance and monitoring, they remain largely undeveloped, and arguably, it is too early to show how effective their operations may prove to be in protecting and promoting human rights. Of continued concern is the large portion of the global population who are not covered by a regional system that has the capacity to receive individual complaints. The system in the Americas perhaps shows the most positive effects in terms of promoting change in member countries, and it is perhaps no coincidence that this system is the one with the most thorough system of monitoring implementation of recommendations. It is also notable that much has been achieved through the joint work with the regional office of the WHO for the Americas, PAHO (Meier and Ayala 2014). Only time will tell if other regions, through working with state parties, NGOs, and UN bodies, will be able to achieve positive human rights outcomes for their populations.

References

Throughout this chapter, in discussing the basic history and structures of human rights systems use has been made of websites and a few key references. The following list provides both sources that have been directly cited in text, and key sources that are not directly referred to.

ACHPR 2001. *Communication 155/96: The Social and Economic Rights Action Center and the Center for Economic and Social Rights/Nigeria*, Banjul: ACHPR. doi.org/10.2307/3070689

ACHPR 2019. *African Commission on Human and Peoples' Rights* [Online], Banjul. Available: www.achpr.org/ [Accessed 03/08/2019].

African Court on Human and Peoples' Rights 2019. *African Court on Human and Peoples' Rights* [Online], Banjul. Available: www.african-court.org/ [Accessed 03/08/2019].

African Union 1988. *African Charter on Human and Peoples' Rights* [Online]. Available: www.achpr.org/instruments/achpr/ [Accessed 13/08/2019].

African Union 2019. *African Union* [Online]. Available: www.achpr.org [Accessed 03/08/2019].

AHRD 2012. *ASEAN Declaration of Human Rights* [Online], Banjul. Available: https://asean.org/asean-human-rights-declaration/ [Accessed 15/03/2019].

Amunwa, B 2011. *Counting the Cost: Corporations and Human Rights Abuses in the Niger Delta*, London: Platform.

An-Na'im, AA 2001. Human rights in the Arab world: A regional perspective, *Human Rights Quarterly*, 23: 701. doi.org/10.1353/hrq.2001.0026

ASEAN 2009. *ASEAN Intergovernmental Commission on Human Rights: Terms of Reference*, Jakarta: ASEAN.

ASEAN 2019. *The Association of Southeast Asian Nations* [Online]. Available: https://asean.org/ [Accessed 03/08/2019].

Baizer, T, & Monk, D 2018. *Instruments of Repression: A Regional Report on the Status of Freedoms of Expression, Peaceful Assembly, and Association in Asia*, Forum-Asia [Online]. Available: www.forum-asia.org/uploads/wp/2019/02/Instruments-of-Repressions-final-edited.pdf [Accessed 21/03/2019].

Cabal, L, Roa, M, & Sepúlveda-Oliva, L 2003. What role can international litigation play in the promotion and advancement of reproductive rights in Latin America?, *Health and Human Rights*, 7(1): 51–88. doi.org/10.2307/4065417

Cairo Institute for Human Rights Studies 2019. *Cairo Institute for Human Rights Studies* [Online]. Available: www.cihrs.org/ [Accessed 12/08/2019].

CIHRS 2008. *Human Rights in the Arab Region: Annual Report 2008*, Cairo: Cairo Institute for Human Rights Studies.

CIHRS 2018. *The Militarization of Politics and an Authoritarian Revival: The Eighth Annual CIHRS Report on Human Rights in the Arab Region*, Cairo: Cairo Institute for Human Rights Studies.

Council of Europe 1950. *Convention for the Protection of Human Rights and Fundamental Freedoms* [Online]. Available: www.echr.coe.int/Documents/Convention_ENG.pdf

Council of Europe 2019. *The European Convention on Human Rights* [Online]. Available: www.coe.int/en/web/human-rights-convention/landmark-judgments

EU 2000. Charter of fundamental rights of the European Union, *Official Journal of the European Communities*, C364: 1–22.

EU Network 2006. *Commentary of the Charter of Fundamental Rights on the European Union*, Brussels: EU Network of Independent Experts on Human Rights.

European Commission 2019. *EU Charter of Fundamental Rights* [Online]. Available: https://ec.europa.eu/info/aid-development-cooperation-fundamental-rights/your-rights-eu/eu-charter-fundamental-rights_en [Accessed 12/08/2019].

European Court of Human Rights 2019. *European Court of Human Rights* [Online]. Available: www.echr.coe.int/ECHR/ [Accessed 12/08/2019].

European Union Agency for Fundamental Rights 2019. *European Union Agency for Fundamental Rights* [Online]. Available: http://fra.europa.eu/fraWebsite/home/home_en.htm [Accessed 12/08/2019].

Evans, M, & Murray, R 2008. *The African Charter on Human and Peoples' Rights: The System in Practice 1986–2006*, Cambridge, UK, Cambridge University Press.

Federal Ministry of Justice 2008. *Nigeria's Third Periodic Country Report 2005–2008 on the Implementation of the African Charter on Human and Peoples' Rights in Nigeria*, Abuja: Federal Ministry of Justice Nigeria.

Federal Ministry of Justice 2017. *Nigeria's Third Periodic Country Report 2015–2016 on the Implementation of the African Charter on Human and Peoples' Rights in Nigeria*, Abuja: Federal Ministry of Justice Nigeria.

Forum-Asia 2018. *Sustainable Development Goals: A Human Rights-Based Approach*, Working Paper Series Number 4, Forum-Asia. Available: www.forum-asia.org/uploads/wp/2018/10/FINAL-WEB-Forum-Asia-Working-Paper-Series-No-4-Web-File-21-9-2018.pdf [Accessed 03/08/2019].

Forum-Asia 2019. *Asian Forum for Human Rights and Development* [Online], Geneva. Available: www.forum-asia.org/ [Accessed 03/08/2019].

FRA 2010. *European Union Agency for Fundamental Rights Annual Report 2010, Conference Edition*, Vienna: FRA.

FRA 2018. *Fundamental Rights Report 2018*, European Union Agency for Fundamental Rights. Available: http://fra.europa.eu/en/publication/2018/fundamental-rights-report-2018 [Accessed 20/03/2019].

Goldhaber, MD 2007. *A People's History of the European Court of Human Rights*, New Brunswick, NJ: Rutgers University Press.

Greer, SC 2006. *The European Convention on Human Rights: Achievements, Problems and Prospects*, Cambridge, UK, Cambridge University Press.

Hanung, CD, Ginting, MS, & Judhistari, RA 2018. *Reasonable Doubt: The Journey within: A Report on the Annual Performance of the ASEAN Human Rights Mechanisms in 2017* [Online], Asian Form for Human Rights and Development. Available: www.forum-asia.org/?p=27616 [Accessed 19/03/2019].

Helfer, LR 1993. Consensus, coherence and the European convention on human rights, *Cornell International Law Journal*, 26: 133–165.

Heyns, C 2003. The African regional human rights system: The African Charter, *Penn State Law Review*, 108: 679.

IACHR 2001. *Report Nº 29/01 Case 12.249 Jorge Odir Miranda Cortez et al. El Salvador March 7, 2001*, Washington, DC: OAS.

IACHR 2009a. *Indigenous and Tribal Peoples' Rights over Their Ancestral Lands and Natural Resources: Norms and Jurisprudence of the Inter-American Human Rights System*, Washington, DC: OAS.

IACHR 2009b. *Report Nº 27/09 Case 12.249 Jorge Odir Miranda Cortez et al. El Salvador Merits Report, March 20, 2009*, Washington, DC: OAS.

IACHR 2010. *Access to Maternal Health Services from a Human Rights Perspective*, Washington, DC: OAS.

IACHR 2011. *Annual Report of the Inter-American Commission on Human Rights 2010*, Washington, DC: Inter-American Commission on Human Rights.

IACHR 2016. *Annual Report of the Inter-American Commission on Human Rights 2016*, Washington, DC: Inter-American Commission on Human Rights.

IACHR 2017. *Indigenous Women and Their Human Rights in the Americas*, Washington, DC: Inter-American Commission on Human Rights/Organization of American States.

IACHR 2018a. *Annual Report 2018* [Online]. Available: www.oas.org/en/iachr/docs/annual/2018/TOC.asp [Accessed 03/08/2019].

IACHR 2018b. *Annual Report of the Inter-American Court of Human Rights 2017*, San Jose, Costa Rica: Organization of American States.

IACHR 2019. *Inter-American Court of Human Rights* [Online]. Available: www.oas.org/en/iachr/default.asp [Accessed 03/08/2019].

Jirasek, J 2008. *Application of the Charter of Fundamental Rights of the EU in the United Kingdom and Poland According to the Lisbon Treaty*. Available: www.law.muni.cz/sborniky/cofola2008/files/pdf/evropa/jirasek_jan.pdf [Accessed 03/08/2019].

Keller, H, & Sweet, AS (eds.) 2008. *The Reception of the ECHR in the Member States*, Oxford: Oxford University Press.

Kufuor, K 2010. *The African Human Rights System: Origin and Evolution*, Springer. doi.org/10.1057/9780230106543

Magliveras, KD 2017. Completing the institutional mechanism of the Arab human rights system, *International Human Rights Law Review*, 6(1): 30–52. doi.org/10.1163/22131035-00601003

Mann, S 2004. "Modernizing" the Arab rights charter, *Respect, The Human Rights Newsletter*, 20(201): 5.

Mayer, AE 2018. *Islam and Human Rights: Tradition and Politics*, 5th edn, New York/London: Routledge. doi.org/10.4324/9780429495120

McHale, J 2010. Fundamental rights and health care, in E Mossialos, G Permanad, R Baeten, & T Hervey (eds.) *Health Systems Governance in Europe: The Role of European Union Law and Policy*, Cambridge: Cambridge University Press.

Meier, BM, & Ayala, AS 2014. The Pan American Health Organization and the Mainstreaming of Human Rights in Regional Health Governance, *Journal of Law, Medicine and Ethics*, 42(3): 356–374. doi.org/10.1111/jlme.12152

OAS 2019. *Organisation of American States* [Online]. Available: www.oas.org [Accessed 03/08/2019].

Organisation of Islamic Cooperation 2019. *Organization of Islamic Cooperation* [Online]. Available: www.oic-oci.org/ [Accessed 12/08/2019].

Organisation of Islamic Cooperation 2019. *Independent Permanent Human Rights Commission (IPHRC)* [Online]. Available: www.oic-iphrc.org/en/home [Accessed 12/08/2019].

Peers, S, & Ward, A 2004. *The EU Charter of Fundamental Rights: Politics, Law and Policy*, Oxford: Hart.

Pernice, I 2008. *The Treaty of Lisbon and Fundamental Rights, Walter Hallstein-Institut für Europäisches Verfassungsrecht Humboldt-Universität zu Berlin WHI – Paper 7/08* [Online]. Available: www.judicialstudies.unr.edu/JS_Summer09/JSP_Week_1/Pernice%20Fundamental%20Rights.pdf [Accessed 06/07/2011].

Phan, HD 2019. Promotional versus protective design: The case of the ASEAN intergovernmental commission on human rights, *International Journal of Human Rights*. doi:10.1080/13642987.2018.1562919

Rishmawi, M 2010. The Arab Charter on human rights and the league of Arab states: An update, *Human Rights Law Review*, 10(1): 169–178. doi.org/10.1093/hrlr/ngp043

Rishmawi, M 2015. *The League of Arab States Human Rights Standards and Mechanisms: Towards Further Civil Society Engagement: A Manual for Practitioners* [Online], Open Society Foundations and Cairo Institute for Human Rights Studies. Available: www.cihrs.org/wp-content/uploads/2015/12/league-arab-states-manual-en-20151125.pdf [Accessed 20/03/2019].

SAPATFAHR 2010. *Hiding Behind Its Limits: A Performance Report of the First Year of the ASEAN Intergovernmental Commission on Human Rights 2009–2010*, Bangkok: Forum-Asia, Asian Forum for Human Rights and Development.

Ssenyonjo, M 2012. *The African Regional Human Rights System: 30 Years after the African Charter on Human and Peoples' Rights*, Leiden: Brill.

Trubek, DM, & Trubek, LG 2005. Hard and soft law in the construction of social Europe: The role of the open method of co-ordination, *European Law Journal*, 11(3): 343–364. doi.org/10.1111/j.1468-0386.2005.00263.x

Umozurike, UO 1983. The African Charter on human and peoples' rights, *American Journal of International Law*, 77(4): 902–912.

UNEP 2011. *Environmental Assessment of Ogoniland*, Nairobi: UNEP.

Yen, Y-M 2011. The formation of the ASEAN Intergovernmental Commission on Human Rights: A protracted journey, *Journal of Human Rights*, 10(3): 393–413. doi.org/10.1080/14754835.2011.596070

4

NATIONAL AND SUBNATIONAL HUMAN RIGHTS SYSTEMS

Ann Taket and Fiona H. McKay

Introduction

This chapter turns to the question of national and subnational systems for protection and promotion of human rights. There is incredible diversity here, and the chapter cannot attempt to cover every country and its system in detail. Instead, it discusses five countries to illustrate some of the different approaches and structures, and in each case to explore links to health and health policy.

Most national systems are based around a form of national human rights institution (NHRI), in some cases more than one. The present concept and status of NHRIs developed over fifty years and is closely linked to the growth and development of international human rights, in particular based around the United Nations (UN) system (Pohjolainen 2006). This evolution can be divided into three broad stages: the introduction and development of the idea (1946–1978), the 'popularisation' of the concept (1978–1990), and the expansion of NHRI from 1990 onwards.

The end of the Cold War, and the collapse of communism were significant factors in the developmental process of NHRI, it was only in the early 1990s that governments came to accept the principle that all national institutions should fulfil certain minimum criteria (Pohjolainen 2006). A crucial step in this process came in 1993 when the World Conference on Human Rights endorsed the establishment of national institutions (UN General Assembly 1993) and the use of the 'Principles relating to the status of national institutions' that had been formulated in 1991 in Paris, generally known as the Paris Principles (see Table 4.1 for a summary of the principles). The UN has played an important role in the development and establishment of national human rights structures, by functioning both as an arena for intergovernmental debate and dialogue, and as a human rights actor; while the UN has not worked in a vacuum, its role has been decisive (Pohjolainen 2006). A collection of papers edited by Lindsnaes et al. (2000), and published by the NHRI for Denmark, the Danish Centre for Human Rights, offers an interesting analysis of the early years of experience gained in developing institutions in line with the Paris Principles and illustrates some of the challenges institutions face in ensuring independence, sufficient budget, and public awareness of their existence.

TABLE 4.1 Main features of the Paris Principles for NHRIs

---

1. Has a broadly defined mandate with emphasis on the national implementation of international human rights standards
2. Is established by legislative means
3. Is independent of the state in decision-making procedures
4. Has a pluralist representation of civil society and vulnerable groups in its governing body/bodies
5. Handles complaints from individuals

Source: derived from chapter 1 of Lindsnaes et al. (2000)

In the early 1990s there were only relatively few NHRIs (Pohjolainen 2006). By mid-2019, there were 149 NHRIs listed on the database of the National Human Rights Institutions Forum (NHRI 2019). According to Pohjolainen (2006), four broad categories of NHRI can be distinguished: the human rights commission model, the advisory committee model, the ombudsman model, and the human rights institute model. She also distinguishes four different functions that NHRIs may have: *monitoring* of observance of human rights, including sometimes the investigation of complaints; *advisory*, providing advice to the government and sometimes to other relevant actors; *education and information*, including awareness-raising, education and training; and finally, *research*, undertaking specific investigations, studies, and sometimes public inquiries.

The role of the NHRI depend on the position of human rights within the country concerned. In some countries the right to health or similar rights have been established in national constitutions, however, others have utilised non-binding policies, limiting recourse to national courts. Each of the four regions distinguished by the OHCHR incorporate a different type of institution: mainly statute-based commissions are found in the Asia Pacific and Europe; the ombudsman model being common in Eastern Europe; constitutionally based commissions are most common in Africa; and constitutionally based ombuds-institutions are common in the Americas (OHCHR 2009).

The next section presents five different national human rights systems, the examples chosen to illustrate the variety in the ways in which different countries have chosen to establish such systems. The chapter then moves on to look at the question of linking NHRIs into the UN system, including a brief discussion of the role of the GANHRI, the Global Alliance of NHRIs. The chapter concludes with an examination of the success of national human rights systems in terms of the promotion and protection of human rights.

Contrasts and convergences

This section considers five countries: Sweden, Ghana, Australia, India, and Japan. These countries have been chosen to illustrate some of the different mandates, structures, and implementation mechanisms in existence. In each case the latest annual report of the relevant national agency, if available, has been used to give an illustration of the scope and activities of the agency.

Sweden: precursor of modern NHRIs

The Swedish system, based on the Swedish Ombudsman, is the precursor of all modern NHRIs (Carver 2010). The Swedish Ombudsman was established in 1809, when the Swedish

Parliament created a new official, the Justitie-Ombudsman, which loosely translates to the 'citizen's defender' or 'representative of the people'. The responsibility of the Justitie-Ombudsman was to ensure that public authorities and their staff comply with the laws and other statutes governing their actions. This supervision was exercised by evaluating and investigating complaints from the general public, by making inspections of the various authorities, and by conducting other forms of inquiry that they initiate themselves. In Swedish the word 'ombudsman' is without gender.

Since May 2009, a single agency, the Equality Ombudsman (DO) has sought to combat discrimination and promote equal rights and opportunities for everyone. Before this time, the Swedish national human rights system was based around four different ombudsmen: the Children's Ombudsman, the Swedish Ombudsman against Ethnic Discrimination, the Swedish Disability Ombudsman, and the Ombudsman for Equal Rights. The DO is primarily concerned with ensuring compliance with the Discrimination Act (Equality Ombudsman 2011). This law prohibits discrimination related to a person's sex, transgender identity or expression, ethnicity, religion or other belief, disability, sexual orientation, or age. The head of the agency is appointed by the government.

The Ombudsman registers and investigates complaints based on the law's prohibition of discrimination and harassment, and can represent victims in court free of charge. The Ombudsman also investigates complaints from employees on parental leave who feel they have been treated unfairly for having taken such leave. In addition, the Ombudsman exercises supervision by monitoring how employers, higher education institutions, and schools live up to the provisions of the Discrimination Act requiring active measures against discrimination. The Ombudsman's other duties include raising awareness and disseminating knowledge and information about discrimination and about the prohibitions against discrimination, both among those who risk discriminating against others and those who risk being subjected to discrimination. This means that the agency offers guidance to employers, higher education institutions, schools, and others, and helps develop useful methods on their behalf. A further task is to ensure, through awareness-raising initiatives, that everyone knows their rights. In addition, the Ombudsman is required to draw attention and create debate around human rights issues. The DO also has special responsibility for reporting on new research and international developments in the human rights and discrimination field.

One particular issue addressed is that of national minorities, and in particular, the Sámi people. The situation of the Sámi were raised at both the first and second the Universal Periodic Review of Sweden at the UN (OHCHR 2019). The Sámi were recognised by Sweden as an Indigenous people in 1977, and as such should enjoy certain additional rights under Swedish national law and international law (Pikkarainen and Brodin 2008a). Research commissioned by the Ombudsman against Ethnic Discrimination (reported in Pikkarainen and Brodin 2008a) revealed that the Sámi continue to experience discrimination in all areas of society, including in access to health and health services, and that institutionalised racism or structural discrimination exists widely. Recommendations proposed by the Equality Ombudsman were directed to the Swedish government and include the ratification of relevant conventions on Indigenous peoples. A second report (Pikkarainen and Brodin 2008b) examined discrimination against national minorities in the education system, and put forward a similarly wide ranging set of recommendations to address the issue, both inside and outside the education system.

In January 2009, Sweden became the first country in the world to introduce a legal ban on discrimination associated with gender identity or gender expression (Equality Ombudsman 2019). Previous anti-discrimination legislation only protected the right of trans people not to be subjected to discrimination. The new ground of discrimination was introduced to ensure comprehensive protection against discrimination for all people on any gender identity of expression. Later Swedish legislation, introduced in 2013 removed the requirement for patients to be unmarried and sterile to obtain access to assisted reproductive technologies, supporting the reproductive rights of people of all gender identities and sexualities (Erbenius and Payne 2018).

Ghana: linking human rights and anti-corruption

The Commission on Human Rights and Administrative Justice (CHRAJ) is an independent organisation for the safeguarding of human rights in Ghana. It was established in 1993 by an act of the Parliament of Ghana (1993) as directed by Article 216 of the 1992 Ghana Constitution. The CHRAJ is a constitutional body and can formulate its own rules of procedure (Quashigah 2000).

Since its inception, cases handled by CHRAJ have ranged from human rights abuses and corruption to administrative injustice (Asibuo 2001). Asibuo's scrutiny of the Commission's performance over the period 1993 to 1999 leads to the conclusion that it has been successful in terms of keeping the executive arm of government working to address both human rights and public accountability. He also notes that CHRAJ has been ambitious both in creating a nationwide network of offices and in taking on a broad array of issues.

In 2013 the Commission received 11,035 cases, 10,576 of which related to human rights. It concluded 10,694 cases, 10,219 of which related to human rights. CHRAJ (2013a) details a range of activities in delivering human rights education to a variety of audiences. CHRAJ (2013b) reports on an enquiry into the state of human rights in the country in 2013, focusing in particular on economic, social, and cultural rights, including the right to health.

Australia: 'human rights: everyone, everywhere, everyday'

Australia provides an interesting example of a country that has in-country regional differences in relation to human rights. Australia is a federal system with some variation between states; one of the complexities of life in Australia is disentangling federal from state responsibilities in areas including health and human services provision. The Australian Constitution does not guarantee human rights; successive Australian governments have argued in the various periodic reports submitted to the UN that separate legislation covers these adequately. A Human Rights and Equal Opportunity Commission was established in 1986 by an act of federal Parliament. The Commission is an independent statutory organisation and reports to the federal Parliament through the Attorney-General. Over the period 2008–2009 the Human Rights and Equal Opportunity Commission changed its name to the Australian Human Rights Commission, with the vision of 'Human rights: everyone, everywhere, everyday'. The act was modified in April 2017, introducing changes to complaint handling processes to ensure that unmeritorious complaints could be dismissed at an early stage in the process.

Complaints can be brought in relation to 'discrimination, harassment, or bullying' and in relation to breach of human rights by the Commonwealth and its agencies. There are no provisions for complaints to be brought under the national system in relation to human rights breaches (apart from discrimination) by private companies or other levels of government or individuals, as the Commission explicitly points out in its annual report (AHRC 2010), thus falling somewhat short of the scope implied by the Commission's vision. The Commission offers a conciliation process for complaints. If the complaint is not resolved by conciliation, and the President of the Commission is satisfied that a complaint cannot be resolved, the complaint will be terminated. In some cases, the complainant can then make an application within the next sixty days for the Federal Magistrates Court or the Federal Court of Australia for the court to hear the allegations in the complaint. Complaints lodged under the Australian Human Rights Commission Act, which allege a breach of human rights or discrimination in employment by or on behalf of the Commonwealth, cannot be taken to court for deter- mination. If conciliation is unsuccessful or inappropriate, and the Commission finds that there has been a breach of human rights or workplace discrimination has occurred, then the Commission can prepare a report of the complaint, including recommendations for action, for the Attorney General. The reports must be tabled in Parliament, and are available on the Commission's website.

In 2017–2018, the Commission received 2,046 complaints and finalised 2,111. The Com- mission conducted 1,262 conciliations and resolved 931 complaints, 74 percent (AHRC 2018). The Commission reports a range of other activities for the year 2017–2018, including the commencement of the Wiyi Yani U Thangani (Women's Voices) project of national con- sultations with Aboriginal and Torres Strait Islander women and girls about their rights. This is the first dedicated consultation on these issues in thirty years and has reinvigorated debate about the important role of women in Indigenous communities (AHRC 2018). The other key area of work is reported in the *Change the course* report (AHRC 2017) on experiences of sexual assault and sexual harassment in university settings, leading to a significant re-appraisal of the systems and policies across all thirty-nine Australian universities.

Two Australian states, Victoria and Queensland, and one Australian territory, the Austra- lian Capital Territory (ACT), have introduced specific rights legislation. In Victoria a Charter of Human Rights and Responsibilities has been enacted and is discussed further below. In the ACT a Human Rights Act was passed in 2004 and the ACT Human Rights Commission exists to resolve complaints and promote rights. Queensland enacted legislation on 27 Febru- ary 2019. In two further states, Tasmania and Western Australia, public consultation processes have been held which resulted in recommendations for a Charter of Human Rights at state level, these have not yet been implemented.

CASE STUDY: VICTORIA, STATE BASED HUMAN RIGHTS IN A COUNTRY WITHOUT A BILL OF RIGHTS

The main human rights body at state level in Victoria is the Victorian Equal Opportu- nity and Human Rights Commission (VEOHRC), an independent statutory body with responsibilities under three laws: the Equal Opportunity Act (1995 and 2011), the Racial and Religious Tolerance Act 2001, and the Charter of Human Rights and Respon- sibilities Act 2006. The Equal Opportunity Acts (1995 and 2011) prohibit discriminate against people on the basis of a number of different personal characteristics. The Racial and Religious Tolerance Act 2001 makes it against the law to vilify people because of their race or religion. Under the Equal Opportunity Acts (1995 and 2011) and the Racial and Religious Tolerance Act 2001, the Commission helps people resolve complaints of discrimination, sexual harassment and racial or religious vilification through a free and impartial complaint resolution service, with the aim of achieving a mutual agreement.

TABLE 4.2 Twenty Rights in the Victorian Charter of Rights and Responsibilities

Freedom	Dignity
Freedom from forced work (section 11)	Protection from torture and cruel, inhuman or degrading treatment (section 10)
Freedom of movement (section 12)	Privacy and reputation (section 13)
Freedom of thought, conscience, religion and belief (section 14)	Appropriate treatment of children in the criminal process (section 23)
Freedom of expression (section 15)	Right to a fair hearing (section 24)
Peaceful assembly and freedom of association (section 16)	Rights in criminal proceedings (section 25)
Property rights (section 20)	Right not to be tried or punished more than once (section 26)
Right to liberty and security of person (section 21)	Right not to be prosecuted or punished for things that were not criminal offences at the time they were committed (section 27)
Humane treatment when deprived of liberty (section 22)	

Respect	Equality
Right to life (section 9)	Recognition and equality before the law (section 8)
Protection of families and children (section 17)	Taking part in public life (section 18)
Cultural rights (section 19)	

Source: summarised from Department of Justice (2006)

The Victorian Charter of Human Rights and Responsibilities (Department of Justice 2006) includes twenty specific rights. A comparison of Table 4.2 in relation to the UDHR, ICCPR and ICESCR shows that the Victorian Charter is much more limited, for example rights to education, health, and employment are not covered. The Charter means that government and public bodies must consider human rights when making laws and providing services. The Commission's role is to educate people about the rights and responsibilities contained in the Charter and to report annually to the government about the operation of the Charter. The Commission does not handle complaints related to the Charter. Complaints about breaches of the Charter can be made to the Victorian Ombudsman if the complaint involves government departments, statutory authorities, local councils, or a private agency that carries out statutory responsibilities of government. If the complaint is not covered by the ombudsman, the website directs the reader to a list which, as at 26 March 2019, contains seventeen other Victorian complaint and dispute resolution bodies, four Federal complaint and dispute resolution bodies, two specialist police bodies, four Victorian courts and tribunals, and eight Commonwealth and interstate Ombudsman offices. This certainly does not represent a simple or straightforward system.

In relation to human rights, the VEOHRC reports annually on the operation of the Charter, and carries out a range of advocacy functions, as well as running an advice line and offering training and consultancy. From its latest annual report the Commission delivers a picture of mixed progress, reporting positive change occurring across government agencies, resulting in positive outcomes for Victorians, but identifying that the impact of the Charter across government and local government is inconsistent and that there are instances where, despite policy and legislation complying with human rights obligations, practical implementation and service delivery fail to live up to these (VEOHRC 2018). With particular relevance to health they report on an investigation into discrimination on the grounds of mental health in travel insurance, which has already seen major insurers change their policies to reduce such discrimination (VEOHRC 2018).

Under the Act establishing the Charter are requirements for four- and eight-year reviews of its operation. In July 2016, the Attorney-General announced the Victorian Government's response to the Eight-Year Review of the Charter, which included funding for the Commission and Department of Justice and Regulation's Human Rights Unit (HRU) to develop human rights resources and deliver education across the public sector and 'further embed and improve the human rights culture in Victoria' (VEOHRC 2018: 14).

India: the potential of national litigation

Basic human rights are guaranteed in the Indian Constitution of 1950, and the Protection of Human Rights Act 1993 in Article 2 emphasises that 'human rights means the rights relating to life, liberty, equality and dignity of the individual guaranteed by the Constitution or embodied in the International Covenants and enforceable by courts in India'. The Indian National Human Rights Commission (NHRC), created in 1993 (Sripati 2000) has quasi-jurisdictional competence, that is, powers to compel the appearance of witnesses and the production of evidence under the Protection of Human Rights Act 1993. The founding statutes of the Indian NHRC explicitly provide that the human rights in their mandate are those derived from international sources, from treaties ratified by the state and incorporated into domestic law. This excludes economic, social, and cultural rights, which are not protected in the constitutional Bill of Rights, but have a secondary status as non–enforceable 'directive principles of state policy'. However, according to Kumar (2006), the NHRC has followed the Supreme Court in taking an expansive approach to both the use of treaties as sources of law at the municipal level and in developing the application of economic, social, and cultural rights. The Commission itself also reports its role in 'studying treaties and other international instruments on human rights, and making recommendations for their effective implementation' (NHRC 2006: 7). NHRC (2009: 2) reports its view that the right to life with dignity means that 'it is essential for the Commission to focus, in equal measure, on economic, social and cultural rights, just as it does on civil and political rights'. Its latest annual report (NHRC 2016) reinforces this, identifying the necessity for state governments to take action to protect and promote these rights.

The Human Rights Protection Act of 1993 also provided for State Human Rights Commissions to be created to deal with complaints (NHRC 2006). The NHRC has been pursuing this with the state governments, since its inception, however, it reports that not all states have functioning commissions (NHRC 2009). Complaints may be brought to the commission by individuals or may be raised by the Commissions themselves on the basis of a media report. The Commission can make recommendations and award compensation. One of the functions of the Commission is increasing human rights literacy and promoting knowledge about mechanisms available for rights protection. Two other crucial functions of the Commission linked to its role as a protector are the power to intervene in legal proceedings that involve the violation of any fundamental rights and the power of initiating new litigation (Sripati 2000).

India provides an excellent example of the potential of the use of national litigation to support directly the right to health. Article 21 of the Indian Constitution guarantees an individual's right to life and is enforceable in court. Although the article does not contain any explicit reference to a right to health, in 1981, the Indian Supreme Court signalled its intention to make the right to health enforceable by inference from the right to life. As Sharma (2003) reports, the Supreme Court, following a review of conditions in a number of mental hospitals gave the Commission the responsibility of monitoring implementation of its recommendations regarding change in three mental hospitals. A sequence of cases (twenty-two separate cases over the period 1980 to 2002 are described in Singh et al. 2007) has resulted in courts directing provision of particular services to disadvantaged groups in the population and health promoting changes in workplaces and working conditions, including:

- installation of safety measures in state-run pencil factories;
- improvements in working conditions in state and private run asbestos industry;
- provision of health services to convicted criminals;
- provision of emergency medical care to all free of charge.

CASE STUDY: ACCESS TO PALLIATIVE CARE IN INDIA

In 2008, Human Rights Watch undertook research into the experiences of those in India requiring palliative care (HRW 2009), interviewing more than 100 people across India, including patients with advanced life-threatening or debilitating illnesses, healthcare experts and volunteers, and government health officials. Their research identified that only five of approximately 300 medical colleges in the entire country have integrated any instruction into their curricula on palliative care. Consequently, the vast majority of medical doctors in India are unfamiliar with even the most basic tenets of palliative care. In many cases, patients are denied treatment and suffer severe pain, often for weeks or months on end. Many patients told Human Rights Watch that their suffering was so severe that they wanted to die. Some said they had contemplated or attempted suicide. The report also documented the difference that palliative care made to recipients' quality of life.

The report was published in October 2009. This was followed by activities in partnership with Pallium India and the Pain Relief and Palliative Care Society of Hyderabad, and the creation of detailed proposals for how doctors specialising in palliative care should be trained. These proposals were submitted to the Medical Council of India.

Human Rights Watch also began advising the plaintiffs in a case on palliative care still being heard by India's Supreme Court on how international standards could be used to strengthen their case. This case, brought by the Indian Association of Palliative Care and others, would oblige the government to introduce palliative care training for healthcare providers and to eliminate drug laws that impede the availability of essential pain medicine.

In January 2011, years of joint advocacy by Human Rights Watch and Indian palliative care groups culminated in the Medical Council of India recognising palliative care as a specialisation of medicine and approving an MD Palliative Care program.

Source: Human Rights Watch www.hrw.org/en/news/2011/02/14/upholding-right-health

India is a federal country with twenty-eight states and seven union territories; average figures for India hide a great deal of variation in the performance of different states in relation to health (Bajpai et al. 2010) and human rights violations (Beer and Mitchell 2006). Prakasam et al. (2010) gives an interesting collection of papers presented at the Sixth National Conference of the Indian Association for Social Sciences and Health on the theme 'Health, Equity and Human Rights' 2009; these illustrate that the issue of human rights argumentation in support of public health goals has been taken up very broadly in India, addressing health inequities, maternal health, gender dimensions of health, the reduction of vulnerability, nutrition and health, and finally social aspects of health.

Japan: a system characterised by absence of an NHRI

The 1946 Constitution of Japan (*Nihon Koku Kenpo*) adopted human rights, with a provision on 'fundamental human rights' in Article 11. The 1946 Constitution also provides for women's suffrage and the separation of state powers as a principle of democratic Japanese government. As Holland (2009) identifies, the (American) framers of the constitution intended that individual rights would receive protection through the Supreme Court, who have explicit power of judicial review.

Japan has no NHRI. The Japanese government undertakes human rights promotion and protection work through two major, parallel systems: the Human Rights Bureau under the Ministry of Justice and the Human Rights Volunteers. The Human Rights Bureau works along with eight Human Rights Departments under the Ministry of Justice's Legal Bureaus located in eight major cities in the country. These government human rights bodies deal with 'human rights infringements' which are defined as not only against the law but also against the spirit of respecting human rights, which is the basic principle of the Constitution of Japan and the UDHR. These bodies can undertake 'voluntary' investigation to determine whether or not human rights infringement has occurred based on 'requests' for relief from victims or based on report of newspapers and magazines. Once a human rights infringement has been confirmed, relief measures can be provided including legal advice, conciliation, strict warning to the perpetrator, and assistance to the victim.

Parallel to the existence of the Human Rights Bureau, are Japan's Human Rights Volunteers (around 14,000 volunteers in total) who are appointed by the Minister of Justice. They are lay people who work to encourage respect for human rights, make efforts to avoid infringements of the rights of residents and to protect human rights in their local community. From among the Human Rights Volunteers, some are appointed as conciliators under the 'Human Rights Conciliator System'. Some are appointed by the Minister of Justice as Volunteers for Children's Rights Protection to deal with problems affecting child rights. The latter collect information on children's rights in addition to promoting cooperation with the PTA (Parents-Teachers Association), *kodomokai* (Children's Neighbourhood Associations), and the Commissioner for Children to identify signs of abuse as soon as possible.

In the most recent review reporting to the UPR, Japan reported that the Act on the Promotion of Efforts to Eliminate Unfair Discriminatory Speech and Behavior against Persons Originating from Outside Japan came into force in June 2016 (Government of Japan 2017). This Act allows for action to ensure children's rights; and identifies work undertaken on elimination of discriminatory treatment on the grounds of sexual orientation and gender identity. Outstanding problems on all of these issues were noted in the published summary of stakeholders' submissions on Japan (OHCHR 2017). Japanese human rights organisations (OHCHR 2017) have criticised the government for failing to establish an independent NHRI. They also cite the inadequacy of the current human rights mechanism in the country. The bill aimed at establishing an independent NHRI discussed during the previous UPR failed to be enacted (Government of Japan 2017).

Japan thus sits in a very different position in terms of its human rights system than many other countries, and it is therefore of interest to examine the extent to which international systems have an impact within Japan. Iida (2004) presents an analysis of the impact of international human rights law on Japan for three different topics, commercial sexual exploitation of children, eugenics and wartime sexual slavery, and the measures taken to remedy them. The analysis finds that although international human rights law and norms played a major role in each of these episodes, its influence was uneven. To explain this variation, the analysis focused on the domestic balance of power in Japan and identifies three significant factors: shared common interests between pro-human rights constituencies and their political opponents; consensual decision making; and transnational coalition-building through international conferences. In terms of the outcomes, Japan was successful in terms of passing a law to tackle commercial sexual exploitation of children, and following this through to prosecution, through an alignment of these three factors. For eugenics, human rights campaigners were targeting Japan's 1948 'Eugenics Protection Law' that legalised forced sterilisation of the mentally ill and those with hereditary diseases; however, the issue was complicated by the inclusion in the same bill of legalisation of abortion on grounds of 'economic hardship', which became the focus of interest of women's rights groups looking to strengthen women's reproductive rights. This divergence of interest groups meant that the use of international forums by pro-rights groups became crucial in leading to the replacement of the Eugenic Protection Law by the Maternal Body Protection Law in 1996.

A further example is provided in the exploration by Tsutsui and Shin (2008) of the position regarding the human rights of Korean resident in Japan. In this case global human rights norms provide vocabulary that helped to construct cohesive activism within the country, and proved a more successful basis to argue for change than a basis in citizenship rights. International forums and pressure from outside Japan, from networks of international human rights activists, also created pressure on the Japanese government, contributing to successful change within Japan. Holland's examination of role of the Japanese Supreme Court (Holland 2009: 79), finds it to be a 'timid and largely deferential institution', acting as a brake on the lower courts whenever judges attempt to challenge a law or action on human rights grounds, and largely upholding government policies that are being challenged on rights grounds. He argues that this has led to the development of rights-oriented NGOs within Japan and the use of human rights defenders. Holland (2009) does however find signs that the stance of the Supreme Court may change in the future, consequent on pressures on Japan's leadership role within the region, and the arrival of a new generation of lawyers in the Supreme Court, as well as increasing international pressure on its human rights policies.

Linking national human rights institutions into the UN system

At the International Conference held in Tunis in 1993, NHRIs established the International Coordinating Committee of NHRIs (ICC) to help coordinate the activities of the NHRI network. In 1998, rules of procedures were developed for the ICC and its membership was enlarged to sixteen members, four from each of the geographical regions. At that same meeting, the ICC resolved to create a process for accrediting institutions. In 2008, the ICC discussed governance issues, including incorporation of the ICC in order to better cope with the changing environment including the developing role of NHRIs in the international human rights system. The ICC decided to incorporate itself as a legal entity under Swiss law, with a Bureau of 16 voting members representing the four regions of the ICC.

The ICC also decided to streamline rules of procedures and to clearly define its membership and the role and governance of its annual meeting and international conferences. In 2009, the ICC discussed matters related to the Committee's governance working group and the working group on sustainable funding and the Subcommittee on Accreditation. General Meetings of the ICC, meetings of the ICC Bureau and of the Subcommittee on Accreditation, as well as International Conferences of the ICC, are held under the auspices of, and in cooperation with, OHCHR. The ICC links NHRIs directly into the UN system. The accreditation system governs access to UN committees. Institutions accredited by the ICC with 'A status', meaning full compliance with the Paris Principles, are usually accorded speaking rights and seating at human rights treaty bodies and other UN organs. The ICC representative often presents statements on behalf of individual NHRIs or the regional groups. In 2016 the ICC changed its name to Global Alliance of National Human Rights Institutions (GANHRI). GANHRI has a web portal maintained on its behalf by the OHCHR. As at March 2019, it shows a list of 149 national institutions. Of those, seventy-eight are currently accredited with 'A status' by the ICC, and are thus entitled to vote or hold office in GANHRI or its regional groups.

GANHRI has one member of staff representing it at the UN in Geneva. Secretariat support is provided to the GANHRI by the National Institutions and Regional Mechanisms (NIRM) Unit of the Field Operations and Technical Cooperation Division of the OHCHR. Additional work devolves on the NHRI elected to chair the network, currently the German Institute for Human Rights, and the chairs of the GANHRI's four regional networks. The peer review process for initial accreditation, and reaccreditation every five years, is managed by a subcommittee consisting of one representative of each of the regional networks. GANRHI holds annual general meetings (usually in Geneva in March, coinciding with the UN Human Rights Council session) and a biennial thematic conference. GANHRI also works closely with its four regional NHRI networks: the Asia Pacific Forum (APF), the European

Network of National Human Rights Institutions, the Network of African National Human Rights Institutions (NANHRI), and the Red de Instituciones Nacionales para la Promoción y Protección de los Derechos Humanos del Continente Americano (RINDHCA) (GANRHI 2018). Two of the latest pieces of work undertaken by GANHRI examine NHRIs work on migrants human rights (Kämpf 2019) and preventing all forms of violence against women and children (Bouchard et al. 2019).

The Asia Pacific Forum of National Human Rights Institutions (APF) is the largest (in terms of number of members of national human rights institutions that comply with the Paris Principles) regional human rights organisation in the Asia Pacific. It was established in 1996 to support the establishment and strengthening of national human rights institutions in the region. Current members are national institutions in fifteen different countries across the Asia-Pacific region: Afghanistan, Australia, India, Indonesia, Jordan, Malaysia, Mongolia, Nepal, New Zealand, Palestine Territories, Philippines, Qatar, Republic of Korea, Thailand, and Timor Leste. The APF provides a framework for national human rights institutions to work together and cooperate on a regional basis through a wide range of services, including training, capacity building, networks, and staff exchanges.

In Sweden, the agency represented by the Equality Ombudsman, discussed above, is not accredited by the ICC (GANRHI 2018), although the predecessor Ombudsman for Equal Rights did have A status accreditation which lapsed at the end of 2008 (FRA 2010). Ghana's CHRAJ is accorded A status by the ICC, as is Australia's AHRC and India's NHRC (GANRHI 2018). Japan has no NHRI listed on the ICC system (GANRHI 2018).

Later treaties in the UN human rights system have been formulated with an explicit role for NHRIs in their implementation or monitoring, namely the Optional Protocol to the Convention Against Torture (OPCAT), which entered into force in June 2006 and the Convention on the Rights of Persons with Disabilities (CRPD), which entered into force in May 2008. Pohjolainen (2006) sees this as a return of an idea circulating in the earliest years of the UN, that national committees should be established to monitor compliance with the UDHR.

Protecting and promoting human rights: how successful are national human rights systems?

The examples of the different countries considered here demonstrate the variety that exists in structure, organisation, mandate, and functioning of the different national human rights systems. Given this variety, and the highly diverse economic and socio-political contexts of different countries, it should come as no surprise that there is considerable variation of achievements of the different systems in terms of protecting and promoting human rights within countries.

One factor worthy of consideration is the question of whether at the country level a single institution or multiple human rights institutions is to be preferred. Carver (2011) provides an analysis, identifying that there is no guidance on this point within international and regional human rights standards. The Paris Principles give no explicit guidance, although they do state that an NHRI should be 'be given as broad a mandate as possible' (OHCHR 1993, para 2). After a detailed consideration of the arguments both for and against single institutions, Carver (2011) concludes that arguments of both pragmatism and effectiveness are 'overwhelmingly' in favour of a single institution, noting that a number of countries have at different times decided in favour of a merger of different national institutions, Australia (in 1986), the UK (in 2006) and Sweden (in 2008). Not all countries have chosen to do this however. Hungary maintains four separate, but connected ombudsman institutions, and Lithuania has three ombudsman institutions that operate almost entirely separately (Carver 2011).

Shown here, the outcomes from the different national systems are extremely varied, and direct comparison is impossible given the many and diverse factors affecting achievement, including resourcing, timelines, simplicity, or access to proceedings, but also the variation in socio-political context. Elsewhere, in the research literature, is an examination of what has been achieved within national systems broadly, and particularly in relation to the right to health. As Finnegan et al. (2010) point out; the United States has maintained an ambivalent relationship with the discourse of international human rights. The United States has ratified less than a third of the international human rights instruments. Finnegan et al. (2010) explore how US human rights activists conceptualise, relate to, and utilise the human rights framework, finding that activists contend with substantial political obstacles, including the US government's perceived exploitations of the human rights framework. Activists considered that deep-seated American cultural identities of liberalism, meritocracy, and exceptionalism acted as strong barriers to the use of a human rights framework, however, grassroots approaches remain a potential avenue for future human rights organising in the context of the United States.

A review by Hogerzeil et al. (2006) examined completed court cases in low- and middle-income countries where individuals or groups had sought access to essential medicines, with reference to the right to health. The review identified successful cases in ten countries, eight countries in Central and Latin America, plus India and South Africa. Their findings suggest that litigation can help ensure that governments fulfil their human rights obligations, but they suggest that the courts should be used as a last resort and that it is better to ensure that human rights considerations are planned into policy and programs. The review by Singh et al. (2007) highlights the positive health reforms that have been achieved in four different countries, Argentina, Ecuador, South Africa, and India, by use of legal measures. They identify four factors as responsible for the extensive successes in South Africa and India: intense and sustained pressure by strong and competent civil society organisations in those countries; fairly independent, competent, and progressive judicial authorities; governments having respect for the rule of law; and use of medical evidence to support legal arguments.

Looking specifically at the right to health, the South East Asian Regional Office of WHO (SEARO 2011), has summarised the positioning of the right to health in the constitutions of the eleven countries contained in this WHO region. This finds the right positively stated in six countries (DPR Korea, Indonesia, Maldives, Nepal, Thailand and Timor-Leste), while the remaining five countries (Bhutan, Bangladesh, India, Myanmar and Sri Lanka) do not explicitly state this as a positive right but nonetheless compel the state to provide health services and in some cases to improve public health (SEARO 2011). However, as highlighted in the discussion on India, lack of statement of a positive right to health in the constitution has not prevented this right being inferred from others that are constitutionally mandated. Presence of the right to health in the constitution is also a long way from a guarantee that the right will be implemented. Finally, and most comprehensively of all, Backman et al. (2008) propose seventy-two indicators that reflect some of the health system features associated with the right to health and uses globally processed data on these indicators for 194 countries as well as national data for five other countries to assess the state of achievement of the right to health, finding a very mixed picture of achievement.

As yet, there is no comprehensive overview of the functioning and effectiveness of national systems and NHRIs. A set of benchmarks and indicators has been produced (ICHRP 2005), but these have not been yet been taken up in a comprehensive fashion. Some are reflected in the OHCHR survey on NHRIs mentioned at the beginning of the chapter (OHCHR 2009) which provides some insight into the factors that NHRIs themselves consider impinge on their effectiveness. Factors identified include: limited capacity to follow up on recommendations, a particular issue in Africa and the Americas; lack of diversity in the composition of governing bodies; lack of sufficient resources or materials to carry out human rights education and research in many cases where there was the mandate to carry out this function; and finally, the need to strengthen relationships with relevant national stakeholders, particularly public bodies such as the executive, parliament and the judiciary. The Asian NGO network on NHRIs, ANNI, report on the performance and establishment of NHRIs in Asia (ANNI 2018). The report presents a chapter on each of thirteen countries in the region, only one of which (Taiwan) does not yet have an NHRI.

Within the European Union, the European Agency for Fundamental Rights (FRA) reports on NHRIs in EU member states (FRA 2010), with the intention of identifying gaps and concerns in what it calls the fundamental rights architecture of the EU, looking at data protection bodies, equality bodies and NHRIs. This identifies that in many of the EU member states without an NHRI fully compliant with the Paris Principles (currently seventeen of the twenty-seven member states), human rights education and awareness-raising, promotion of human rights, and interaction with civil society are either not mandated, or not carried out due to resource constraints. Their report recommends that the Paris Principles should be seen as the very minimum standards for NHRIs in the European Union.

Perhaps it is not surprising that the picture given of the performance and achievements of national human rights systems is somewhat patchy, given that in many countries, the NHRIs concerned, if they exist, are relatively young. As has already been noted, an increasing role may be played by these institutions in terms of monitoring human rights compliance at the country level.

References

Throughout this chapter, in discussing the basic history and structures of human rights systems use has been made of websites and a few key references. The following list provides both sources that have been directly cited in text, and key sources that are not directly referred to.

AHRC 2010. *Australian Human Rights Commission Annual Report 2009–2010*, Sydney: Australian Human Rights Commission.
AHRC 2017. *Change the Course: National Report on Sexual Assault and Sexual Harassment at Australian Universities*, Sydney: AHRC.
AHRC 2018. *Australian Human Rights Commission Annual Report 2017–2018*, Sydney: AHRC.
AHRC 2019. *Australian Human Rights Commission* [Online], Sydney. Available: www.humanrights.gov.au [Accessed 03/08/2019].
ANNI 2018. *On the Performance and Establishment of NHRIs in Asia*, Bangkok: Asian Forum for Human Rights and Development (FORUM-ASIA).
Asia-Pacific Human Rights Information Center 2019. [Online], Osaka. Available: www.hurights.or.jp/english/ [Accessed 03/08/2019].

Asibuo, SK 2001. *The Role of the Commission on Human Rights and Administrative Justice (CHRAJ) in Promoting Public Service Accountability under Ghana's Fourth Republic*, Tangier: African Training and Research Centre in Administration for Development.

Backman, G, Hunt, P, Khosla, R, Jaramillo-Strouss, C, Fikre, BM, Rumble, C, Pevalin, D, Páez, DA, Pineda, MA, Frisancho, A, Tarco, D, Motlagh, M, Farcasanu, D, & Vladescu, C 2008. Health systems and the right to health: An assessment of 194 countries, *The Lancet*, 372(9655): 2047–2085. doi. org/10.1016/S0140-6736(08)61781-X

Bajpai, N, Sachs, JD, & Dholakia, RH 2010. *Improving Access and Efficiency in Public Health Services: Mid-Term Evaluation of India's National Rural Health Mission*, New Delhi: Sage.

Beer, C, & Mitchell, NJ 2006. Comparing nations and states: Human rights and democracy in India, *Comparative Political Studies*, 39(8): 996–1018. doi.org/10.1177/0010414005282392

Bouchard, A, Jesudasam, NC, Lalonde, J, Ishoq, BM, Trilsch, M, & Blard, L 2019. *Preventing and Eliminating All Forms of Violence against Women and Girls: The Role of National Human Rights Institutions* [Online], GANHRI/The German Institute for Human Rights. Available: https://nhri.ohchr.org/EN/Pages/ExternalPublications.aspx [Accessed 28/03/2019].

Carver, R 2010. A new answer to an old question: National human rights institutions and the domestication of international law, *Human Rights Law Review*, 10(1): 1–32. doi.org/10.1093/hrlr/ngp040

Carver, R 2011. One NHRI or many? How many institutions does it take to protect human rights? Lessons from the European experience, *Journal of Human Rights Practice*, 3(1): 1–24. doi.org/10.1093/jhuman/hur005

Chappell, L, Chesterman, J, & Hill, L 2009. *The Politics of Human Rights in Australia*, Port Melbourne: Cambridge University Press.

CHRAJ 2013a. *2013 State of the Human Rights Report*, Accra: CHRAJ.

CHRAJ 2013b. *2013 Annual Report*, Accra: CHRAJ.

CHRAJ 2019. *Commission on Human Rights and Administrative Justice Ghana* [Online], Accra. Available: https://chraj.gov.gh/ [Accessed 03/08/2019].

Department of Justice 2006. *The Charter of Human Rights and Responsibilities*, Victoria: State Government.

Equality Ombudsman 2019. *Gender Equity in Sweden* [Online], Stockholm. Available: https://sweden. se/society/gender-equality-in-sweden/ [Accessed 03/08/2019].

Equality Ombudsman 2011. *About the Equality Ombudsman* [Online], Stockholm. Available: www.do.se/other-languages/english/ [Accessed 03/08/2019].

Erbenius, T, & Payne, JG 2018. Unlearning cis-normativity in the clinic: Enacting transgender reproductive rights in everyday patient encounters, *Journal of International Women's Studies*, 20(1): 27–39.

Finnegan, AC, Saltsman, AP, & White, SK 2010. Negotiating politics and culture: The utility of human rights for activist organizing in the United States, *Journal of Human Rights Practice*, 2(3): 307–33. doi. org/10.1093/jhuman/huq009

FRA 2010. *National Human Rights Institutions in the EU Member States: Strengthening the Fundamental Rights Architecture in the EU I*, Luxembourg: Publication Office of the EU.

GANRHI 2018. *2018 Annual Report: 25 Years Advancing Human Rights with National Human Rights Institutions and Our Partners* [Online], GANHRI. Available: https://nhri.ohchr.org/EN/AboutUs/GANHRIAnnualReports/Pages/default.aspx [Accessed 25/03/2019].

Government of Japan 2017. *National Report Submitted in Accordance with Paragraph 5 of the Annex to Human Rights Council Resolution 16/21* [Online], A/HRC/WG.6/28/JPN/1. Available: www.ohchr.org/EN/HRBodies/UPR/Pages/JPindex.aspx [Accessed 28/03/2019].

Government of Sweden 2019. *Democracy and Human Rights* [Online], Stockholm. Available: www. government.se/government-policy/democracy-and-human-rights/ [Accessed 03/08/2019].

Hogerzeil, HV, Samson, M, Casanovas, JV, & Rahmani-Ocora, L 2006. Is access to essential medicines as part of the fulfilment of the right to health enforceable through the courts?, *The Lancet*, 368: 305–311. doi.org/10.1016/S0140-6736(06)69076-4

Holland, KM 2009. Rights protection in Japan: The political dimension, *Australian Journal of Political Science*, 44(1): 79–96. doi.org/10.1080/10361140802654992

HRC 2010. *Report of the Working Group on the Universal Periodic Review: Sweden*, A/HRC/15/11, New York: Human Rights Council.

HRW 2009. *Unbearable pain: India's Obligation to Ensure Palliative Care*, New York: Human Rights Watch.

ICHRP 2005. *Assessing the Effectiveness of National Human Rights Institutions*, Geneva: ICHRP/OHCHR.

Iida, K 2004. Human rights and sexual abuse: The impact of international human rights law on Japan, *Human Rights Quarterly*, 26(2): 428–453. doi.org/10.1353/hrq.2004.0022

Kämpf, A 2019. *National Human Rights Institutions and Their Work on Migrants' Human Rights: Results of a Survey among NHRIs* [Online], GANHRI/The German Institute for Human Rights. Available: https://nhri.ohchr.org/EN/Pages/ExternalPublications.aspx [Accessed 28/03/2019].

Kumar, CR 2006. National human rights institutions and economic, social and cultural rights: Towards the institutionalization and developmentalization of human rights, *Human Rights Quarterly*, 28(3): 755–779. doi.org/10.1353/hrq.2006.0035

Lindsnaes, B, Lindholt, L, & Yigen, K (eds.) 2000. *National Human Rights Institutions: Articles and Working Papers*, Copenhagen: Danish Centre for Human Rights.

Ministry of Japan 2019. *Human Rights Bureau* [Online]. Available: www.moj.go.jp/ENGLISH/HB/hb.html [Accessed 03/08/2019].

NHRC 2006. *The National Human Rights Commission*, New Delhi: NHRC.

NHRC 2009. *National Human Rights Commission, Annual Report 2007–2008*, New Delhi: NHRC.

NHRC 2016. *National Human Rights Commission, Annual Report 2015–2016*, New Delhi: NHRC.

NHRI 2019. *National Human Rights Institutions* [Online]. Available: http://nhri.ohchr.org [Accessed 03/08/2019].

OHCHR 1993. *Principles Relating to the Status of National Institutions (The Paris Principles)*, UN General Assembly Resolution 48/134 of 20 December.

OHCHR 2009. *Survey on National Human Rights Institutions: Report on the Findings and Recommendations of a Questionnaire Addressed to NHRIs Worldwide*, Geneva: OHCHR.

OHCHR 2017. *Summary of Stakeholders' Submissions on Japan: Report of the Office of the United Nations High Commissioner for Human Rights* [Online], A/HRC/WG.6/28/JPN/3. Available: www.ohchr.org/EN/HRBodies/UPR/Pages/JPindex.aspx [Accessed 28/03/2019].

OHCHR 2019. *Universal Periodic Review* [Online]. Available: www.ohchr.org/en/hrbodies/upr/pages/uprmain.aspx [Accessed 12/06/2019].

Parliament of Ghana 1993. *Commission of Human Rights Act (Act 456)* [Online]. Available: www.unhcr.org/refworld/docid/44bf7f804.html. [Accessed 25/03/2019].

Pikkarainen, H, & Brodin, B 2008a. *Discrimination of the Sami: The Rights of the Sami from a Discrimination Perspective*, Stockholm: Ombudsmannen mot etnisk diskriminering.

Pikkarainen, H, & Brodin, B 2008b. *Discrimination of National Minorities in the Education System*, Stockholm: Ombudsmannen mot etnisk diskriminering.

Pohjolainen, A 2006. *The Evolution of National Human Rights Institutions: The Role of the United Nations*, Copenhagen: Danish Institute for Human Rights.

Prakasam, PK, Vaidyanathan, KE, Somayajulu, UV, & Audinarayana, N (eds.) 2010. *Health, Equity and Human Rights: Perspectives and Issues*, New Delhi: Serials Publications/Indian Association for Social Sciences and Health.

Quashigah, EK 2000. The Ghana commission on human rights and administrative justice, in B Lindsnaes, L Lindholt, & K Yigen (eds.) *National Human Rights Institutions: Articles and Working Papers*, Copenhagen: Danish Centre for Human Rights.

SEARO 2011. *The Right to Health in the Constitutions of Member States of the World Health Organization South-East Asia Region*, New Delhi: WHO, Regional Office for South-East Asia.

Sharma, S 2003. Human rights of mental patients in India: A global perspective, *Current Opinion in Psychiatry*, 16(5): 547–551. doi.org/10.1097/00001504-200309000-00010

Singh, JA, Govender, M, & Mills, EJ 2007. Do human rights matter to health?, *The Lancet*, 370: 521–527. doi.org/10.1016/S0140-6736(07)61236-7

Sripati, V 2000. India's National Human Rights Commission: Strengths and weaknesses, in B Lindsnaes, L Lindholt, & K Yigen (eds.) *National Human Rights Institutions: Articles and Working Papers*, Copenhagen: Danish Centre for Human Rights.

Tsutsui, K, & Shin, HJ 2008. Global norms, local activism, and social movement outcomes: Global human rights and resident Koreans in Japan, *Social Problems*, 55(3): 391–418. doi.org/10.1525/sp.2008.55.3.391

UN General Assembly 1993. *Report of the World Conference on Human Rights: Report of the Secretary-General*, A/CONF.157/24 (Part I), New York: UN.

UN General Assembly 2010. *Promotion and Protection of Human Rights, Including Ways and Means to Protect the Human Rights of Migrants, Report of the Secretary General*, A/65/156, New York: UN.

VEOHRC 2018. *Annual Report 2017–18: Human Rights Speak to the Heart of What It Means to Be a Fair and Inclusive Community*, Melbourne: VEOHRC.

VEOHRC 2019. *Victorian Equal Opportunity and Human Rights Commission* [Online], Melbourne. Available: www.humanrightscommission.vic.gov.au [Accessed 03/08/2019].

5

HEALTH EQUITY AND HUMAN RIGHTS

Ann Taket and Fiona H. McKay

The links between health and human rights

In understanding the links between health and human rights, it is useful to distinguish three different, but interacting components (WHO 2002a). First, human rights violations can directly affect health: for example, torture, slavery, violence against women and children, and harmful traditional practices. Second, the promotion of human rights, in particular those connected to the social determinants of health, for example rights to education, to food and nutrition, shelter, and employment, lead to reduced vulnerability to ill health and promote health. Third, health development can involve promotion or violation of human rights, depending on how it affects rights such as the right to participation, freedom from discrimination, right to information, and right to privacy. There is a reciprocal impact of health and human rights. The promotion, protection, restriction, or violations of human rights have direct and indirect impacts on health and wellbeing, in the short, medium, and long term.

CASE STUDY: DOMESTIC VIOLENCE – A MAJOR PUBLIC HEALTH AND HUMAN RIGHTS ISSUE

Domestic violence, abuse against women by current or previous intimate partners, is a major public health problem globally (García-Moreno et al. 2005). It occurs in all countries irrespective of culture, socio-economic status, or religion, and occurs in all types of relationships, both same sex and heterosexual (Krug et al. 2002). The context and severity of violence by men against women makes domestic violence against women a much larger problem in public health terms (Krug et al. 2002; WHO 1997). Intimate partner abuse has severe short- and long-term health consequences, both physical and mental, for the partner experiencing abuse, and for any children in the family (Itzin et al. 2010).

A frequent characteristic of domestic violence is that the perpetrator often blames his abuse on the woman and her behaviour, and uses the abuse to assert control over the woman and her life. The woman experiencing abuse is often made to feel inadequate, or a failure, and that she deserves the abuse. Sometimes her movements are curtailed and she is kept a virtual prisoner in the house. These characteristics have led to domestic violence being viewed legally as a human rights issue (Chapman 1990), and to cases being brought under the UN and regional systems for the protection of human rights.

One of the earliest, from 1998, was a petition was presented to the Inter-American Commission on Human Rights (IACHR) bringing the case of a Brazilian woman, Maria da Penha who had suffered years of abuse from her husband. Despite numerous reports to various authorities within the country, no action was taken. As documented by UN Women (2011) in 2006, the Government of Brazil enacted domestic violence legislation, symbolically named the Maria da Penha law on domestic and family violence, mandating preventative measures, special courts, and tough sentences. Two further cases, brought by NGOs against Austria, on behalf of two women murdered by their husbands to the CEDAW Committee under the Optional Protocol. The Committee's decisions on the cases in 2007 were of global significance because they made clear that the state's obligation to protect women from domestic violence extends beyond passing laws. The Committee found that Austria had failed to act with 'due diligence' by not ensuring that the law was implemented properly. In response to the Committee's recommendations and the media attention that surrounded the case, the Austrian Government introduced and accelerated legal reforms to protect women from violence (UN Women 2011: 18).

The UN Special Rapporteur on Violence Against Women from 2009 to 2015, Rashida Manjoo, argued that a UN treaty on violence against women is essential in effectively tackling the issue. See McQuigg (2018) for an exploration on this issue, noting the challenges that would have to be overcome.

Blaker Strand (2019) examines how the European Court of Human Rights has in its interpretations, utilised the normative overlap between the ECHR and CEDAW to strengthen the protection of women's human rights, a process referred to as an 'interpretive widening and thickening'.

As part of a whole of society response, in July 2018, New Zealand passed legislation supporting up to ten days paid leave from work for people experiencing domestic violence, coming into effect in April 2019 (Government of New Zealand 2018). This joins legislation passed in the Philippines, where the Anti-Violence against Women and Their Children Act of 2004 includes provision for victims to take up to ten days special leave. Similar laws also exist in Canada at the provincial level in Manitoba and Ontario.

To illustrate the links between health equity and human rights, two examples are given in the case studies in this chapter, the first above on domestic violence and the second on Indigenous rights. Given the understanding of the close interrelationships between health equity and human rights, it is obviously desirable to ensure that health policies and programs protect and promote rights. This has led for calls for the use of rights-based approaches (RBA) in policy development and implementation, and in the planning and delivery of health programs, understanding RBA to mean approaches that help protect and promote rights. Accepting health equity as a goal of health systems worldwide thus necessitates a focus on human rights, and indeed vice versa. This chapter sets out to explore in more detail what is meant by the term 'rights-based approach' and how effective this can be in moving towards health equity and social justice.

CASE STUDY: HEALTH OF INDIGENOUS AUSTRALIANS – THE IMPORTANCE OF PROTECTING AND PROMOTING RIGHTS

The health status of Indigenous Australians is shaped by the legacy of centuries of social disadvantage, dispossession, discrimination, and colonialism. The current position is still characterised by social disadvantage in many areas including education, housing, employment, and income. Life expectancy of Indigenous men is 67.2 (compared to non-Indigenous men 78.7) and of Indigenous women is 72.9 (compared to non-Indigenous 82.6) (ABS 2009).

In 2007, in response to the report of an inquiry into child sexual abuse in Indigenous communities in the Northern Territory (Wild and Anderson 2007), the Australian federal government introduced the Northern Territory Emergency Response (NTER, often known as 'the intervention'), a package of eleven emergency measures including compulsory child health checks and significant welfare reforms. Legislation was introduced to do this, and provisions in three of the Acts were deemed to be 'special measures', allowing the suspension of part of the Racial Discrimination Act. There was much concern about this, about many aspects of the processes through which the NTER was developed and implemented, and about some of its major provisions, including: the use of the Australian Army to lead implementation; the acquisition of land title in prescribed communities; compulsory income management for all adults in prescribed communities who were receiving welfare payments; and, compulsory health checks for children. In addition, the measures in the NTER were not well matched with the recommendations from the inquiry itself.

An independent review of the NTER measures was set up by the Australian Government in June 2008, involving consultation with those affected by the measures. The review's overarching recommendations were (Yu et al. 2008):

- that the Federal and Northern Territory Governments recognise as a matter of urgent national significance the continuing need to address the unacceptably high level of disadvantage and social dislocation being experienced by Aboriginal Australians living in remote communities throughout the Northern Territory;
- in addressing these needs both Governments acknowledge the requirement to re-set their relationship with Indigenous people based on genuine consultation, engagement, and partnership;
- and that Government actions affecting Indigenous communities respect Australia's human rights obligations and conform with the Racial Discrimination Act 1975.

The Australian Government accepted the review's overarching recommendations and commenced action to give effect to them. In June 2010, the Parliament passed legislation to reinstate the Racial Discrimination Act 1975 in relation to the NTER and make necessary changes to the NTER laws.

A health impact assessment of the NTER was undertaken, with a human rights component, by the Australian Indigenous Doctors' Association (AIDA) in collaboration with the Centre for Health Equity Training, Research and Evaluation at the University of New

South Wales (CHETRE). This began in late 2007 and the full report was published in 2010 (AIDA and CHETRE 2010). The assessment concludes that 'the intended health outcomes of the NTER (improved health and wellbeing, and ultimately, life expectancy) are unlikely to be fully achieved. It is predicted that it will leave a negative legacy on the psychological and social wellbeing, on the spirituality and cultural integrity of the prescribed communities. However, it may be possible to minimise or mitigate these negative impacts if the Australian and Northern Territory governments commit to and invest in taking the steps necessary to work in respectful partnership with the Aboriginal leaders and organisations responsible for the governance of the prescribed communities in the NT. The principal recommendations arising from the HIA are based on the evidence (from communities, stakeholders and experts) that it is essential to find ways to work together as equals' (AIDA and CHETRE 2010: 55). Later studies, for example Cobb-Clark et al. (2017), demonstrated that income management has not impacted positively on truancy rates.

There is ongoing debate as to whether the Australian government's response has fully taken on board all the points raised and debate continues, see for example papers within the Universal Periodic Review of Australia in 2016 (OHCHR 2019).

Health equity and the health system

Although the social determinants of health are very important in affecting health equity, the health system also has a major part to play. Comprehensive primary health care in the sense described in the 1978 Alma Ata Declaration, and reaffirmed in the 2018 Astana Declaration, is foundational to achieving shared global goals in Universal Health Coverage (UHC) and the health-related Sustainable Development Goals (SDGs) (WHO and UNICEF 2018). As we saw in Chapter 2 these are an important part of the right to health. To achieve the right to health, secondary and tertiary health services are important and need to be available, accessible, acceptable, and of high quality. The achievements of rights-based approaches to health systems are considered later in this chapter in terms of their effects on health equity.

Rights-based approaches to health policy and practice

The first thing to consider is what exactly should be understood by a rights-based approach to health. According to WHO (2002a) this has three components, it refers to the processes of: using human rights as a framework for health development; assessing and addressing the human rights implications of any health policy, program or legislation; and, making human rights an integral dimension of the design, implementation, monitoring, and evaluation of health-related policies and programs in all spheres, including political, economic, and social. Singh (2010) identifies four key features or principles of RBAs: the realisation of rights without discrimination; the principle of accountability to rights holders by duty bearers; a recognition of the importance of participation in process; and, finally adaptation to the local context. An expansion of these in the context of a human rights based approach to development programming is provided by Silva (2003) reporting on the common understanding achieved among the different UN agencies working in the field, although some have criticised this. For example, Gruskin and colleagues (2010: 134), refer to it as 'a lowest common denominator approach'. A review by Nyamu-Musembi and Cornwall (2004) of the different methodologies associated with RBAs in the field of development, argue that RBAs would mean little if they have no potential to achieve a positive transformation of power relations among the various development actors. Gruskin et al. (2010) offer a four-question framework for assessing RBAs to health (with a further set of at least four questions embedded in one of the questions); most importantly, they draw attention to a minimum list of principles that must be included: participation; non-discrimination; service availability, accessibility, acceptability; quality; transparency; and accountability.

The past thirty years has seen the development of a wealth of different approaches and assessment tools for assisting in the task of ensuring that health policies and programs respect, protect and promote human rights. Worm (2010) examines 17 different approaches to impact assessment in the field of human rights and gender equality, although not all of these explicitly draw on international human rights standards in their conceptual frameworks. The case study below presents an analysis of the evidence of the impact of a human rights-based approach to the health of women and children.

CASE STUDY: IMPLEMENTING A HUMAN RIGHTS-BASED APPROACH TO THE HEALTH OF WOMEN AND CHILDREN

Funded by the Deutsche Gesellschaft für Internationale Zusammenarbeit (Silberhorn 2015), WHO published a monograph reporting on a project to consider the evidence that adopting a RBA to women and children's health is effective. The project examined four countries: Brazil, Italy, Malawi, and Nepal. Two distinct questions were explored: has a RBA explicitly shaped the laws, policies, and programs related to women's and children's health; and, if so, what is the evidence that these explicitly human rights-shaped interventions have contributed to improvements in women's and children's health. Each of the four countries adopted a different theme for examination. Sexual, reproductive, and maternal health was the focus in Brazil, women's and children's health in Italy, children's health in Malawi, and maternal and child health in Nepal.

In each of the four countries human rights have, to varying degrees, explicitly shaped the laws, policies, and programs related to women's and children's health. The studies do not however attribute improvements exclusively to the use of a RBA.

The project also examined the academic literature on participation, human rights, and women's and children's health to explore whether women's participation in design, implementation, management, and/or evaluation of community health services/systems leads to greater access to, and use of, acceptable and quality reproductive, maternal, and child health services, and/or improved outcomes. The review found evidence of an association between women's participation and improved health and health-related outcomes, and drew attention to additional RBA principles alongside participation.

Find more in Bustreo et al. (2013).

In the remainder of this chapter, the use of RBAs is discussed by means of a range of different examples concerned with changing policy and/or practice. They are organised into six different sections. The first looks at policy advocacy and considers two episodes in the history of response to the challenge of HIV/AIDS where RBA has been influential in driving forward change. The second section focuses on RBA to program planning. The third section turns to the use of RBA in health and other health-related systems. The fourth considers practice in individual care and looks as some examples of RBAs in individual interactions between health/welfare professionals and patients/clients examining how rights-based approaches support health equity. The fifth section examines human rights education, focusing in particular on rights-based rights education as empowerment education. The sixth section addresses individual and business behaviours in terms of their effects on human rights. The chapter concludes with a brief reflection on the current state of the growing RBA industry.

Policy advocacy

The earliest significant body of work using RBAs for health policy advocacy purposes was in the field of HIV/AIDS, where the work carried out demonstrated the power of rights-based argumentation in securing appropriate treatment and resources for people living with HIV/AIDS. Later in this section, two of the episodes from this history are examined, exploring action taken to seek improved access to essential medicines, and antiretrovirals (ARVs) in particular.

The various human rights treaties assign governments the role of ensuring the right to health and discussions on the right to health are often implicitly based on an assumption that the government is the sole or major provider of health services, or at least that services reside in the not-for-profit sector. Apart from attention to the pharmaceutical industry and action to try and improve access to essential medicines, very little attention has been given to the role of for-profit enterprise in the realisation of the right to health. One exception is McBeth (2004) who considers what happens to the state's human rights duties when services are privatised. Considering three specific areas where this experience is common – health, education and prisons – he argues that such private providers of social services have human rights obligations, and at the same time, that the state's obligations change in nature from a duty of action to one of supervision, and, if necessary, intervention. Another exception is the work by Kinney (2010), who examines how for-profit enterprise has worked at cross-purposes with the achievement of the right to health, and explores a number of principles that might assist private for-profit enterprises in adopting a supportive role. Steendam (2019) presents a collation of the global evidence that points to deleterious effects of market-led approaches in service provision: higher inequality in access to care; higher health care costs; loss of efficiency; loss of quality; less public control; and lower availability of health workers and poorer working conditions for them. A further example of rights-based policy advocacy is provided by De Negri Filho (2008). Drawing on work on Latin American social medicine in Brazil, Colombia, and Venezuela, he discusses new ways of thinking about social fragility (instead of risks) and developing intersectoral programming to improve care, as well as to reduce inequalities among population groups. The article argues that a right-based approach can be a concrete tool for restructuring both public polices and action.

Donald and Mottershaw (2009), conducted an analysis, commissioned by the UK's NHRI (the Equality and Human Rights Commission), of cases brought to court under the UK's

Human Rights Act, which came into force in 2000, or the European Convention on Human Rights. They were concerned to examine the impact on policy and practice among public authorities in England and Wales. The UK's Human Rights Act provides for cases that breach the European Convention to be heard in UK courts and made it unlawful for a public authority, such as government departments, local authorities, or the police, to act in a way that is incompatible with a Convention right. They analysed ten selected cases, all of which involved civil and political rights, and several of which also involve economic and social rights through addressing health, housing, or destitution. They used a range of methods to trace the impact of the decisions into policy and practice; a detailed analysis of each case can be found in Donald et al. (2009). Their research finds some evidence of direct impact on policy and practice; however, they note the methodological difficulties of establishing this. They argue that one factor hindering impact was the absence of a body like the Equality and Human Rights Commission, which only came into being in 2007, and which might draw out the implications of court cases for policy and practice, and promote the necessary changes. They identify a particularly significant role for advocacy from service users and advocacy organisations.

HIV/AIDS – struggles over access to essential medicines

As an exploration of the role of RBAs in health policy, this section looks at two distinct episodes in the history of the global response to HIV/AIDS, and in particular at the issue of trying to ensure access to essential medicines. A more extended treatment of this history was given in the first edition of this book (Taket 2012).

In 1997 the South African Medicines and Related Substances Control Amendment Act was introduced; this aimed to increase the availability of affordable medicines via provisions including generic substitution of off-patent medicine, transparent pricing for all medicines and the parallel importing of patented medicines (Fisher and Rigamonti 2005). This was challenged in the South African High Court, in a case filed in 1998 by a consortium of pharmaceutical companies. Their challenge was on the basis that the act amounted to a violation of the World Trade Organization (WTO) TRIPS (Trade-Related Aspects of Intellectual Property Rights) Agreement, which sought to provide minimum levels of intellectual property protection in all WTO member states and of the South African constitution. The nub of the argument to be considered in the Court was whether South Africa was misusing the flexibilities within TRIPS.

Before the case came to court, a dirty fight started, aiming to influence the outcome in the pharmaceutical companies' favour. The United States put pressure on South Africa by withholding trade benefits and threatening further trade sanctions. AIDS activists in the United States then entered the fray, on the side of increased access to medicines, and as a result of increasing public pressure the United States changed its stance by the end of 1999 ('t Hoen 2005). In 2000, the case was heard by the South African High Court (case no 4183/98). By this point, public opinion was against the position of the pharmaceutical companies. Several governments and the European Parliament demanded that the companies withdraw; which they eventually did unconditionally in April 2001 (Fisher and Rigamonti 2005).

These events raised two important issues. First, the interpretation of the flexibilities of TRIPS and their use for public health purposes needed clarification if low income countries were to be able to use the provisions without threat of legal or political challenges. Secondly, it became clear that high-income countries that exercised trade pressures to defend the interests of their multinational industries needed to recognise that this would result in counter-pressure being exerted by NGOs and public health/human rights activists ('t Hoen 2005).

A second episode, the case of US versus Brazil begun in the mid-1990s when Brazil offered comprehensive AIDS care including universal access to ARV treatment; succeeding in reducing AIDS-related mortality and morbidity dramatically from the late 1990s (Nunn et al. 2009). One reason behind this success was Brazil's ability to produce medicines locally. Generic competition resulted in reductions in prices of ARV and lower prices for patented drugs being negotiated using the threat of production under compulsory licence, a possibility created by Article 68 of the Brazilian patent law, allowing a patent to be used without the consent of the patent holder. Additionally Brazil offered a cooperation agreement including technology transfer to low income countries for the production of generic ARV drugs ('t Hoen 2005). In February 2001, the United States took action against Brazil at WTO Dispute Settlement Body, arguing that Article 68 discriminated against American owners of Brazilian patents, curtailed patent holders' rights, and was in violation of TRIPS articles. The US action came under immediate and fierce pressure from the international NGO community, and five months later, in June 2001, the United States withdrew ('t Hoen 2005). Later episodes in the struggle for essential medicines and Brazil's pivotal role in this are covered by Nunn et al. (2009) and Greco (2016), who provide a useful summary of thirty years of confronting the AIDS epidemic in Brazil.

In both these examples, NGOs played a key role in advancing human rights argumentation and drawing attention to the flexibilities potentially available within TRIPS, (for example, see www.msfaccess.org; this website, run by MSF's Campaign for Access to Essential Medicines, is an excellent source of information on the ongoing struggles in both courts and policy arena to ensure access to medicines globally). But there were other players who were also important, including the public health community ('t Hoen 2005). For trade agreements going into the future it is important to ensure that a balance is struck in negotiations that genuinely fosters innovation while ensuring patients' expedited access to affordable drugs (Jorge 2018).

Rights-based approaches to program planning

This section turns to an examination of program planning using RBAs. There are a number of manuals and tool kits. Jonsson (2003) describes UNICEF's rights-based approach to development programming, and Chopra and Ford (2005) consider a human rights approach to health promotion, drawing on the UNICEF approach. A resource pack has been produced by ActionAid International in collaboration with a number of NGOs in Ghana, Uganda, and Brazil (Chapman and Mancini 2006). There is also UNFPA's Human Rights-Based Approach to Programming (UNFPA and Harvard School of Public Health 2010) which discusses their culturally sensitive, gender-responsive, human rights-based approach to programming; this deals particularly with UNFPA's three main areas of work: population and development, reproductive health, and gender; it also covers humanitarian emergencies.

The detailed example of CARE International, which took up the challenge of incorporating a RBA into all their work, is presented in Chapter 12. This is of particular interest since their work was conducted all over the world, and they subjected the approach they produced to evaluation. Further documentation of CARE's RBA can be found in other projects and settings: work on the prevention of female genital cutting in Ethiopia and Kenya in East Africa (Igras et al. 2004); work on the right to health in Peru (Frisancho and Goulden 2008), in collaboration with Forosalud, a civil society network; and later work carried out by CARE USA and Oxfam America described by Rand and Watson (2008). Sarelin (2007) discusses a needs-based study carried out by CARE International in Malawi to establish the impact of HIV/AIDS on agricultural production and rural livelihoods, as well as to identify measures that could be taken to alleviate the situation. Her analysis highlights differences and similarities between needs-based and RBAs, an essential difference being that rights-based analysis necessitates consideration of power, politics, and struggles over resources.

Increasingly, the literature is reflecting different applications of RBAs to program design and planning. There is not space here for an exhaustive review; instead, a selection of the literature is discussed, focusing on those publications that have included some type of assessment or evaluation of the impacts of the use of RBAs.

Berman (2008) reports on lessons learnt from documenting experiences and programs that incorporated RBAs in several Asia-Pacific countries from 2004 to 2008, involving fourteen projects in Bangladesh, India, Nepal, Cambodia, Indonesia, Laos, Vietnam, the Philippines, and Fiji under the aegis of the Asia-Pacific UN Inter-Agency Lessons Learned Project (LLP) on the RBA to Development. WHO (2008) brings together a range of examples of a RBA to the health components of poverty reduction strategies. Both of these demonstrate different success stories through the projects included, and to the limited extent that they offer conclusions across the different projects, they reinforce the findings from CARE International's evaluation discussed in Chapter 12.

Successful uses of RBA are also reported in a wide variety of projects working with different marginalised or disadvantaged groups. Pillai et al. (2008) provide an example of successful rights-based HIV/AIDS work with people in prostitution and sex workers in rural India. Perkins (2009), discusses the RBA used by a drop-in centre for vulnerable women in Cairo, including women who have low income, or are displaced or refugees, an approach that has helped women access basic health determinants like clean water, sewerage and electrical power. Paiva et al. (2010) document the success of a multicultural RBA in working on HIV prevention for young people with different religious communities (Catholic, Evangelical, and Afro-Brazilian) in Brazil. Their analysis demonstrated success of the RBA in increasing inter-religious tolerance and building a common understanding of the sexuality and prevention needs of youth. This analysis is deepened in Paiva and Silva (2015) to explore the response to the emergence of Catholic fundamentalist movements since 2011, putting into question the public acceptability of sexuality education in schools that the human rights perspectives had established. They focus on how an explicitly multicultural RBA diffused the resistance to sexuality education, successfully sustaining notions of equality and protection of the right to a comprehensive sexuality education that is explicitly accepting of differences. In this way, they succeeded in changing a backlash into an opportunity to develop productive resistance and innovation.

Williams and Brian (2012), demonstrate the use of General Comment 14 on the right to health (discussed in Chapter 2) to produce a simple rights-based tool to assess the design of health-related program activities proposed for Papua New Guinea by a consortium of NGOs. They present a case study illustrating how failures to address the indicators that make up this tool will result in simplistic program designs that may win political or financial support but cannot deliver quality services, available, accessible, and acceptable to all.

The need for a RBA to infectious disease epidemics has also received particular attention. Pearson (2018) analyses the outbreak of Ebola Virus Disease in March 2014, examining how the health standards and containment measures employed during the course of the outbreak and resolution measured against states' obligations in international human rights law. The analysis argues that a rights-based response facilitates a more effective, comprehensive, and inclusive recovery, and that a new set of guidelines for a rights-based response to epidemics would therefore be valuable.

WHO (2016) produced Innov8, an eight-step approach for reviewing national health programs in order to produce recommendations to make them more equity-oriented, rights-based, and gender-responsive, while addressing critical social determinants of health. Koller et al. (2018) discuss how the approach was used in Indonesia in 2014–2015, led by the Indonesian Ministry of Health with support from WHO. During 2015–2017, components of the Innov8 approach were integrated into some planning processes at district level. Koller et al. (2018) report that the Innov8 approach can help operationalise the SDG commitment to leave no one behind.

Rights-based approaches in health and other health-related systems

There are a number of different examples of RBAs across a range of different countries. Mayhew et al. (2006) argue that NGOs need to be seen as duty bearers who are required to uphold rights through their services, activities, and principles of operation. They describe the difficulties this may cause in terms of funding policies that mitigate against adopting such a position. NGOs must ensure their three-way accountability: to government, to their clients, and to other civil society groups working in the area. Mayhew et al. (2006) discuss their work in collaboration with NGOs delivering HIV-related services to prisoners and injecting drug users in Malawi and Pakistan, and the framework for rights-based work for health that resulted, demonstrating how it helped the NGOs to develop their practice as well as monitoring their accountability.

In England, the Department of Health (2007), identified five key aims of a RBA to health care: putting human rights principles and standards at the heart of policy and planning; empowering staff and patients with knowledge, skills, and organisational leadership and commitment to achieve human rights-based approaches; enabling meaningful involvement and participation of all key stakeholders; ensuring clear accountability throughout the organisation; and finally, non-discrimination and attention to vulnerable groups. Dyer (2015) presents an analysis of the Human Rights in Healthcare Programme in England and Wales, which worked with eight National Health Service (NHS) trusts to use a RBA to place human rights at the centre of healthcare. The program was successful in showing the benefits possible from the use of a RBA, and in the development and testing of a range of practical human rights-based resources to assist the spread of good practice (NHS 2019). Limited resources and health service reorganisation constrained the extent to which the program could demonstrate health impact let alone greater cost-effectiveness.

When considering RBAs in health service provision, Simonelli and Fernandes Guerreiro (2010) report on an initiative of the International Network of Health Promoting Hospitals and Health Services to promote respect for children's rights in hospital, usually based around a charter for children's rights. From an application of their self-evaluation model in seventeen hospitals across nine countries in Europe plus Australia, they identify many aspects of good practice that demonstrate that respecting children's rights in hospital can result in a positive influence on both quality of service provision and health outcomes. However, they also identify a need for awareness raising and training around rights in hospital staff, and report particular challenges in terms of lack of attention given to the right of children to information and participation. There are also examples of specific programs developed for children. Ala-Luhtala et al. (2015) describe a human rights-based emotional and safety skills program that trains workers in health, social care, and education sectors to help children learn and apply emotional and safety skills. This program draws on earlier work on human rights education for children (Flowers 2009).

The Scottish Human Rights Commission (the national human rights institution for Scotland) has published the results of its independent evaluation of a human rights-based approach used in the high-security forensic mental health institution for Scotland and Northern Ireland (SHRC 2009). The results provide practical lessons for other public authorities in the health and other sectors, as well as evidence of the value of adopting a RBA in three different areas. First, it led to improvements for staff and patients, namely a more constructive atmosphere with reduced staff stress, anxiety, and fear. There was also a reduction in blanket policies and increased individual assessment of rights and risks, and a more proportionate use of measures such as seclusion. The use of a RBA reduced risks, including organisational risks such as litigation. Finally, the RBA laid the foundation for integrating all other duties, including new equality, mental health, and freedom of information laws. Among the key factors identified as responsible for success in adoption were: top-level buy-in and leadership; involving human rights expertise in all stages of audit and review; a participatory approach; and finally, the focus on everyone's rights, including those of staff. Finally, Morgaine (2011), using the critique and experiences of women of colour, identifies the challenges within the mainstream domestic violence movement in the United States and concludes that a human rights approach could address some of these concerns by supporting the necessary holistic approach to domestic violence and increasing coalition building and community engagement.

Managing the potential tensions between priority setting across the whole spectrum of health issues and expenditure and assuring the right to health for particular individuals or groups deserves some comment. Arising from an international workshop, Rumbold et al. (2017) put forward a three-step process by which decision makers can reconcile these tensions: first, coverage should be on the basis of need; second, one aim should be to generate the greatest total improvement in health; and third, contributions should be based on ability to pay. More recently is the framework put forward by Friedmann (2019) who provides a set of seven principles, which form a RBA that is applicable in all health programs, in all sectors at all levels.

Practice in individual care: rights-based approaches in individual interactions between health/welfare professionals and patients/clients

The use of RBAs in the practice of individual health and welfare professionals is a topic that deserves a book in itself, however, here it will be restricted to a short review only. There is considerable overlap with different codes of professional ethics. For example the 'Principles of the Ethical Practice of Public Health' of the American Public Health Association (Public Health Leadership Society 2002) start with a reference to the UDHR. Nixon and Forman (2008) explore complementary features of human rights and public health ethics, finding that each has something to offer to the other, and that they can thus act synergistically.

Curtice and Exworthy (2010) delineate a simple mnemonic encapsulating what they see as the RBA: human rights can be protected in clinical and organisational practice by adherence to the underlying core values of fairness, respect, equality, dignity, and autonomy (FREDA). Their paper goes on to demonstrate that these principles are the basics of good clinical care as set out in professional standards, such as the third edition of Good Psychiatric Practice (Royal College of Psychiatrists 2009), relating this to examples of clinical practice in the context of the UK's 1998 Human Rights Act and relevant decisions of the European Court of Human Rights. Asher and colleagues (2007), in a publication on 'the right to health' produced for the British Medical Association and Commonwealth Medical Trust, include a section on a RBA for professional practice. However, there can be tensions between ethical and human rights standards, London (2008) discusses the experience in South Africa, arguing that unless the complementarities and differences in ethical and human rights standards, particularly acute in the problems of dual loyalty faced by clinicians, providers, and policy makers, are recognised, insufficient use of rights-based approaches will be made to impact the health of the most vulnerable in society.

Professional practice in disciplines such as occupational therapy, disability and social work is increasingly being focused around strengths-based and person-centred approaches that embrace shared decision-making (Pepin et al. 2010; Coulter and Collins 2011), and medical and other health professional practice increasingly focuses on patient-centred care recognising its links to improved quality of life and reduced morbidity (Bauman et al. 2003). These approaches are highly correlated with rights-based approaches, although this link is not always explicitly made, and where it is, the discussion often be in terms of 'patient rights' without making explicit connections to 'human rights' (see for example Groene (2011) and McClimans et al. (2011), for a discussion of the links to clinical ethics). Ward and Moreton (2008) provide a very interesting discussion of a framework for addressing victimisation issues with sexual offenders, drawing on the resources of human rights theory and strengths-based treatment approaches. Birgden and Cucolo (2011), provide a discussion of the treatment of sex offenders more generally, argue that underpinning treatment approaches with human rights and professional ethics in a 'treatment as rehabilitation' approach is more effective than a 'treatment as management' approach.

Within the disability field, professional practice has developed over the last three decades in order to respond to the demands of practice free from discrimination. The development of the International Classification of Functioning, Disability and Health or ICFDH (WHO 2001) has helped support this change. The ICFDH provides a common language for discussion of functioning, activity, and participation in relation to a diverse spectrum of health conditions and can be applied to any individual; it avoids the need for the labelling of an individual as disabled or non-disabled, and recognises the importance of environment and social context in supporting or hindering participation in different activities.

The Centre for Human Rights (1994) and Ife (2008) consider how a human rights perspective can provide a unifying framework within which social work can be incorporated, while still accommodating cultural, national, and political difference. Ife (2008) argues that a human rights perspective can strengthen social work, providing a strong base for practice that seeks to realise the social justice goals of social workers.

Empowerment education

Where, after all, do universal human rights begin? In small places, close to home – so close and so small that they cannot be seen on any map of the world. Yet they are the world of the individual person: the neighborhood he lives in; the school or college he attends; the factory, farm or office where he works. Such are the places where every man, woman, and child seeks equal justice, equal opportunity, equal dignity without discrimination. Unless these rights have meaning there, they have little meaning anywhere. Without concerted citizen action to uphold them close to home, we shall look in vain for progress in the larger world.

Eleanor Roosevelt (1958)

This section focuses on human rights education, referred to here as empowerment education owing to the aim of such work to provide people with the tools to take control of their own lives and to participate in the different sectors of society, in the way described by Eleanor Roosevelt in the quote above. These approaches are concerned with making rights accessible to all, and concentrate on work with individuals or groups, often networked into and through different NGOs. The first section looks at a UK-based program, called 'Active Learning for Active Citizenship'; although this was an explicitly RBA, note that the title of the program focused on active citizenship. Then a section on human rights education considers programs that have been explicitly labelled as such, including the WHO cartoons on the right to health and HIV/AIDS.

Active Learning for Active Citizenship

Active Learning for Active Citizenship (ALAC) was a UK government-funded program that took place over the period 2004–2006, during which seven regional 'hubs' experimented with a variety of approaches to citizenship learning for adults. The work of the hubs was presented in detail in Taket (2012). Here the focus is on program outcomes, drawing on the report by the external evaluators (Mayo and Rooke 2006), as well as the Take Part program that followed ALAC, based on the national framework for active learning for active citizenship (Bedford et al. 2006) and its evaluation (Miller and Hatamian 2010, 2011). A book on the program is also available (Annette and Mayo 2010), including chapters by the evaluators, from the facilitators, and from the different regional hubs; the external evaluators have also written a paper (Mayo and Rooke 2008) which focuses on the participatory approach to evaluation that was adopted.

ALAC started by recognising and valuing local expertise, knowledge and experience and emphasising the development of sustainable partnerships for the longer term. ALAC was a community development-based approach, working towards empowerment, supporting organisations and groups within communities, and pursuing agendas for equity and social justice. Within the program, there were seven different teams, each based in a different geographical location and each working with different constellations of groups and individuals. The seven teams formed the nucleus of seven regional hubs. The hubs organised into a network to learn from each other's experience, and an external team of evaluators was engaged.

Citizenship education was to start from local people's own perceptions of their issues and their learning priorities, negotiated in dialogue rather than imposed from outside. The hubs were intended as local people's provision – their provision, based in accessible premises, with a variety of programs and activities tailored to local people's interests, driven by the priorities and aspirations of the learners themselves. Learner participation was to be central at every stage in the process. Whilst the forms and levels of ALAC provision varied enormously across the hubs, there were a number of shared principles and approaches. Starting from people's own priorities and needs, ALAC emphasised experiential learning, processes of critical reflection and dialogue rooted in people's own experiences, both individually and collectively, through collective action. This drew upon the methods and approaches developed by the Brazilian educator, Paulo Freire (1972), facilitating the development of critical consciousness and understanding, through cycles of action, reflection, and then further action. In this model of learning, defined in terms of collective and critical reflection and dialogue, learners and learning providers learn together.

The ALAC evaluation demonstrated a wide range of positive outcomes. Participants in the program gained increased confidence and skills in tackling local issues with service providers, and reported positive change in health and wellbeing within their families. Individuals and groups became involved in service development and/or volunteering as trainers, became involved in formal volunteering and local networks, and also became more organised and involved in structured grassroots community activity. Participants learnt about and became more involved in governance structures. ALAC's wide range of outcomes included some that were planned, and a variety of multiplier effects of these, as active learning impacted not only upon individuals but also cascaded to impact upon their friends, families, and communities. ALAC has led to beneficial ripple effects on services and service provision and the development of more effective forums and partnerships. In some of the evaluation workshops, participants mapped their influence at different levels: self, family, neighbourhood and community, local, regional, national, and global.

The evaluation of the ALAC program produced findings with a considerable overlap with those from CARE's evaluation covered in Chapter 12. First, they noted the time and support that this work takes. Secondly, the importance of involving key stakeholders was stressed. Thirdly, it required variety and flexibility in use of methods. Fourth is the need for careful attention to systematic analysis of inequities. Finally, tactical decisions were required as to the extent to use rights and rights language explicitly.

Over the two years of its life, the ALAC program thus demonstrated promising signs of change; in particular marginalized groups were becoming no longer voiceless or faceless. Questions remained about its sustainable impact however, as funding for continuation in the same form was not forthcoming. The work and its positive evaluation led to the production of a national framework for active learning for active citizenship (Bedford et al. 2006), and a further funded national program, the Take Part program and associated network was created to continue the process of sharing resources and experience. Funding for Take Part was secured for 2009 to 2011, along with an evaluation.

The interim evaluation of ALAC (Miller and Hatamian 2010) and final evaluation (Miller and Hatamian 2011) offer a number of important conclusions. Firstly, the Take Part style of learning is most effective when developed in response to people's own issues and concerns, that is, when the community development principle of starting where people are is followed. Learning is most successful when it is participatory and includes an element of critical reflection; there is a strong emphasis on increasing levels of civic participation through Take Part, which is seen as requiring long-term support structures. Where local government has a working relationship with the organisation or group facilitating Take Part, there is increased coordination of empowerment activities. Potential barriers and risks to the remainder of the program include limited networking between organisations or groups at both regional and national levels.

Human rights education

Turning now to human rights education that is explicitly labelled as such, first of all the two cartoon books produced by WHO are considered. These were both produced in the UN Decade on Human Rights Education (1995–2004), which argued that people need to be more aware of their rights so that they can take more control over their lives and hold governments, and other powerful actors, accountable. The first of the cartoon books, on the right to health (WHO 2002b) aimed at making the right to health more widely known and understood as an instrument to empower those most in need, in recognition of the fact that improving awareness and understanding the right to health is an essential prerequisite to operationalising this right. The second book, 'HIV/AIDS Stand Up for Human Rights' (WHO 2003, updated in 2010) was launched by the United Nations Office for the High Commissioner for Human Rights (OHCHR), the United Nations Joint Programme for HIV/AIDS (UNAIDS) and the World Health Organization (WHO). This second cartoon book was designed to empower young people to promote human rights in relation to HIV/AIDS, to raise awareness of the key linkages between HIV/AIDS and human rights, to demystify HIV/AIDS and to combat the myths and taboos associated with HIV and AIDS. More recently the cartoon books have been replaced with a series of infographics about standing up against human rights abuses, the right to health and more (WHO 2019).

A growing amount of research demonstrates the value of human rights education. Kapoor (2007) demonstrates the significant role of human rights in addressing gender-caste discrimination in the state of Orissa in India, empowering the Dalit community, and Dalit women in particular to take action. These activities have resulted in improvements at the local level, in terms of initiatives such as better legal aid/support, and the establishment of police stations run by women, which will permit women to more easily report assaults against them, and advocate for further change at state and national level. Kapoor (2007: 283) notes how human rights education, for the Dalit communities he discusses, changed 'their view of themselves and what is possible'. Also in India, Bajaj (2012) in a study of school-based human rights education in Tamil Nadu illustrates the power of human rights education in government schools to bring about change in terms of pupils' agency and actions at school, home and in the community, while Kaushik et al. (2006) discusses activities at an institution of higher education for women demonstrating the links between improvements in women's education, human rights and life chances. Ramasubban (2008) examines the intersections between HIV/AIDS, sexuality, and human rights in a paper on the history of resistance to the anti-sodomy law in India. This demonstrates how the struggle around a particular piece of legislation has acted to mobilise disparate alternative sexualities grouped around a common strategy, thereby creating a loosely connected 'community' or prototype social movement. This work argues that going beyond legal reform in the direction of sexual rights, however, requires a broader coalition of groups, and a broad-based political agenda of sexual rights for all, which must critique patriarchy, dominant masculinity, and sexual violence – forces that together govern both the subordination of women and repression of alternative sexualities.

Hopkins (2011) presents an analysis of the difference between two contrasting approaches to human rights education: curriculum-based and experiential learning. The two programs compared are both delivered by Amnesty International: a curriculum-based program in Washington, D.C., in the US, and experiential learning in Ouagadougou, Burkina Faso. She finds both methods were successful in empowering participants and increasing their impact as effective activists. She further argues that the effectiveness of these approaches can be enhanced by incorporating peer education approaches within both models.

Morals, ethics, and human rights

Given the increasing globalisation inherent in neoliberal capitalism, individual behaviour choices in terms of purchasing, saving, and investment decisions carry human rights implications both locally at the point of decision-making and distally at the point of production. This has been taken up in two interrelated ways, firstly, demands that businesses be held to account for the human rights effects of their business practices, and secondly, campaigns to influence individual choice towards options that promote, or at least do not damage, human rights. Campaigns around fair trade (Frye 2015), environmental sustainability (Thangavel and Sridevi 2014), blood diamonds (Bieri 2016), and ethical/sustainable investment are growing nationally and internationally to address these issues.

In 2014, the Human Rights Council established (by a vote of 20 to 14, with 13 abstentions) an open-ended intergovernmental working group on transnational and other business enterprises with respect to human rights. The group's mandate is 'to elaborate an international legally binding instrument to regulate, in international human rights law, the activities of transnational corporations and other business enterprises' (A/HRC/RES/26/9). The UK, US, France, and Germany all voted against the resolution. ESCR-Net (the International Network for Economic, Social and Cultural Rights) is a collaborative initiative of groups and individuals from around the world working to secure economic and social justice through human rights. One area of their work is corporate accountability. This includes work towards a treaty on human rights and business, work on identifying business strategies that have adverse effects on human rights, and case support to provide technical support to organisations or grassroots groups tackling human rights violations caused by corporate actions. In particular, ESCR-Net has worked closely with the intergovernmental working group. A draft of the treaty and an associated optional protocol is currently (as of April 2019) under consideration.

As a detailed example of work carried out in this field in the absence of such a treaty, Khoo (2012) presents a detailed case study of the Consumers' Association of Penang in Malaysia and their involvement in networked consumer campaigns around the marketing of breast milk substitutes. This was linked into campaigns around health, environment, and development that also tackled concerns about pesticides and drugs transmissible through breast milk. Khoo (2012: 18) concludes that 'rights-based approaches to health and consumer activism are both relevant to contesting and transcending the neoliberal social contract, when they enable people to claim health necessities and preserve health as public goods'. In terms of resources to support future work in this field, the website of the Business and Human Rights Resource Centre track the human rights performance of over 8,000 companies worldwide and assists in helping the vulnerable challenge abuse of their human rights.

Rights-based approaches: a growing industry

The examples discussed in this chapter demonstrate the positive effects that can result from the use of RBAs. This does not mean that RBAs represent some sort of 'magic bullet', a panacea for all ills. As the examples of ALAC above and Care International in Chapter 12 illustrate, not all contexts or situations are suitable for advocacy that is explicitly based in human rights.

A number of the examples discussed have highlighted the importance of power relations, calling for explicit attention to an examination of these as part of any rights-based approach. This remains an important area for further development as to different methods and tools that can assist in this process. One very helpful example to illustrate the possibilities is provided by Surjadjaja and Mayhew (2011), in their analysis of policy change in relation to abortion over the period 2004 to 2006, using stakeholder analysis frameworks to analyse the power, networking and political will of key actors, and how this influenced and was influenced by the framing of the issue as a health issue and/or a rights issue by the different stakeholder groups. In more recent work, Hernández et al. (2019) analyse a range of citizen-led initiatives for the right to health of Indigenous populations in rural Guatemala. Their findings reinforce the value of network building and participatory monitoring, alongside persistence in demands, demonstrating the potential of collective power to hold authorities accountable for health systems failures. The question of suitable indicators for use in measuring progress is one that is being taken up more and more (for example Williams and Brian 2012; Bustreo et al. 2013; Dyer 2015; Gruskin et al. 2017; Skempes et al. 2018), and is an area where we can expect future developments. The challenge will be to ensure that the drive for quantitative measurement does not overtake the need to pay close attention to context in making effective use of RBAs.

References

ABS 2009. *Experimental Life Tables for Aboriginal and Torres Strait Islander Australians, 2005–2007*, 3302.0.55.003, Canberra: Australian Bureau of Statistics.

AIDA and CHETRE 2010. *Health Impact Assessment of the Northern Territory Emergency Response*, Canberra: Australian Indigenous Doctors' Association.

Ala-Luhtala, R, Lottes, L, Valkama, S, & Liimatainen, L 2015. A human rights-based emotional and safety skills programme for children in Finland, *International Journal of Children's Rights*, 23(4): 687–704. doi.org/10.1163/15718182-02304004

Annette, J, & Mayo, M (eds.) 2010. *Taking Part? Active Learning for Active Citizenship, and Beyond*, London: NIACE.

Asher, J, Hamm, D, & Sheather, J 2007. *The Right to Health: A Toolkit for Health Professionals*, London: British Medical Association.

Bajaj, M 2012. From "time pass" to transformative force: School-based human rights education in Tamil Nadu, India, *International Journal of Educational Development*, 32(1): 72–80. doi.org/10.1016/j.ijedudev.2010.10.001

Bauman, AE, Fardy, HJ, & Harris, PG 2003. Getting it right: Why bother with patient-centred care? *Medical Journal of Australia*, 179(5): 253–256. doi:10.5694/j.1326-5377.2003.tb05532.x

Bedford, J, Marsh, H, & Wright, D 2006. *The National Framework for Active Learning for Active Citizenship*, London: Togetherwecan.

Berman, G 2008. *Undertaking a Human Rights-Based Approach: A Guide for Basic Programming: Documenting Lessons Learned for Human Rights-Based Programming: An Asia-Pacific Perspective: Implications for Policy, Planning and Programming*, Bangkok: UNESCO.

Bieri, F 2016. *From Blood Diamonds to the Kimberley Process: How NGOs Cleaned Up the Global Diamond Industry*, London/New York: Routledge. doi.org/10.4324/9781315583280

Birgden, A, & Cucolo, H 2011. The treatment of sex offenders: Evidence, ethics and human rights, *Sexual Abuse: Journal of Research and Treatment*, 23(3): 295–313. doi.org/10.1177/1079063210381412

Blaker Strand, V 2019. Interpreting the ECHR in its normative environment: Interaction between the ECHR, the UN convention on the elimination of all forms of discrimination against women and the UN convention on the rights of the child, *The International Journal of Human Rights*, 1–14. doi.org/10.1080/13642987.2019.1574423

Bustreo, F, Hunt, P, Gruskin, S, Eide, A, McGoey, L, Rao, S, Songane, F, Tarantola, D, Unnithan, M, Yamin, AE, van Bolhuis, A, Ferguson, L, Halliday, E, Kuruvilla, S, Popay, J, & Sander, G 2013. *Women's and Children's Health: Evidence of Impact of Human Rights*, Geneva: World Health Organization.

Centre for Human Rights 1994. *Human Rights and Social Work: A Manual for Schools of Social Work and the Social Work Profession*, Professional Training Series, 1, Geneva: United Nations.

Chapman, J 1990. Violence against women as a violation of human rights, *Social Justice*, 17(2).

Chapman, J, & Mancini, A (eds.) 2006. *Critical Webs of Power and Change: A Resource Pack for Planning, Assessment and Learning in People-Centred Advocacy*, Johannesburg: ActionAid.

Chopra, M, & Ford, N 2005. Scaling up health promotion interventions in the era of HIV/AIDS: Challenges for a rights-based approach, *Health Promotion International*, 20(4): 383–390. doi.org/10.1093/heapro/dai018

Cobb-Clark, DA, Kettlewell, N, Schurer, S, & Silburn, S 2017. *The Effect of Quarantining Welfare on School Attendance in Indigenous Communities*, Life Course Centre Working Paper 2017–22 [Online]. Available: www.lifecoursecentre.org.au/wp-content/uploads/2018/06/2017-22-LCC-Working-Paper-Cobb-Clark-et-al.pdf [Accessed 02/04/2019].

Coulter, A, & Collins, A 2011. *Making Shared Decision-Making a Reality: No Decision About Me, Without Me*, London: King's Fund.

Curtice, MJ, & Exworthy, T 2010. FREDA: A human rights-based approach to healthcare, *Psychiatrist*, 34(4): 150–156. doi.org/10.1192/pb.bp.108.024083

De Negri Filho, A 2008. A human rights approach to quality of life and health: Applications to public health programming, *Health and Human Rights*, 10(1): 93–101. doi.org/10.2307/20460090

Department of Health 2007. *Human Rights in Healthcare: A Framework for Local Action*, London: Department of Health.

Donald, A, & Mottershaw, E 2009. Evaluating the impact of human rights litigation on policy and practice: A case study of the UK, *Journal of Human Rights Practice*, 1(3): 339–361. doi.org/10.1093/jhuman/hup019

Donald, A, Mottershaw, E, Leach, P, & Watson, J 2009. *Evaluating the Impact of Selected Cases under the Human Rights Act on Public Services Provision*, London: Equality and Human Rights Commission.

Dyer, L 2015. A review of the impact of the human rights in healthcare programme in England and Wales, *Health and Human Rights*, 17(2): 111–122.

Fisher, WW, & Rigamonti, CP 2005. The South Africa AIDS controversy: A case study in patent law and policy, in Harvard Law School, *The Law and Business of Patents* [Online]. Available: http://cyber.law.harvard.edu/people/tfisher/South%20Africa.pdf [Accessed 01/09/2011].

Flowers, N (ed.) 2009. *Compasito, Manual on Human Rights Education for Children*, 2nd edn, Budapest: Directorate of Youth and Sport of the Council of Europe.

Freire, P 1972. *Pedagogy of the Oppressed*, London: Sheed & Ward.

Friedmann, EA 2019. *Health Equity Programs of Action: An Implementation Framework*, Georgetown: O'Neill Institute.

Frisancho, A, & Goulden, J 2008. Rights-based approaches to improve people's health in Peru, *The Lancet*, 372(9655): 2007–2008. doi.org/10.1016/S0140-6736(08)61785-7

Frye, JJ 2015. Re-conceptualizing the global fair-trade movement, *Journal of Social Justice*, 5: 1–25.

García-Moreno, G, Jansen, HAFM, Ellsberg, M, Heise, L, & Watts, C 2005. *WHO Multi-Country Study on Women's Health and Domestic Violence against Women*, Geneva: World Health Organization.

Government of New Zealand 2018. *Domestic Violence: Victims' Protection Bill* [Online], Auckland. Available: www.legislation.govt.nz/bill/member/2016/0215/latest/whole.html [Accessed 04/08/2019].

Greco, DB 2016. Thirty years of confronting the AIDS epidemic in Brazil, 1985–2015, *Ciencia e Saude Coletiva*, 21(5): 1553–1564. doi.org/10.1590/1413-81232015215.04402016

Groene, O 2011. Patient centredness and quality improvement efforts in hospitals: Rationale, measurement, implementation, *International Journal for Quality in Health Care*, 23(5): 531–537. doi.org/10.1093/intqhc/mzr058

Gruskin, S, Bogecho, D, & Ferguson, L 2010. Rights-based approaches to health policies and programs: Articulations, ambiguities, and assessment, *Journal of Public Health Policy*, 31(2): 129–145. doi.org/10.1057/jphp.2010.7

Gruskin, S, Ferguson, L, Kumar, S, Nicholson, A, Al, M, & Khosla, R 2017. A novel methodology for strengthening human rights-based monitoring in public health: Family planning indicators as an illustrative example, *PLoS One*, 12(12). doi.org/10.1371/journal.pone.0186330

Hernández, A, Ruano, AL, Hurtig, A-K, Goicolea, I, San Sebastián, M, & Flores, W 2019. Pathways to accountability in rural Guatemala: A qualitative comparative analysis of citizen-led initiatives for the right to health of indigenous populations, *World Development*, 113: 392–401. doi.org/10.1016/j.worlddev.2018.09.020

Hopkins, K 2011. Amnesty international's methods of engaging youth in human rights education: Curriculum in the United States and experiential learning in Burkina Faso, *Journal of Human Rights Practice*, 3(1): 71–92. doi.org/10.1093/jhuman/hur007

Ife, J 2008. *Human Rights and Social Work: Towards Rights-Based Practice*, 2nd edn, Cambridge: Cambridge University Press. doi.org/10.1017/CBO9780511808326

Igras, S, Mutteshi, J, Wolde Mariam, A, & Ali, S 2004. Integrating rights-based approaches into community-based health projects: Experiences from the prevention of female genital cutting project in East Africa, *Health and Human Rights*, 7(2): 251–271. doi.org/10.2307/4065358

Itzin, C, Taket, A, & Barter-Godfrey, S (eds.) 2010. *Domestic and Sexual Violence and Abuse: Tackling the Health and Mental Health Effects*, London: Routledge. doi.org/10.4324/9780203842201

Jonsson, U 2003. *Human Rights Approach to Development Programming*, Nairobi: UNICEF.

Jorge, MF 2018. Tough medicine: Ensuring access to affordable drugs requires fixing trade agreements starting with NAFTA, *Journal of Generic Medicines*, 14(4): 160–166. doi.org/10.1177/1741134318810061

Kapoor, D 2007. Gendered-caste discrimination, human rights education, and the enforcement of the prevention of atrocities act in India, *Alberta Journal of Educational Research*, 53(3): 273–286.

Kaushik, SK, Kaushik, S, & Kaushik, S 2006. How higher education in rural India helps human rights and entrepreneurship, *Journal of Asian Economics*, 17(1): 29–34. doi.org/10.1016/j.asieco.2006.01.004

Khoo, SM 2012. Re-interpreting the citizen consumer: Alternative consumer activism and the rights to health and development, *Social Science and Medicine*, 74(1): 14–19. doi.org/10.1016/j.socscimed.2011.02.048

Kinney, ED 2010. Realizing the international human right to health: The challenge of for profit health care, *West Virginia Law Review*, 113: 49–66.

Koller, TS, Saint, V, Floranita, R, Koemara Sakti, GM, Pambudi, I, Hermawan, L, Briot, B, Frenz, P, Solar, O, Campos, P, Villar, E, & Magar, V 2018. Applying the Innov8 approach for reviewing national health programmes to leave no one behind: Lessons learnt from Indonesia, *Global Health Action*, 11. doi.org/10.1080/16549716.2018.1423744

Krug, EG, Dahlberg, LL, Mercy, JA, Zwi, AB, & Lozano, R (eds.) 2002. *World Report on Violence and Health*, Geneva: World Health Organization. doi.org/10.1016/S0140-6736(02)11133-0

London, L 2008. What is a human rights-based approach to health and does it matter?, *Health and Human Rights*, 10(1): 65–80. doi.org/10.2307/20460088

Mayhew, S, Douthwaite, M, & Hammer, M 2006. Balancing protection and pragmatism: A framework for NGO accountability in rights-based approaches, *Health and Human Rights*, 9(2): 180–206. doi.org/10.2307/4065407

Mayo, M, & Rooke, A 2006. *Active Learning for Active Citizenship: An Evaluation Report*, London: Togetherwecan.

Mayo, M, & Rooke, A 2008. Active learning for active citizenship: Participatory approaches to evaluating a programme to promote citizen participation in England, *Community Development Journal*, 43(3): 371–381. doi.org/10.1093/cdj/bsn013

McBeth, A 2004. Privatising human rights: What happens to the state's duties when services are privatised?, *Melbourne Journal of International Law*, 5: 133–154.

McClimans, LM, Dunn, M, & Slowther, A 2011. Health policy, patient-centred care and clinical ethics, *Journal of Evaluation in Clinical Practice*, 17(5): 913–919. doi.org/10.1111/j.1365-2753.2011.01726.x

McQuigg, RJA 2018. Is it time for a UN treaty on violence against women?, *International Journal of Human Rights*, 22(3): 305–324. doi.org/10.1080/13642987.2017.1359552

Miller, S, & Hatamian, A 2010. *Take Part Interim Report: Second Year Evaluation of the Take Part Programme*, London: Community Development Foundation.

Miller, S, & Hatamian, A 2011. *Take Part Final Report*, London: Community Development Foundation.

Morgaine, K 2011. 'How would that help our work?': The intersection of domestic violence and human rights in the United States, *Violence against Women*, 17(1): 6–27. doi.org/10.1177/1077801209347749

NHS 2019. *Human Rights in Healthcare* [Online]. Available: www.humanrightsinhealthcare.nhs.uk [Accessed 04/08/2019].

Nixon, S, & Forman, L 2008. Exploring synergies between human rights and public health ethics: A whole greater than the sum of its parts, *BMC International Health and Human Rights*, 8(special section): 1–9. doi.org/10.1186/1472-698X-8-2

Nunn, A, Da Fonesca, E, & Gruskin, S 2009. Changing global essential medicines norms to improve access to AIDS treatment: Lessons from Brazil, *Global Public Health*, 4: 131–149. doi.org/10.1080/17441690802684067

Nyamu-Musembi, C, & Cornwall, A 2004. *What Is the 'Rights-Based Approach' All About? Perspectives from International Development Agencies*, IDS Working Paper No. 234, Brighton: Institute of Development Studies.

OHCHR 2019. *Universal Periodic Review* [Online]. Available: www.ohchr.org/en/hrbodies/upr/pages/uprmain.aspx [Accessed 12/06/2019].

Paiva, V, Garcia, J, Rios, LF, Santos, AO, Terto, V, & Munoz-Laboy, M 2010. Religious communities and HIV prevention: An intervention study using a human rights-based approach, *Global Public Health*, 5(3): 280–294. doi.org/10.1080/17441691003677421

Paiva, V, & Silva, VN 2015. Facing negative reactions to sexuality education through a multicultural human rights framework, *Reproductive Health Matters*, 23(46): 96–106. doi.org/10.1016/j.rhm.2015.11.015

Pearson, E 2018. Towards human rights-based guidelines for the response to infectious disease epidemics: Righting the response, *Australian Journal of Human Rights*, 24(2): 201–222. doi.org/10.1080/1323238X.2018.1485443

Pepin, G, Watson, J, Hagiliassis, N, & Larkin, H 2010. Ethical and supported decision making, in K Stagnitti, A Schoo, & D Welch (eds.) *Clinical and Fieldwork Placement in the Health Professions*, Melbourne: Oxford University Press.

Perkins, F 2009. A rights-based approach to accessing health determinants, *Global Health Promotion*, 16(1): 61–64. doi.org/10.1177/1757975908100753

Pillai, S, Seshu, M, & Shivdas, M 2008. Embracing the rights of people in prostitution and sex workers, to address HIV and AIDS effectively, *Gender and Development*, 16(2): 313–326. doi.org/10.1080/13552070802120491

Public Health Leadership Society 2002. *Principles of the Ethical Practice of Public Health*, New Orleans: Public Health Leadership Society.

Ramasubban, R 2008. Political intersections between HIV/AIDS, sexuality and human rights: A history of resistance to the anti-sodomy law in India, *Global Public Health*, 3(Suppl. 2): 22–38. doi.org/10.1080/17441690801990655

Rand, J, & Watson, G 2008. *Rights-Based Approaches: Learning Project*, Boston, MA/Atlanta, GA, USA: Oxfam America/Care.

Roosevelt, E 1958. *In Your Hands: A Guide for Community Action for the Tenth Anniversary of the Universal Declaration of Human Rights*, New York: United Nations.

Royal College of Psychiatrists 2009. *Good Psychiatric Practice*, 3rd edn, College Report CR154, London: Royal College of Psychiatrists.

Rumbold, B, Baker, R, Ferraz, O, Hawkes, S, Krubiner, C, Littlejohns, P, Norheim, OF, Pegram, T, Rid, A, Venkatapuram, S, Voorhoeve, A, Wang, D, Weale, A, Wilson, J, Yamin, AE, & Hunt, P 2017. Universal health coverage, priority setting, and the human right to health, *The Lancet*, 390: 721–714. doi.org/10.1016/S0140-6736(17)30931-5

Sarelin, AL 2007. Human rights-based approaches to development cooperation, HIV/AIDS, and food security, *Human Rights Quarterly*, 29(2): 460–488. doi.org/10.1353/hrq.2007.0022

SHRC 2009. *Human Rights in a Health Care Setting: Making It Work*, Glasgow: Scottish Human Rights Commission.

Silberhorn, T 2015. Germany's experience in supporting and implementing human rights-based approaches to health, plus challenges and successes in demonstrating impact on health outcomes, *Health and Human Rights*, 17(2): 21–29.

Silva, M-L 2003. *The Human Rights-Based Approach to Development Cooperation Towards a Common Understanding among UN Agencies*, Geneva: Office of the High Commissioner for Human Rights.

Simonelli, F, & Fernandes Guerreiro, AI 2010. *Final Report on the Implementation Process of the Self-Evaluation Model and Tool on the Respect of Children's Rights in Hospital*, Florence: International Network of Health Promoting Hospitals and Health Services.

Singh, A 2010. Commentary: Rights-based approaches to health policies and programmes: why are they important to use, *Journal of Public Health Policy*, 31(2): 146–149. doi.org/10.1057/jphp.2010.11

Skempes, D, Melvin, J, Von Groote, P, Stucki, G, & Bickenbach, J 2018. Using concept mapping to develop a human rights-based indicator framework to assess country efforts to strengthen rehabilitation provision and policy: The Rehabilitation System Diagnosis and Dialogue framework (RESYST), 16 Studies in Human Society 1605 Policy and Administration 18 Law and Legal Studies 1801 Law, *Globalization and Health*, 14(1). doi.org/10.1186/s12992-018-0410-5

Steendam, J 2019. *Why Public Health Care Is Better*. Viva Salud. Available: https://en.vivasalud.be/news/paper-why-public-health-care-better.

Surjadjaja, C, & Mayhew, SH 2011. Can policy analysis theories predict and inform policy change? Reflections on the battle for legal abortion in Indonesia, *Health Policy and Planning*, 26(5): 373–384. doi.org/10.1093/heapol/czq079

Taket, A 2012. *Health Equity, Social Justice and Human Rights*, London: Routledge. doi.org/10.4324/9780203119242

Thangavel, P, & Sridevi, G (eds.) 2014. *Environmental Sustainability: Role of Green Technologies*, New Delhi: Springer. doi.org/10.1007/978-81-322-2056-5

't Hoen, E 2005. TRIPS, pharmaceuticals, patents and access to essential medicines: A long way from Seattle to Doha, in S Gruskin, M Grodin, S Marks and G Annas (eds.) *Perspectives on Health and Human Rights*, New York: Routledge.

UNFPA and Harvard School of Public Health 2010. *A Human Rights-Based Approach to Programming: Practical Information and Training Materials*, New York: UNFPA.

UN Women 2011. *Progress of the World's Women 2011–2012: In Pursuit of Justice*, New York: UN Women.

Ward, T, & Moreton, G 2008. Moral repair with offenders: Ethical issues arising from victimization experiences, *Sexual Abuse: Journal of Research and Treatment*, 20(3): 305–322. doi.org/10.1177/1079063208322423

WHO 1997. *Violence against Women: A Health Priority Issue, FRH/WHD/97.8*, Geneva: WHO.

WHO 2001. *International Classification of Functioning, Disability and Health*, Geneva: WHO.

WHO 2002a. *25 Questions and Answers on Health and Human Rights* [Online], Geneva: WHO. Available: https://apps.who.int/medicinedocs/documents/s21768en/s21768en.pdf [Accessed 21/08/2019].

WHO 2002b. *The Right to Health*, Geneva: WHO.

WHO 2003. *HIV/AIDS: Stand Up for Human Rights*, Geneva: WHO.

WHO 2008. *Human Rights, Health and Poverty Reduction Strategies*, Geneva: WHO/OHCHR.

WHO 2016. *Innov8 Approach for Reviewing National Health Programmes*, Geneva: WHO.

WHO 2019. *Human Rights and Health Infographics* [Online], Geneva. Available: www.who.int/gender-equity-rights/knowledge/hr-and-health-infographics/en/ [Accessed 04/08/2019].

WHO & UNICEF 2018. *A Vision for Primary Health Care in the 21st Century: Towards Universal Health Coverage and the Sustainable Development Goals*, Geneva: WHO and UNICEF.

Wild, R, & Anderson, P 2007. *Ampe akelyernemane meke mekarle: Little Children Are Sacred: Report of the Northern Territory Board of Inquiry into the Protection of Aboriginal Children from Sexual Abuse*, Darwin: Northern Territory Government.

Williams, C, & Brian, G 2012. Using health rights to improve programme design: A Papua New Guinea case study, *International Journal of Health Planning and Management*, 27(3): 246–256. doi.org/10.1002/hpm.2103

Worm, I 2010. *Human Rights and Gender Equality and Health: Overview of Impact Assessment Tools*, Health and Human Rights Working Paper Series, 7 [Online], Geneva: WHO. Available: www.who.int/ hhr/information/mapping_impact_assessment.pdf [Accessed 21/08/2019].

Yu, P, Duncan, ME, & Gray, B 2008. *Northern Territory Emergency Response: Report of the NTER Review Board*, Canberra: Attorney-General's Department.

6

THE RIGHTS OF THE CHILD

Fiona H. McKay and Ann Taket

Introduction

The Universal Declaration of Human Rights (UDHR), adopted in 1948, described the rights applicable to everyone, regardless of nationality, gender, or age. However, in recognition of their vulnerability, children have been provided with special protections since the beginning of the nineteenth century. Despite over a century of various protections, in 2017 over 5 million children died prematurely of preventable diseases (WHO 2019), while many millions more experience a range of human rights abuses including unnecessary disease, lack of education, neglect, or separation from their parents.

This chapter will introduce a range of child's rights, discuss the history of child's rights, the development of, and some of the detail of the Convention on the Rights of the Child (CRC), and provide some examples of how and when these rights are infringed.

A short history of the rights of the child

One of the first legally binding treaties relating to the rights of children was introduced in 1919. The 1919 treaty described the conditions under which children could work and prevented their employment in workplaces that would be dangerous or hazardous (Fass 2011). While some people were concerned with the welfare of children prior to this time, particularly those who worked directly with children: magistrates, educators, and teachers; much of this concern was directed at children who were considered 'at risk' (Moody 2015). At risk children included those who were homeless or abandoned, those who were working, or those considered 'delinquent' children.

With the creation of the League of Nations at the conclusion of the First World War, many individuals and groups became actively involved in issues related to the conditions and welfare of children. The First World War resulted in millions of orphans, refugees, and displaced children who soon became the concern of western nations, primarily Western Europe. One challenge at the time for many of these nations was the discovery of children in their care who were nationals of former, but recent, enemies, or the realisation that western countries were taking actions that were actively disadvantaging these children (including for example, preventing supplies travelling to enemy nations in the post-war period). While some leaders and politicians sought to maintain that the children of an enemy were also an enemy, Eglantyne Jebb, a British woman and the founder of the NGO Save the Children, took the position that children should not be subjected to the consequences of the crimes and hatred of adults (Moody 2015). Jebb led a vocal group of humanitarians and social reformers who successfully petitioned for the first session of the General Assembly of the League of Nations in 1920 to be dedicated to making child welfare for victims of war a priority (Marshall 1999).

A result of the calls for greater attention to child welfare was the adoption, in 1924, by the League of Nations, of the non-binding Declaration of the Rights of the Child (often termed the Geneva Declaration of the Rights of the Child). This Declaration was the first declaration on human rights adopted by any intergovernmental organisation (Buck and Lee 2014). The Declaration contained five key principles (see Table 6.1) that were directed at creating conditions to enable the protection of children and allow them to develop into adults who could contribute to their society (League of Nations 1924). Given its adoption in the period immediately following the First World War, and the significant disadvantages experienced by children at this time, the 1924 Declaration refers mainly to the fate of children affected by the war, see for example Principle 3 which suggests that children should get relief first in times of distress, and protecting children who were employed (see Principle 4) (Marshall 1999).

While the Declaration of 1924 recognised 'personhood' for children, it stopped at allowing children to participate in decision making or be engaged in self-determination. Furthermore, the intention during the discussions on this declaration was not to create a binding treaty, but rather to create guiding principles for those working in international child welfare (Buck and Lee 2014).

After the League of Nations was dissolved in the aftermath of the Second World War, and the United Nations (UN) took its place, the 1924 Declaration was revisited, and then revised. In 1959 the UN endorsed the non-binding Declaration on the Rights of the Child (UN General Assembly 1959). This Declaration, adopted unanimously by all 78 Member states of the UN General Assembly, set out ten principles for the care and protection of children (UN General Assembly 1959). In addition to the five aspects included in the 1924 Declaration (although, slightly modified), the 1959 Declaration included entitlements to name and nationality; efforts that sought to ensure that children grew up in loving and understanding homes with an opportunity for play and recreation; and provisions for free and compulsory primary level education (Holcomb 2016). Like the 1924 Declaration, the 1959 Declaration was aspirational and, as a Declaration and not a Convention, it was not legally binding. The

TABLE 6.1 Text of the 1924, Declaration of the Rights of the Child (League of Nations 1924)

1. The child must be given the means requisite for its normal development, both materially and spiritually.
2. The child that is hungry must be fed, the child that is sick must be nursed, the child that is backward must be helped, the delinquent child must be reclaimed, and the orphan and the waif must be sheltered and succored.
3. The child must be the first to receive relief in times of distress.
4. The child must be put in a position to earn a livelihood, and must be protected against every form of exploitation.
5. The child must be brought up in the consciousness that its talents must be devoted to the service of its fellow men.

Declaration did include a non–discrimination clause and is premised on the notion that the best interest of the child should be a key consideration (Todres 1998). Despite its non-binding nature, it represented the most comprehensive international statement on children's rights to that point (Bennett Jr 1987).

To commemorate the twentieth anniversary of the 1959 Declaration, the UN recognised 1979 as the International Year of the Child. This recognition allowed Poland the opportunity to suggest that the principles identified in the Declaration should be translated into a legally binding Convention (Limber and Flekkoy 1995). This push for a legally binding Convention was based on the observation that children continued to suffer from wars and other forms of aggression, and through colonialism, racism, and apartheid (Detrick 1999). Initially, the Parties involved proposed that the Convention should be based largely on the text of the 1959 Declaration, however, when initial drafts were circulated to member states of the UN, several government representatives objected on the grounds that the language was inappropriate or imprecise or because there was little discussion of implementation (Todres 1998). These disagreements lead to the creation of a working group to focus specifically on the language and items to be included in the final Convention. The working party included representation for all major religions and cultures and operated on the basis that only those ideas agreed on by all members could be included (Bennett Jr 1987). The CRC emerged from this drafting process as a comprehensive treaty on the rights of the child, including provisions related to civil and political rights, as well as economic, social, and cultural rights. It was opened for signature in 1989, the thirtieth anniversary of the 1959 Declaration, and came into force in 1990.

The Convention on the Rights of the Child and the role of UNICEF

The CRC is the most extensively ratified human rights treaty in the world, with all but one country, the United States, having ratified the Convention. In principle, the rights set out in other human rights documents, including the UDHR, and the International Covenant on Economic, Social and Cultural Rights (ICESCR) and International Covenant on Civil and Political Rights (ICCPR) apply to both adults and children, however, a recognition by member states that children experience special vulnerably lead to the creation of the Convention to provide specific protections for children (Detrick 1999). The CRC was the first treaty document to consider a range of rights (Wilcox and Nalmark 1991), with previous international instruments considering civil and political rights (often put forward by Western nations), to be separate from economic, social, and cultural rights (traditionally advanced by nations of the former Eastern Bloc) (Limber and Flekkoy 1995). Under the CRC, children are seen as individual rights-holders, meaning that they are entitled to the same human rights and fundamental freedoms as adults, and where possible, should be involved in decisions that affect them (Liefaard and Sloth-Nielsen 2017).

The CRC lists the obligations of states both to undertake specific actions on behalf of protected individuals and to refrain from taking actions that might harm them (Limber and Flekkoy 1995). These obligations require states to 'respect and ensure the rights set forth' in the Convention on behalf of every child within their jurisdiction (UN General Assembly 1989).

The CRC contains a preamble and fifty-four Articles; however, the contents are often considered within nine themes (see Table 6.2). Each State Party must submit a report to the Committee on the Rights of the Child on their progress in realising these rights (Committee

TABLE 6.2 Nine thematic areas of the CRC

1. Implementation of the CRC
2. Definition of a child
3. General Principles
4. Civil rights and freedoms
5. Prevention of violence against children
6. The family environment and alternative care
7. The rights related to disability, basic health, and welfare
8. Education, leisure, and cultural activities.
9. Special protection measures for children in especially vulnerable situations

on the Rights of the Child 2010). The Committee requests that states make their report, not in sequential order of the fifty-four Articles, but in order of these themes, with equal weight given to each Article, and with a recognition that these rights are indivisible and interrelated (Detrick 1999).

The first theme is concerned with the implementation of the CRC and consists of Article 4, the requirement of states to implement the rights that they have agreed to; Article 42; that states make the provisions within the CRC publicly known; and Article 44, that states report back to the committee on their progress in realising these rights. The second theme relates to the definition of a child, found in Article 1 as someone who is under eighteen years of age, unless a country has a specific policy that allows individuals to reach the age of maturity earlier. This is followed by the general principles. These include the right to non-discrimination (Article 2), the guarantee that decisions made will be in the best interests of the child (Article 3), the right to life, survival, and development (Article 6), and the right for the child's views to be respected (Article 12). This is followed by a number of civil rights and freedoms. These include the right to a name and nationality (Article 7), the perseveration of identity (Article 8), freedom of expression (Article 13), religion (Article 14), and association (Article 15), the protection of privacy (Article 16), and access to appropriate information (Article 17).

The next theme is related to the prevention of violence against children. This set of rights includes the prevention of abuse and neglect (Article 19), measures that prohibit and eliminate all forms of harmful practices, including, but not limited to, female genital mutilation and early and forced marriages (Article 24), sexual exploitation and sexual abuse (Article 34), the right not to be subjected to torture or other cruel, inhuman or degrading treatments or punishments, including corporal punishment (Article 37(a) and Article 28(2)), the right to physical and psychological recovery and social reintegration of children who do experience harm (Article 39), and the availability of helplines for children (found in General comment No 8, 2006).

The next thematic area includes the articles and provisions related to the family environment and alternative care. This includes parental guidance (Article 5), and the right that describes the parental responsibility in the development of the child (Article 18). This set of rights also describes situations when children are separated from their parents (Article 9) or are deprived of the family environment (Article 20) and the possibility of family reunification (Article 10), while prohibiting illicit transfer and non-return, particularly in the situation when parents live in different countries (Article 11). Also important under this theme are the requirements for financial maintenance for children (Article 27), and the situation where children are removed from their family (Article 25), or when their family members are incarcerated, highlighting the possibility that a child may live in a prison with their mothers (General comments No 7, 2005). The CRC also identifies a number of conditions around adoption, with the preference that children remain with their family in their country of origin where possible (Article 21).

The seventh thematic area refers to those rights related to disability, basic health, and welfare. These articles are concerned with ensuring that children have access to social security (Article 26), and that measures are taken to ensure that children with disabilities are able to maintain dignity, self-reliance, and be active members of their community (Article 23). States are required to ensure the survival and development of children (Article 6), and that primary health care (Article 24) and physical (including reproductive) and mental health and wellbeing of children are promoted; measures are also to be taken to prevent communicable and non-communicable diseases, and children are to be protected against substance abuse (Article 33). Finally, there is the right to adequate nutrition, clothing, and housing to ensure children's physical, mental, spiritual, moral, and social development, and to reduce poverty and inequality (Article 27).

Theme eight is concerned with education, leisure, and cultural activities. This includes the right to education, including vocational training and guidance (Article 28), the right to a broad and quality education (Article 29), a recognition of the cultural rights of children belonging to Indigenous and minority groups (Article 30), and the right to rest, play, leisure, recreation and cultural and artistic activities (Article 31). The final thematic area relates to the special protection measures for children in especially vulnerable situations. These rights seek to protect children outside their country of origin seeking refugee protection (Article 22), children belonging to a minority or an Indigenous group (Article 30), to prevent economic exploitation, including child labour (Article 32) and the use of children in the illicit production and trafficking of narcotic drugs and psychotropic substances (Article 33). This theme also includes the prevention of sexual exploitation and sexual abuse (Article 34), and the sale, trafficking, and abduction of children (Article 35), or other forms of exploitation (Article 36). This area also seeks to ensure that children are provided with appropriate justice (Article 40), followed by rehabilitation (Article 39), and that if they are deprived of their liberty, that any arrest, detention, or imprisonment of a child shall be used as a measure of last resort and for the shortest amount of time with the prompt provision of legal and other assistance, and that capital punishment or life imprisonment are avoided (Article 37).

Different countries interpret these principles in different ways, depending on the context and history of the country (Roose and Bouverne-de Bie 2007). For example, countries that experience conflict tend to focus on the protection of children, since giving children the same rights and responsibility as adults can be fatal in situations of warfare (Cohn 1991). While higher income countries, not experiencing conflict, are more often engaged in issues of participation rights for children (Howe 2001).

Optional protocols to and general comments on the Convention

There are currently three optional protocols to the CRC. These optional protocols have been adopted to clarify or to make stronger points of the CRC.

The text of the first prohibits children from taking part in armed conflicts. While the CRC does prevent children under the age of 15 from taking a direct part in armed conflict (Article 38), it did not prohibit children being employed as spies, porters, informers, or in other supportive roles. The Optional Protocol to the Convention on the Rights of the Child on the Involvement of Children in Armed Conflict (OPAC), adopted in 2000, seeks to prevent such activities. The OPAC treaty has been widely ratified, with 168 states having ratified or acceded to the treaty by the end of 2018; a further eleven states have signed but not yet ratified the Protocol (United Nations 2019c).

The second optional protocol is related to the sale of children, child prostitution, and child pornography. This protocol builds on a number of previous instruments, including the 1926 Slavery Convention, and the Convention for the Suppression of the Traffic in Persons and of the Exploitation of the Prostitution of Others (Pais 2010). While there are provisions in the CRC to protect children from exploitation (Article 34), there were concerns that this article did not go far enough to protect children. The Protocol, for the first time defines the 'sale of children', 'child pornography', and 'child prostitution' with the aim of making justice clearer and more straightforward for victims of these crimes (Dennis 2000). The protocol has been ratified by 176 states, with 9 having signed but not yet ratified the Protocol (United Nations 2019c).

The third optional protocol is concerned with ensuring appropriate communication and a complaints mechanism. While the CRC has been adopted by almost all nations, and many achievements in child rights have been realised, a number of violations of the CRC persist. A lack of mechanism to report violations and seek remedies was identified as in part responsible for this and for the, often, weak enforcement (Lee 2010). The Optional Protocol to the Convention on the Rights of the Child on a Communications Procedure, adopted in 2014, allowing children or their representatives to file complaints against the Convention. The protocol has been ratified by only forty-three State Parties, with nineteen parties having signed but not ratified the Protocol (United Nations 2019c).

General Comments are provided by all treaty bodies. General comments contain the interpretation of the provisions by the treaty body and cover a range of subjects, from the comprehensive interpretation of substantive provisions, to general guidance on the information that should be submitted in state reports relating to specific articles of the treaties (United Nations 2019a). General comments do not have the same weight as Articles, but rather provide guidance to the treaty. The CRC has eighteen General Comments on a range of issues.

CASE STUDY 1: CHILD LABOUR

It is estimated that globally, around one in four children (aged five to seventeen) in the world's poorest countries are engaged in child labour; this equates to around 168 million children (UNICEF 2017). Most child labourers are located in West and Central Africa (32 percent of children aged five to seventeen), and Sub Saharan Africa (29 percent of children aged five to seventeen). The Middle East and North Africa both have around 7 percent of children aged five to seventeen working, while around 11 percent of the population of children aged five to seventeen age in Latin America are working (UNICEF

2017). The main cause of child labour is poverty, a lack of educational opportunities, inadequate industrial technology, and traditional attitudes toward the participation of children in employment (ILO 2017a). While some of these children are employed in factories, most are employed by their family at home, on the family farm, or in the family business (Edmonds 2007).

Child labour is guided by two main international conventions along with the CRC. The first is the International Labour Organization (ILO) Convention concerning minimum age for employment, and the suggestion that states should provide for poverty so that children are not required to work (Convention No. 138 and Recommendation No. 146), this Convention has been ratified by 171 states (ILO 2017b). The second is ILO Convention No. 182 Concerning the Prohibition and Immediate Action for the Elimination of the Worst Forms of Child Labour, and Recommendation No. 190 concerned specifically with hazardous work (1999), this Convention has been ratified by 184 states (ILO 2017b). These conventions frame the concept of child labour and form the basis for child labour legislation.

As a way to decrease the demand for child labour, the last decade has seen an increase in discussion around providing consumers with information on the supply chains of a number of key products including diamonds, gold, silver, chocolate, and clothing. Several codes of practice have been drafted that allow consumers to understand the supply chain of the goods that they have purchased, to enable the purchase of goods that follow good human rights practices (Human Rights Watch 2018). Few industries, however, have taken up these transparency procedures, and while they remain voluntary, few others will do so.

There are also moves to limit the number of children working in tobacco farms and fields. Agriculture is the largest employer of children, with 60 percent of child labourers worldwide working in the agriculture industry, the majority are unpaid and work for family members (ILO 2017a). Many of these children work in tobacco farms, picking and tending tobacco plants. In the United States, weak child labour laws mean that children as young as twelve can work an unlimited number of hours, so long as they are not absent from any school, while children in other countries such as Indonesia and Zimbabwe often work alongside their parents all day on dangerous tobacco fields. The government of Brazil has recently adopted policies that prevent children under the age of eighteen from any work with tobacco, with penalties for both the farmers and the companies who purchase the goods if these conditions are breached. The effect of this change in policy has been a decrease in the number of children working with tobacco and this suggests a model for the elimination of children in tobacco farming for other countries (Wurth and Buchanan 2018).

UNICEF

In the aftermath of the Second World War, with many thousands of casualties and a large number of children experiencing famine and disease, the UN created the United Nations International Children's Emergency Fund, or UNICEF, to provide emergency food and health care to children and mothers (Skelton 2007). While initially conceived to be a temporary agency, in 1953 it gained permanent status in the UN system, allowing the organisation to play a key role first in the establishment of the Declaration and then the Convention. In recognition of its permanent status, and not that of a body responsible for responding to emergencies, it was renamed to the United Nations Children's Fund (but kept original acronym, UNICEF). The mandate of UNICEF is to advocate for children's rights and to strive to create a better world for all children.

UNICEF now works in 190 countries and territories, focusing on vaccination and providing health services, advocating for education and gender equality, and working to see human rights realised for all children (UNICEF 2018). The work of UNICEF is entirely funded through donations from private donors and governments. The US government is the largest donor; however, in recent years, UNICEF has sought sponsorship to divest its reliance on government finding. For example, in 2006, Spanish Football Club FC Barcelona began a partnership with UNICEF that sees the club donate €1.5 million per year and feature the logo on the front of their jersey (UNICEF 2006). Since this initial signing, UNICEF has continued to partner with sporting clubs and other social groups through a form of sponsorship that has the added bonus of giving UNICEF free advertising in areas its message would not normally reach.

Rights of the child in the United States

The US government played an active role in drafting the CRC, including commenting on or proposing many articles – some of which came directly from the US Constitution; however, the United States remains the only country that has not ratified the Convention. While the United States signed the CRC in 1995, the ratification process in the United States is complicated and can be difficult to achieve; as such, ratification has not been progressed. Under the US Constitution, ratification of a treaty involves first signing the treaty by the president. The president must then advise the Senate of the treaty and the implications for the country. If the Senate approves ratification by a two-thirds majority, then the president can ratify the treaty. In recent years, both President Bill Clinton and President Barack Obama were supportive of ratification; however, they were unable to persuade Senators of the benefits.

Much of the opposition to the ratification of the CRC comes from religious groups and political conservatives who claim that the CRC is in conflict with the US Constitution, and that through ratification, US parents would lose authority over decisions relating to their children (Gunn 2006). Those in opposition have two main arguments. The first is against human rights treaties and the UN in general, suggesting that ratification of any treaty would see the United States surrender their sovereignty to a power that was not elected by US citizens (Kilbourne 1998b). The second argument relates more to the content of the Convention, and largely with the suggestion that the Convention seeks to diminish the rights of parents when dealing with their children (Kilbourne 1998a).

Other areas of concern for many in the United States include firstly the limits suggested by the CRC on adoption (found in Article 21), with UNICEF (2015) specifically discouraging intercountry adoption where other arrangements can be made, and secondly the prohibition of capital punishment or life sentencing for individuals under eighteen years (Article 37 and Article 40). While the United States does comply with parts of these Articles, they do not comply entirely. For example, since 2005 individuals under the age of eighteen cannot be subject to capital punishment, however, they continue to be committed to prison for life without parole (Feld 2008).

CASE STUDY 2: THE RIGHT TO AN EDUCATION

Article 28 of the CRC outlines a child's right to an education, with the further stipulation that education at an elementary or primary level needs to be free and available to all. However, as a result of poverty and marginalization, estimates suggest that 100 million children around the world are unschooled (Human Rights Watch 2019b), many of these children live in the poorest parts of the world; including Sub Saharan Africa, and Central and East Asia.

There are also a large number of children who experience education poverty, that is, children who are attending some school, but typically are only able to receive 4 or fewer years of education. Millions stop going to school because they need to work long hours or cannot afford school fees, they experience violence or abuse from teachers or fellow students or find their schools the target of armed attack (Human Rights Watch 2019b). Gender also plays a role in education and school completion. Families often do not send girls to school, force them out of school to marry, or deny them an education when they become pregnant. For example, Pakistan has been described as among the worse countries for education. In Pakistan, 32 percent of primary school aged girls are not in school compared with 21 percent of boys, by the end of grade six, this is closer to 60 percent of girls and 50 percent of boys (Human Rights Watch 2019b).

Attacks on education occur around the world, both inside and outside of situations of armed conflict, with some armed groups intentionally targeting schools, teachers, and students (Human Rights Watch 2019a). In addition to putting children and teachers at risk of injury or death, these attacks violate the rights of the child, minimising the chance that they will be able to complete their education. Recent conflicts in Syria, Cameroon, and Pakistan have all seen schools the target of deliberate attacks, resulting in the deaths of hundreds of children and teachers, and limiting the opportunity for education for many thousands of other children (Human Rights Watch 2019a).

Challenges with the CRC

While the CRC is largely celebrated as having made positive changes to the lives of many thousands of children across the world, there are a number of areas where the CRC is described as insufficient (Freeman 2018). One such example is how to resolve a situation when two or more principles are in conflict. For example, what if a child (or their parent on their behalf) refuses medical treatment, but the child will suffer harm if the treatment is not given (Walker and Doyon 2001). The CRC somewhat addresses this problem in three Articles: Article 3 says that all decisions relating to children must be made 'within the best interest of the child', Article 6 specifies that children have a right to life and that the state must ensure the survival and development of the child, and Article 13 ensures the right to seek, receive, and impart information. Together, these three articles suggest that while a child does have the right to make a decision about themselves, and that they should be provided with the highest standard of care, these decisions must be considered in light of the developmental capacity of the child (Walker and Doyon 2001). As a result, in most cases (unless the child is close to the age of maturity), authority is provided to the parent or guardian to make decisions in the best interest of the child, regardless of whether the child is in agreement or not (Salter 2012). Another, albeit less common, example of this, is the case of the conjoined twins in the UK in 2000. The parents in this case refused to have their conjoined daughters separated as one twin would not survive the operation, despite medical advice suggesting that without the operation, both twins would die. The law in the UK prohibits the deliberate causing of death, leaving the courts in a difficult position of ruling that one or both twins would die (Rennie and Leigh 2008). In the end, it was decided that as one child had no chance of survival with or without the surgery, the treating medical team should try to save the stronger child. The twins were separated shortly after this decision and the weaker twin died.

Another area of uncertainty in the CRC is related to the point where life begins. Like most other international treaties or pieces of international law, the CRC says little about abortion. The absence of any discussion of where the rights of the child begin, before or after birth, is usually attributed to a compromise made during the drafting of the CRC (Alston 1990). While Article 1 states that a child is defined as any person below the age of 18 years, there is no clear designation of when childhood begins; at fertilisation, conception, at birth, or at some other point (Janoff 2004). The lack of definition of the beginning of life means that there is some ambiguity when discussing the right to abortion under the CRC. According to Janoff (2004), if an unborn foetus is a child for the purposes of the CRC, then, it would have 'the inherent right to life' (Article 6). But, if the foetus's right to life conflicts with the rights guaranteed to a pregnant girl which safeguard her right to health (Article 24) and to consideration of her best interests (Article 3), there remain questions regarding whose rights are protected or considered first. In response to this ambiguity, the Committee on the Rights to the Child released General Comment 15 in 2013. This comment says that:

States should review and consider allowing children to consent to certain medical treatments and interventions without the permission of a parent, caregiver, or guardian, such as HIV testing and sexual and reproductive health services, including education and guidance on sexual health, contraception, and safe abortion.

While the General Comment also suggests that safe abortion should still be available whether it is legal in the country or not, states are under no obligation to provide abortion services (United Nations 2013). As a result, individual states make decisions around abortion based on domestic law and customs.

Finally, are the gaps in the CRC around gender. For example, gay, transgender, and intersex children, and to some extent girl children are not specifically mentioned in the CRC. While the CRC was intended to be 'gender blind' there are areas where the rights of boy children appear to have received greater protections. For example, boy children are more likely to be recruited as child soldiers, a situation covered in Article 38, however, conditions that are more likely to impact girl children, such as child marriage, are not included (Askari 1998).

Each year, around 12 million girls are married before the age of eighteen (Girls not Brides 2019). In response UNICEF, working with other NGOs, has launched the Global Programme to Accelerate Action to End Child Marriage. This program seeks to encourage and empower governments around the world to eliminate child marriage through legislation and changes to culture. The Human Rights Council, during session 26 in 2014, raised concerns over the existence of child marriage, and highlighted that, according to the second Protocol to the CRC, child marriage might be considered as the 'sale of children'. Many countries have enacted legislation making illegal the marriage of anyone below the age of eighteen years, however, a large number of countries allow a child to marry with the consent of their parents. Despite positive gains in the number of countries that prevent child marriage, there remain approximately one in five women who are married before their eighteenth birthday (UNICEF 2019).

Monitoring children's rights

Each state that ratifies the CRC is required to provide a report detailing how it is fulfilling its human rights obligations to the convention and the two optional Protocols. The report is submitted to a body of eighteen independent experts called the Committee on the Rights of the Child (the Committee). States must submit a report two years after they ratify the Convention. After that, progress reports are made every five years. The Committee can also hear individual complaints against the CRC and the two optional protocols by those states who are party to the third optional protocol, the committee can also carry out its own independent investigation into grave or serious breaches of the CRC or protocols (United Nations 2019b).

Rights of the child in the twenty-first century

While the realisation of the child's rights has come a long way since a time when it was expected that children would work long days alongside parents on farms or in mines, there remains a long way to go. Many children continue to be denied a formal education, child marriage exists in many counties, and despite greater transparency around child labour, many children continue to work long hours in dangerous employment. Greater awareness and enforcement of the rights of the child is needed for these rights to be realised for all children.

References

Alston, P 1990. The unborn child and abortion under the draft Convention on the Rights of the Child, *Human Rights Quarterly*, 12(1): 156–178. doi.org/10.2307/762174

Askari, L 1998. The Convention on the Rights of the Child: The necessity of adding a provision to ban child marriages, *ILSA Journal of International and Comparative Law*, 5: 123.

Bennett Jr, WH 1987. A critique of the emerging convention on the rights of the child, *Cornell International Law Journal*, 20(1).

Buck, T, & Lee, F 2014. *International Child Law*, London, UK: Routledge. doi.org/10.4324/9780203538135

Cohn, I 1991. The convention on the rights of the child: What it means for children in war, *International Journal of Refugee Law*, 3(1): 100–111. doi.org/10.1093/ijrl/3.1.100

Committee on the Rights of the Child 2010. Treaty-specific guidelines regarding the form and content of periodic reports to be submitted by states parties under article 44, paragraph 1 (b), of the Convention on the Rights of the Child, Geneva.

Dennis, MJ 2000. Newly adopted protocols to the Convention on the Rights of the Child, *American Journal of International Law*, 94(4): 789–796. doi.org/10.2307/2589806

Detrick, S 1999. *A Commentary on the United Nations Convention on the Rights of the Child*, Leiden, Netherlands: Martinus Nijhoff Publishers.

Edmonds, EV 2007. Child labor, *Handbook of Development Economics*, 4: 3607–3709. doi.org/10.1016/S1573-4471(07)04057-0

Fass, PS 2011. A historical context for the United Nations Convention on the Rights of the Child, *The Annals of the American Academy of Political and Social Science*, 633(1): 17–29. doi: 10.1177/0002716210382388

Feld, BC 2008. A slower form of death: Implications of Roper v. Simmons for juveniles sentenced to life without parole, *Notre Dame Journal of Law, Ethics & Public Policy*, 22(9). doi.org/10.1163/9789004358829

Freeman, M 2018. *Children's Rights: New Issues, New Themes, New Perspectives*, Leiden, Netherlands: Brill.

Girls not Brides 2019. *Child Marriage* [Online], London. Available: www.girlsnotbrides.org/about-child-marriage/ [Accessed 15/04/2019].

Gunn, TJ 2006. The religious right and the opposition to US ratification of the Convention on the Rights of the Child, *Emory International Law Review*, 20: 111.

Holcomb, J 2016. Children's rights, *Encyclopedia of Family Studies*: 1–6. doi.org/10.1002/9781119085621. wbefs144

Howe, RB 2001. Do parents have fundamental rights?, *Journal of Canadian Studies*, 36(3): 61–78. doi. org/10.3138/jcs.36.3.61

Human Rights Watch 2018. *Child Labor* [Online], New York. Available: www.hrw.org/topic/childrens-rights/child-labor [Accessed 15/04/2019].

Human Rights Watch 2019a. *Attacks on Education* [Online]. Available: www.hrw.org/topic/childrens-rights/attacks-education [Accessed 15/04/2019].

Human Rights Watch 2019b. *Education* [Online]. Available: www.hrw.org/topic/childrens-rights/education

ILO 2017a. *Child Labour in Agriculture* [Online]. Available: www.ilo.org/ipec/areas/Agriculture/lang-en/index.htm [Accessed 15/04/2019].

ILO 2017b. *Conventions* [Online]. Available: www.ilo.org/dyn/normlex/en/f?p=1000:12000:::NO::: [Accessed 15/04/2019].

Janoff, AF 2004. Rights of the pregnant child vs. rights of the unborn under the Convention on the Rights of the Child, *Boston University International Law Journal*, 22: 163.

Kilbourne, S 1998a. Opposition to US ratification of the United Nations Convention on the Rights of the Child: Responses to parental rights arguments, *Loyola Poverty Law Journal*, 4(55).

Kilbourne, S 1998b. The Wayward Americans-why the USA has not ratified the UN Convention on the Rights of the Child, *Child and Family Law Quarterly*, 10: 243.

League of Nations 1924. *Geneva Declaration of the Rights of the Child* [Online]. Available: www.un-documents. net/gdrc1924.htm [Accessed 01/04/2019].

Lee, Y 2010. Communications procedure under the Convention on the Rights of the Child: 3rd optional protocol, *The International Journal of Children's Rights*, 18(4): 567–583. doi.org/10.1163/157181810X527239

Liefaard, T, & Sloth-Nielsen, J 2017. 25 years CRC: Reflecting on successes, failures and the future, *The United Nations Convention on the Rights of the Child*: 1–13, Brill Nijhoff. doi.org/10.1163/9789004295056_002

Limber, SP, & Flekkoy, MG 1995. The UN Convention on the Rights of the Child: Its relevance for social scientists, *Social Policy Report*, 9(2): 1–16. doi.org/10.1002/j.2379-3988.1995.tb00034.x

Marshall, D 1999. The construction of children as an object of international relations: The declaration of children's rights and the child welfare committee of league of nations, 1900–1924, *International Journal of Children's Rights*, 7(2): 103–147. doi.org/10.1163/15718189920494309

Moody, Z 2015. The United Nations Declaration of the Rights of the Child (1959): Genesis, transformation and dissemination of a treaty (re) constituting a transnational cause, *Prospects*, 45(1): 15–29. doi.org/10.1007/s11125-015-9343-4

Pais, MS 2010. The protection of children from sexual exploitation Optional Protocol to the Convention on the Rights of the Child on the sale of children, child prostitution and child pornography, *The International Journal of Children's Rights*, 18(4): 551–566. doi.org/10.1163/157181810X536815

Rennie, JM, & Leigh, B 2008. The legal framework for end-of-life decisions in the UK, *Seminars in Fetal and Neonatal Medicine*: 296–300, Elsevier. doi.org/10.1016/j.siny.2008.03.007

Roose, R, & Bouverne-de Bie, M 2007. Do children have rights or do their rights have to be realised? The United Nations Convention on the Rights of the Child as a frame of reference for pedagogical action, *Journal of Philosophy of Education*, 41(3): 431–443. doi.org/10.1111/j.1467-9752.2007.00568.x

Salter, EK 2012. Deciding for a child: A comprehensive analysis of the best interest standard, *Theoretical Medicine and Bioethics*, 33(3): 179–198. doi.org/10.1007/s11017-012-9219-z

Skelton, T 2007. Children, young people, UNICEF and participation, *Children's Geographies*, 5(1–2): 165–181. doi.org/10.1080/14733280601108338

Todres, J 1998. Emerging limitations on the rights of the child: The UN Convention on the Rights of the Child and its early case law, *Columbia Human Rights Law Review*, 30(159).

UN General Assembly 1959. Declaration of the Rights of the Child, *UN Doc A/RES/14/1386*, Geneva.

UN General Assembly 1989. Convention on the Rights of the Child, *United Nations, Treaty Series*, 1577: 3.

UNICEF 2006. *Futbol Club Barcelona, UNICEF Team Up for Children in Global Partnership* [Online], Geneva. Available: www.unicef.org/media/media_35642.html [Accessed 10/04/2019].

UNICEF 2015. *Intercountry Adoption* [Online]. Geneva: UNICEF. Available: https://www.unicef.org/media/intercountry-adoption [Accessed 10/04/2019].

UNICEF 2017. *Child Labour* [Online]. Available: https://data.unicef.org/topic/child-protection/child-labour/ [Accessed 15/04/2019].

UNICEF 2018. *Annual Report, 2017*, New York.

UNICEF 2019. *Child Marriage* [Online]. Available: https://data.unicef.org/topic/child-protection/child-marriage/ [Accessed 15/04/2019].

United Nations 2013. *General Comment No. 15 (2013) on the Right of the Child to the Enjoyment of the Highest Attainable Standard of Health (Art. 24)* [Online]. Available: http://docstore.ohchr.org/SelfServices/FilesHandler.ashx?enc=6QkG1d%2FPPRiCAqhKb7yhsqIkirKQZLK2M58RF%2F5F0vHCIs1B9k1r3x0aA7FYrehlNUfw4dHmlOxmFtmhaiMOkH80ywS3uq6Q3bqZ3A3yQ0%2B4u6214CSatnrBlZT8nZmj [Accessed 15/04/2019].

United Nations 2019a. *Human Rights Treaty Bodies: General Comments* [Online]. Available: www.ohchr.org/en/hrbodies/pages/tbgeneralcomments.aspx [Accessed 15/04/2019].

United Nations 2019b. *Monitoring Children's Rights* [Online]. Available: www.ohchr.org/EN/HRBodies/CRC/Pages/CRCIntro.aspx [Accessed 15/04/2019].

United Nations 2019c. *Treaty Collection* [Online], Geneva. Available: https://treaties.un.org/ [Accessed 08/04/2019].

Walker, NE, & Doyon, T 2001. 'Fairness and reasonableness of the child's decision': A proposed legal standard for children's participation in medical decision making, *Behavioral Sciences & the Law*, 19(5–6): 611–636. doi.org/10.1002/bsl.461

WHO 2019. *Children: Reducing Mortality* [Online], Geneva. Available: www.who.int/en/news-room/fact-sheets/detail/children-reducing-mortality [Accessed 15/04/2019].

Wilcox, BL, & Nalmark, H 1991. The rights of the child: Progress toward human dignity, *American Psychologist*, 46(1): 49. doi.org/10.1037//0003-066X.46.1.49

Wurth, M, & Buchanan, J 2018. *How We Can Fight Child Labour in the Tobacco Industry* [Online]. Available: www.hrw.org/news/2018/06/27/how-we-can-fight-child-labour-tobacco-industry [Accessed 15/04/2019].

7

REFUGEE PROTECTION

Fiona H. McKay and Ann Taket

Introduction

There are a range of rights afforded to individuals who move across borders, including migrants who move for employment or other opportunities, students or tourists temporarily entering a country, or refugees seeking protection. State sovereignty means that states are entitled to exercise jurisdiction over their own territory, and are allowed to decide which non-citizens can enter and remain, who should be refused admission, and who should be compelled to leave (Goodwin-Gill 2014). Given their vulnerability, there are however, exceptions to these laws for those seeking asylum. These exceptions are described in the international law of refugee protection which includes a range of universal and regional conventions or treaties, rules of customary international law, general principles of law, national laws, and the standards and practices of international organisations (Goodwin-Gill 2014). Refugee protection is overseen by the United Nations High Commissioner for Refugees (UNHCR). Refugee protection prescribes the obligations of states and is intended to ensure that no refugee is penalised, expelled, or refouled for seeking protection, while ensuring they are able to enjoy the rights to which they are entitled.

Migration can come with serious obstacles to good health, due to discrimination, issues with access, language and cultural barriers, and other economic and social difficulties (WHO 2003). At the same time, not providing migrants, regardless of their type, with access to suitable and timely health care may have significant public health consequences. This is particularly true for people who have recently fled violence or a situation of conflict, and who may have experienced disrupted health care in their home country. Refuges and people seeking asylum may also experience post-traumatic stress, exacerbated by the conditions of their stay in their country of asylum (WHO 2003).

The global refugee population has grown from around two million in 1951 to over 25 million in 2018 (including over 5 million Palestinians who continue to fall under the responsibility of the United Nations Relief and Works Agency, UNRWA) (UNHCR 2018a). In total there are more than 68.5 million people who are of concern to UNHCR (including asylum seekers, refugees, internally displaced persons, and stateless people), the largest number of people to of concern to UNHCR ever. This chapter will explore the historical context of seeking asylum and the evolution of the Convention Relating to the Status of Refuges, and the human rights specifically afforded to refugees and asylum seekers, it will also include a discussion on the situation of LGBTIQ asylum seekers, and the treatment of asylum seekers in Australia and Germany.

A short history of refugee protection

Current rights and obligations afforded to refugees can be traced back to the period immediately following the First World War. Refugees, at the time termed stateless or Displaced Persons, were principally the concern of humanitarian agencies and non-government organisations (NGOs). However, by the 1920s the number of people forced to flee their homes and seek assistance became so great, that the office of the High Commission for Russian Refugees was established under the League of Nations (White 2017). The Commissioner had a mandate to provide 'material assistance and legal and political protection' to the approximately 1.5 million people who had fled the Russian Revolution and the subsequent Russian Civil War of the early twentieth century (Skran 1995). This legal foundation was not the result of a comprehensive approach to refugee issues, rather it represented an ad hoc response to issues as they arose. It was underpinned by two key principles; the first was that refugees should be considered a special category of migrants who need protection, while the second was that they should not be sent back to a country where they will face persecution (Dörschner and Machts 2011). Within a few years of its creation, the mandate of the Commissioner was extended to other refugee groups including Armenians, Assyrians, Bulgarians, and Assyro-Chaldeans (Holborn 1939). In each of these cases, a refugee was defined as a person in a group for which the Commissioner, under the League of Nations had approved a specific mandate. At this time, refugees were dealt with on an ad hoc basis; there was no general, international, definition for a refugee.

At the end of the Second World War, the League of Nations was disbanded and replaced by the United Nations (UN). At this time, the large number of refugees in Europe and Asia lead to the establishment of the International Refugee Organization (IRO) under the UN, as the body responsible for resolving the refugee situation created by the Second World War. Political and diplomatic challenges at the time meant the IRO was not well supported by member states of the UN and was soon disbanded. Despite its short life, the IRO was able to assist hundreds of thousands of refugees and displaced persons to return home or to find safety in a new country (Goodwin-Gill 2014). As the refugee population grew in the years after the Second World War, and the situations for refugees became increasingly complex, the UN came under pressure to find a solution to problems relating to refugees more generally. In 1951, the Office of the United Nations High Commissioner for Refugees (UNHCR) became the principle agency concerned with the protection of refugees.

The Refugee Convention

From its creation, the work of UNHCR was intended to be complimented by a treaty and a formal definition of a refugee. Building on Article 14 of the Universal Deceleration of Human Rights (UDHR), which recognises the right of people to seek asylum from persecution in other countries, a Convention Relating to the Status of Refugees (the Convention) was adopted in 1951. The Convention was developed to combine and extend existing international instruments relating to refugees, to regulate the legal systems (Weiss 1954), and for the first time, it offered a definition of a refugee and conferred the rights and protections available to a person falling within the definition. The definition, found in Article 1A(2) of the Convention, is as follows:

> As a result of events occurring before 1 January 1951 and owing to well-founded fear of being persecuted for reasons of race, religion, nationality, membership of a particular social group or political opinion, is outside the country of his nationality and is unable or, owing to such fear, is unwilling to avail himself of the protection of that country; or who, not having a nationality and being outside the country of his former habitual residence as a result of such events, is unable or, owing to such fear, is unwilling to return to it.
>
> *(UNHCR 1951)*

The Convention limits states' obligations to those who became refugees before 1951; States also had the option to restrict their assistance to refugees as a result of events occurring in Europe (found in Article 1B). As the number of refugees needing assistance increased, these temporal and geographical limitations proved unworkable, and in 1967, a Protocol relating to the Status of Refugees (the Protocol) was enacted to remove these restrictions. The Protocol also has a provision allowing ratifying countries to agree to the Convention without further action. These two documents are the core international legal instruments relating to refugee protection and asylum. The Convention and the Protocol have been ratified by 146 nations (United Nations 2019).

In addition to being outside their country of 'former habitual residence', usually understood to mean citizenship, to be a refugee, one must be in fear of being persecuted, and this fear must be 'well founded'. While there is no definition of persecution with the Convention, several Articles refer to threats to life or freedom, as such, it is generally understood that persecution refers to a threat of death, torture, or cruel, inhumane, or degrading treatment or punishment (Goodwin–Gill 2014). In addition to the fear being well founded, it must also be a future risk. While a refugee may have experienced persecution in the past, to be recognised under the Convention, there must be a real risk of future persecution if the refugee returns home (McAdam and Chong 2014). Finally, while there are a number of situations where an individual may fear that they are at risk of persecution from government or non–government actor, a refugee must be unable or unwilling to receive help or protection from their state.

The Convention has a number of objectives. In addition to describing the characteristics of a refugee; the Convention is clear on who cannot access its protection. For political reasons, the Convention excludes Palestinian refugees from protection by UNHCR and does not deal with those who are stateless. Anyone who is believed to have committed a crime against peace, a war crime, a crime against humanity, or a serious non–political crime outside the country of refuge prior to admission to that country as a refugee, or has been guilty of acts contrary to the purposes and principles of the UN are excluded (Article 1F). An individual is also excluded from the protection if they voluntarily return to their country of origin or if the situation in their county becomes stable enough for their claim no longer to be valid (Article 1C).

The Convention also describes the responsibilities of the state. States are obliged grant refugee status to someone who meets the definition regardless of any reciprocity from the refugee's home country (Article 7). States must respect a refugee's personal status, for example, their marriage in another country (Article 12), and provide refugees with identity (Article 27) and travel identification papers (Article 28). States must provide free access to courts (Article 16), and the possibility of assimilation and naturalization to refugees (Article 34). States are required to ensure that refugees do not face discrimination (Article 3), and that they are able to enjoy religious freedom (Article 4), they are prevented from expecting refugees to pay taxes different to those of nationals (Article 29), or imposing penalties on refugees who entered illegally in search of asylum if they present themselves without delay (Article 31).

Possibly the most important article is Article 33. Article 33 stipulates that states cannot return or expel persons to the frontiers of territories where their 'life or freedom' would be threatened on account of one of the five Convention areas – race, religion, nationality, membership of a particular group, or political opinion. This principal is termed *non-refoulement*. While Article 1 provides a definition of who a refugee is, it is the inclusion of *non-refoulement* in Article 33 that protects refugees from being returned to persecution. Article 33 is the most fundamental right of a refugee and is often described as the cornerstone of the Convention; furthermore, as it is understood to be a part of customary international law it also applies to asylum seekers while they wait for their refugee status to be decided, and to countries who have not ratified the Convention. States, however, are under no obligation under the Convention to provide automatic or permanent protection.

The special case of Palestinian refugees

Agreements made after the First World War and the collapse of the Ottoman Empire saw Great Britain take control over Mandatory Palestine, an area that now covers parts of Iraq, Israel, and the occupied West Bank and Gaza Strip. In the early years of British control, thousands of Jewish people fleeing persecution in Eastern and Central Europe migrated to Mandatory Palestine to realise the promise made after the First World War of the establishment in 'Palestine of a national home for the Jewish people' (Kimmerling 2009). While initial immigrants were tolerated by the local Arab population, as the numbers increased, tensions rose, and by the 1930s, the British began to limit Jewish immigration, and place restrictions on the amount of land they could own. With increased persecution of Jewish people in Nazi Germany and surrounding occupied areas in the mid-1930s, a program of clandestine migration began with hundreds of thousands of Jewish migrants from Central Europe traveling to Palestine. The number of migrants, alongside existing tensions led to the formation of Jewish militias to fight both the local Arabs and to resist British rule, and Arab militias to fight the Jewish and the British populations (Kimmerling 2009).

After the Second World War, the UN worked with the international community on the issue of Palestine, and in 1947, the UN General Assembly adopted Resolution 181 (II) which saw the British Palestine Mandate divided into two independent states, a Jewish state, and an Arab state, linked by the city of Jerusalem which would be managed under an international regime (Akram 2014). Partition was designed to be implemented in stages alongside the progressive withdrawal of the British and sought to address the claims of the conflicting Palestinian and Jewish national movements, while encouraging an Economic Union between the states. The plan was accepted by Jewish leaders; but was rejected by Arab leaders from the region who were unwilling to accept any form of territorial division and saw Partition as a form of colonialism, particularly given that many of the surrounding nations had only recently received independence from colonial powers (Kimmerling 2009). Despite this, the UN passed the resolution, and the British began to withdraw from Palestine. Almost immediately, violence between the Palestinians, joined by neighbouring Arab states, and Jewish population began. The war, called the 1948 Arab-Israeli War, was the first of several wars fought in the territory over the following decades. The new state of Israel won this war, claiming greater areas of land than were identified under the UN plan, and leading to thousands of displaced Palestinians inside Palestine and surrounding countries (Bocco 2009).

In response to the large number of people in need, the UN established the United Nations Relief and Works Agency for Palestine (UNRWA) as a specific agency to responded to the refugee problem for a term of three years, and to operate outside of UNHCR. According to UNRWA, a Palestinian refugee is defined as

> persons whose normal place of residence was Palestine during the period 1 June 1946 to 15 May 1948, and who lost both home and means of livelihood as a result of the 1948 conflict.

Unlike other situations that force people to flee their homes, the international community concluded that this refugee crisis was different. In addition to recognising large-scale persecution and expulsion of Palestinians as a people, the international community recognised that, unlike other refugee situations up to that time, the UN itself was partly responsibility for their refugee status (Akram 2002). While the UN recognises that these refugees are persecuted and therefore fall under the definition found in Article 1A(2) of the Convention, they are somewhat different as the obstacle to their repatriation is not that their government cannot protect them, but rather that a member state of the UN prevents their return (Akram 2002).

UNRWA continue to serve those living in its area of operation – Jordan, Lebanon, Syria, the Gaza Strip, and the West Bank, including East Jerusalem; any refugee outside of these areas receives support from UNHCR. To receive UNRWA support, a refugee must meet the definition, be registered, and be found to be in need (UNRWA 2019). The descendants of Palestine refugee males, including adopted children, are also eligible for registration (UNRWA 2019). When UNRWA began operations in 1950, it was responding to the needs of about 750,000 Palestine refugees, the number of those in need is now closer to 5 million (UNRWA 2007, 2019). Of these, around 40 percent live in Jordan, 27 percent in Gaza, 15 percent in the West Bank, 10 percent in Syria, and 9 percent in Lebanon (UNRWA 2019). Almost one third of registered Palestine refugees live in camps. The responsibilities of UNRWA in Palestinian refugee camps is limited to providing services, the host countries are responsible for other functions.

Palestinians have now been in a protracted refugee situation for over seventy years, with the third generation of refugee children becoming adults (UNRWA 2019). With little indication that the situation will change, Palestinian refugees are stuck in a limbo, they are mostly stateless as a result of their forced exile, and with few exceptions, the countries they live in do not afford them meaningful legal protection (Erakat 2014). Morbidity for Palestinians is affected by the increased violence towards children, mental health problems, and poor nutrition, particularly in Gaza (Waterston and Nasser 2017). There are significant health inequalities between the Palestinian populations in the West Bank and Gaza and the population of Israel, with a life expectancy gap of over eight years between the two populations living side by side (WHO 2016), given the ongoing violence and persecution, many Palestinians also suffer significant mental health problems (Canetti et al. 2010).

Human rights of refugees

The obligations of states and entitlements of individuals are based on both the treaties that apply to refugees, but also on broader human rights treaties. In addition to those rights found in the Convention, like all individuals, refugees are entitled to the rights enshrined in the International Covenant on Economic, Social, and Cultural Rights (ICESCR) and the International Covenant on Civil and Political Rights (ICCPR). Some of the rights found in the Convention are applied to an asylum seeker when they arrive in a country. This includes the right to *non-refoulement* and the right to non-discrimination and freedom of religion. Others are afforded when a refugee is lawfully admitted to a country, including access to employment, education, and welfare. The Convention says that a refugee should be entitled to, at minimum, the same standard of treatment as other foreigners in a country, with some rights including the right to protection under the legal system, education, the right to social security, that must be provided at the same level as citizens of the host country.

While the Convention is legally binding, there is no international court or other system of international oversight to enforce the obligations of states toward those seeking asylum, rather, Article 35 of the Convention obliges states to cooperate with UNHCR in the fulfilment of its duties as the agency 'supervising the application' of the Convention. This supervisory role allows UNHCR to give advice and make judgments on states' behaviour under refugee law (Takahashi 2002). UNHCR achieves this through an education and advice capacity, and through persuading states to fully engage in their refugee protection obligations (Loescher 2014). This amounts largely to public shaming of states, which in recent years has done little to change practices. For example, UNHCR regularly condemns Australia for its treatment of people seeking asylum, including practices of mandatory detention and preventing temporary visa holders from employment (UNHCR 2017); recently Nigeria was condemned for forcing refugees back to Cameroon in direct violation of the principle of *non-refoulement* (UNHCR 2018c); and recent changes to US policy related to migrant children and people fleeing persecution in Central and South America have seen UNHCR offer advice and express caution (UNHCR 2018d). While there are avenues for individuals and countries to bring claims against a country who is alleged to be in breach of Convention obligations, these measures have never been taken (O'Byrne 2013). This may suggest that states are not inclined or incentivised to bring international proceedings against other states for noncompliance with refugee obligations (Kidane 2006).

In addition to this supervisory role provided by UNHCR, there are other international mechanism of relevance to the protection of refugees and asylum seekers. This includes the Human Rights Council, specifically around the issue of *non-refoulement* as it relates to the ICCPR (Harvey 2015). The Human Rights Council has also made judgments on the right to education, found in the ICESCR (Willems and Vernimmen 2018). Finally, the Committee on the Elimination of Discrimination against Women (CEDAW) and the Committee on the Elimination of Racial Discrimination (CERD) have heard cases related to the deportation of refugees and asylum seekers relating to specific Articles within the relevant Conventions (Harvey 2015).

Stateless people

The Convention is in place to assist individuals who are unable or unwilling to receive assistance from their government, there are times, however, when a government ceases to exist.

For people in this situation, termed 'stateless', a range of other instruments and associated human rights come into play. In 1954, just three years after the Refugee Convention was adopted, the Convention Relating to the Status of Stateless Persons was agreed upon. Initially designed as a Protocol to the Refugee Convention, it was eventually adopted as a standalone convention (Edwards and Van Waas 2014). The Statelessness Convention establishes the legal definition for stateless persons as 'individuals who are not considered citizens or nationals under the operation of the laws of any country' (UNHCR 2019). The exact number of stateless people are unknown, but UNHCR puts the figure at around 10 million people.

Statelessness may occur for a variety of reasons, including discrimination against ethnic or religious groups or based on gender; the emergence of new states and transfers between existing states; and conflict of nationality laws (UNHCR 2019). Stateless people can be both inside or outside the borders of the country, and statelessness can be passed on; around one third of the stateless population are children as at least twenty-five countries do not allow women to transfer nationality to their children if their fathers are unknown, missing, or deceased (UNHCR 2019). Being stateless can have serious negative impacts on individuals and groups. People who are stateless are often unable to enjoy rights to education, health care, employment, and are often stranded, with no citizenship documents that allow them to travel into other countries (Edwards and Van Waas 2014).

LGBTIQ refugees: an especially vulnerable group

In recent years, there has been an increasing recognition from UNHCR that refugee experiences have been understood through a male and heteronormative framework. This has meant that the claims of women and people who identify as non-heterosexual may have been unfairly assessed (UNHCR 2012). While there have been some calls recently to make changes to the way that the Convention is understood to explicitly include gender and sexuality, it is unlikely to happen soon. Instead, the refugee status determination process has responded by adopting guidelines to fill these gaps (Fiddian-Qasmiyeh 2014). These guidelines recognise the intersectionality of refugees who are also women, lesbian, gay, bisexual, transgender, intersex, and queer (LGBTIQ) individuals (Brotman and Lee 2011). These groups have been identified as an 'especially vulnerable group' who require specific protections as they may be fleeing different types of persecution. As a result, they typically have their refugee status determined through the grounds of their 'membership of a particular social group' within the Convention.

The number of countries decriminalizing or legalising homosexual activity between consenting adults is increasing, however, there remain 70 countries where such activity is illegal (Equaldex 2019). Even in counties where homosexual activity is legal, the situation remains dangerous for many. For example, Brazil hosts the largest Pride Parade in the world and has legalised same-sex marriage, yet also has the world's highest reported rate of homophobic and transphobic murders, and the president, who in 2013 described himself as a 'proud homophobic', while in South Africa, which recognises same-sex marriage, there are reports of 'corrective rape' targeted at lesbians, often going unreported and un-investigated by police (Jordan and Morrissey 2013). There are currently eight UN member states (or parts thereof) where the death penalty occurs as a punishment for same-sex consensual sexual acts, and a further five states where although the death penalty is technically possible it is unused, fourteen other countries carry penalties of up to a life sentence for same-sex consensual sexual acts (Carrol and Mendos 2017).

The assessment of an application based on persecution because of LGBTIQ status is relatively new. The challenges faced by LGBTIQ refugees and asylum seekers can include homophobia, transphobia, the criminalization of same-sex relationships, punishable by imprisonment or death, the promotion of conversion therapy and 'corrective' surgery of intersex individuals and forced sterilisation and marriage (Fiddian-Qasmiyeh 2014). While more LGBTIQ refugees are recognised and afforded refugee status, the pace is slow, with many host countries having little understanding of the nature of LGBTIQ persecution. There remain a number of legal and practical challenges in recognising LGBTIQ persecution. For example, there are difficulties in assessing the claims of applicants who do not disclose their sexual orientation; assessors may rely on stereotypes when making assessments; and human rights information about LGBTIQ individuals from countries of origin is not always available or complete (Jansen 2013). Furthermore, because homophobic and/or transphobic persecution typically occurs in private, the possibility of securing corroborating evidence is limited (Jordan and Morrissey 2013). Finally, with UNHCR promoting voluntary reparation as the most desirable solution to refugee situations, many LGBTIQ refugees will continue to face challenges if they have to return home as the homophobic structures and attitudes underpinning their claim for refugee status may have changed little upon their return (Fiddian-Qasmiyeh 2014).

The health of refugees

Worldwide, most people when fleeing persecution travel to neighbouring countries, given the locations of conflict, most people seeking asylum travel to low and middle income countries for protection, with between just 1 and 2 percent of refugees offered permanent resettlement in a third country (UNHCR 2018b). While the common perception is that refuges live in camps, most live in urban environments; the vast majority will remain in their country of asylum until such a time as it is safe enough to return home, in reality, this can often take years or decades (UNHCR 2018b).

The few refugees resettled in high income countries undergo thorough pre and post arrival screening to identify and treat infectious diseases or other health concerns (Heenan et al. 2019). Refugees may arrive in a country for resettlement mal- or undernourished (Rondinelli et al. 2011), and often due to a lack of culturally appropriate foods, or an inability to source foods, they can gain or lose weight (McKay and Dunn 2015).

Refugees have increased rates of chronic disease in the decades following resettlement (Grigg-Saito et al. 2008), while refugee women have an increased risk of poor health due to higher rates of depression, lower literacy, depression and anxiety, lower social support, violence, and lower reported physical activity than refugee men (Shishehgar et al. 2017). Some research has reported on the growing burden of non-communicable diseases in refugee populations, including cardiovascular disease (Doocy et al. 2015), cancers related to tobacco and alcohol use (Sethi et al. 2017), and diabetes (Rehr et al. 2018).

The World Health Organization (WHO), alongside a number of NGOs, including Médecines Sans Frontières (MSF), the International Committee of the Red Cross and Red Crescent, and Save the Children, work with local governments to provide healthcare and sanitation to displaced populations. This work includes the provision of mobile clinics to test and treat disease, providing medical supplies, particularly in situations of damaged transport infrastructure and bureaucratic roadblocks, and working to restore local health care (WHO 2019). In emergency situations, this work is complemented by the Sphere guidelines aimed at improving the quality of humanitarian assistance (Sphere Association 2018). Sphere provides a set of minimum standards on issues of: water supply and sanitation; food security and nutrition; shelter and settlement; and health. These guidelines have been agreed upon by a number of key NGOs who respond to humanitarian crisis as a way to provide the highest quality health care to forced migrants.

Regardless of where they live, forced displacement places refugees at high risk of poor health and social outcomes (Davies et al. 2009), and compared with non-refugee populations, refugees experience poorer mental and physical health (Hollander 2013). A number of factors contribute to these poor health outcomes. This includes trauma and torture, sometimes leading to post-traumatic stress disorder (PTSD), socio-demographic factors such as being older, a woman, or from a rural background, alongside a range of negative post-displacement experiences such as poor living conditions, and restrictions on employment and education (Silove et al. 2017). There is also an increased risk of infectious diseases in displaced populations. For example, the Rohingya refugees currently living in camps on the Bangladesh border are at increased risk of cholera and diphtheria due to the poor living conditions at the camps, despite many NGOs administering vaccinations against these diseases (Cousins 2018). Large numbers of Syrians living in urban areas in Turkey, Lebanon, and Jordan are at risk of tuberculosis, thanks mainly to the destruction of health care facilities and testing in Syria, and challenges with testing and treating the population in neighbouring countries (Ismail et al. 2018).

Australia: a questionable recent human rights record

Australia has engaged with UNHCR through a formal resettlement program for several decades, allowing for the resettlement in Australia of a small proportion of those forcibly displaced. In the 2017–2018 financial year, the Australian Refugee and Humanitarian Program provided 16,250 humanitarian visas: 14,825 for applicants who applied for their visa from within another country before arriving in Australia, and 1,425 permanent protection visas (DIBP 2018).

Prior to 2001, individuals who arrived in Australia by boat simply had to make it as far as one of Australia's offshore territories, including Ashmore Island, the Cartier Islands, Christmas Island, and the Cocos Islands. In 2001, in an effort to deter asylum seekers from traveling to Australia by boat, these islands, while remaining Australian territory, were removed from the migration zone. This removal lead to an increased number of people seeking asylum who attempted to take the more dangerous journey and reach the Australian mainland. In the six years since 2007, approximately 50,000 people had arrived in Australia by boat, with almost 1,000 perishing at sea while making the journey (McKay et al. 2017). In response to these increased arrivals and deaths, the Australian government removed the Australian mainland from Australia's migration zone in 2013, meaning that even if an asylum seeker made it to an Australian shore by boat, they would not be able to apply for a visa. Australia may grant temporary protection to these individuals but is under no obligation to grant a visa to settle permanently in Australia.

The excision of the Australian mainland from the migration zone is an example of Australia's differing response to asylum seekers who arrive by boat compared to those who arrive by plane. Asylum seekers who arrive by boat with no visa, and asylum seekers who arrive via plane with a valid visa (such as a student, tourist, or work visa) and then seek asylum while in Australia, are referred to as Onshore applicants. Within the category of people identified as Onshore arrivals are those further designated as Illegal Maritime Arrivals (IMAs), a term used to refer to individuals who arrived in Australia after 13 August 2012 via sea and without a valid visa. As a result of policy changes in 2013, IMAs are unable to apply for a permanent protection visa (allowing ongoing residency followed by citizenship) and face a range of exclusionary policy measures such as restrictions on employment and education (McKay et al. 2017).

Australia employs a system of mandatory detention (in one of Australia's processing centres) or temporary housing in the community for people seeking asylum. This policy has seen thousands of asylum seekers moved to immigration detention facilities on Christmas Island, Nauru, and Manus Island (Papua New Guinea). These detention centres were originally opened in 2001 as a part of the Australian government's offshore detention policy and have housed thousands of asylum seekers since this time, most of whom have later been confirmed to be refugees. The centres were closed in 2008, due to public disapproval of detaining asylum seekers and an overall reduction in boat arrivals but were reopened in 2012 when increased boat arrivals put pressure on the government to be seen to be doing something. Current Australian policy says that any asylum seeker who arrives in Australia by boat will be detained and will not be eligible to permanently settle in Australia.

Australia's detention centres exist under strict security procedures, media are unable to lawfully travel to these centres to report on conditions, many politicians are prevented from visiting the centres, and medical professionals who work in the centres are prevented by the Australian government from sharing reports of the conditions of the individuals living there (Woodhead 2015). This means that there is little research investigating the health outcomes of living in prolonged mandatory detention as an asylum seeker beyond an understanding that the detention of asylum seekers is associated with substantial mental health problems (Fazel and Silove 2006; Silove et al. 2001). A study from the Bellevue/NYU Program for Survivors of Torture and Physicians for Human Rights reports high rates for symptoms of depression, anxiety, and PTSD among detained asylum seekers, with mental health worsening the longer they were detained (Physicians for Human Rights 2013). A number of reports have suggested that Australia's system of detention of asylum seekers may amount to torture, particularly as twelve detainees have died while in Australian immigration detention (Sanggaran and Zion 2016). Overall, this research suggests that the mental health impacts of detention are not restricted to the period of detention; rather, the adverse mental health effect of detention may be prolonged, extending well beyond the point of release into the community (Filges et al. 2018).

Differing from the treatment of Onshore arrivals noted above are those humanitarian migrants that have their visa processed Offshore. These applicants are typically from Afghanistan, Myanmar, and Iraq, are only eligible for a visa to Australia if they meet certain requirements (including health, security, and character assessments), and often arrive in Australia after years of screening and processing (Karlsen 2016). Opinion polling and political commentary indicate that much of the Australian population prefer Offshore to Onshore applicants, as they are seen to have 'waited their turn in the asylum-seeking queue' (McKay et al. 2011). Offshore applicants receive significantly more resettlement support, including case management and assistance with housing, education, and employment; services not provided to Onshore applicants (Cook and Sherrell 2018).

The implementation of harsh policies that seek to deter asylum seekers from making the journey to Australia is a cornerstone of Australia's humanitarian program. The intended outcome of these deterrent policies is that other asylum seekers will be encouraged to apply through formal channels for a visa to Australia rather than arriving by boat. This approach has had mixed results. There were no reported asylum seekers arriving by boat between 2015 and 2018, however, almost 60,000 people applied for protection in the same period after arriving in Australia with a temporary visa by plane (Australian Senate 2019). In this time, the number of refugees accepted through the formal UNHCR program has only had modest increases.

While there are many politicians who are proud or supportive of Australia's response to people seeking asylum, both Australia's Human Rights Commission and the UN have described the policy as inhumane and as in breach of human rights. The Australian Human Rights Commission has described the Australian onshore immigration detention system is becoming 'more and more like prison', holding people for longer than any comparable jurisdiction, and in breach of Australia's obligations under the ICCPR and the Convention on the Rights of the Child (Australian Human Rights Commission 2019). The UN Human Rights Council has regularly singled out Australia's policies toward asylum seekers, particularly mandatory and indefinite detention, as cruel and unlawful (OHCHR 2019).

This is supported by a number of cases that have been brought to the Human Rights Committee. One example is the 'Boat-People' case (*A v Australia*) concerning the treatment of asylum seekers in detention. In this case, a Cambodian refugee claimed that Australia breached his rights according to the ICCPR by detaining him. While the Committee did not find that Australia's detention at the time was not per se 'arbitrary' it did suggest that Australia should review the period that a person is detained, and it should be no longer than can be reasonably justified. A full report on the case is found in UN document CCPR/C/59/D/560/1993. In its 2009 Concluding Observations on Australia, the UNHRC criticised Australia's mandatory use of detention in all cases of illegal entry and called for the abolition of mandatory detention. Australia rejected this call and challenged the Committee's interpretation of the ICCPR (Saul 2012).

CASE STUDY: THE RIGHT TO ASYLUM IN GERMANY

The right of asylum for victims of political persecution is included in the Constitution of Germany. During the 1990s, Germany was one of the main asylum destinations in Europe, receiving about half of the asylum seekers arriving in Europe in 1992, mostly from the Former Yugoslavia (Bosswick 2000). The large number of people seeking asylum in Germany at this time resulted in an amendment to the Constitution, known as the 'asylum compromise' (Poutrus 2014). The original statement providing asylum to people who experience political persecution remained, but the compromise was to include a number of restrictions on to whom the protection would be available. The Constitutional change resulted in a decrease in the number of applications, however, since 2008 numbers have begun to rise, with over half a million applications placed in 2015 (UNHCR 2018a).

Despite changes to asylum policy in Germany and some political disagreements relating to Germany's approach to asylum and migration policy, Germany plays a key role in refugee resettlement. Unlike Australia, people seeking asylum in Germany have access to a range of rights and opportunities. In 2018, Germany had over 180,000 applications for asylum, with the majority of claimants from Syria. Despite recently applied restrictive measures, asylum and refugee policy in Germany attempts to process applications quickly, with the average application processed in less than eight months (UNHCR 2018a), and while an application is being processed, the asylum seeker is provided with food and accommodation, and asylum seekers have access to health care and education (Schultz 2019).

The future of seeking asylum

Countries all over the world are making it more difficult for the increasing number of people fleeing persecution to seek asylum. The Trump administration in the United States is making significant changes to the rights and responsibilities of people seeking asylum, Australia again and again is being condemned by various bodies of the UN for its treatment of asylum seekers, and much of Europe has strengthened borders to prevent people from entering and seeking asylum. Given these changes to the approaches that many countries are now taking in response to the presence and arrival of people seeking asylum, it is unsurprising that there are some calls for a re-think of international refugee law, specifically the suitability of the Refugee Convention for twenty-first-century asylum needs.

References

Akram, S 2014. UNRWA and Palestinian refugees, in *The Oxford Handbook of Refugee and Forced Migration Studies* (p. 227), Oxford: Oxford University Press.

Akram, SM 2002. Palestinian refugees and their legal status: Rights, politics, and implications for a just solution, *Journal of Palestine Studies*, 31(3): 36–51. doi.org/10.1525/jps.2002.31.3.36

Australian Human Rights Commission 2019. *Risk Management in Immigration Detention*, Sydney: Australian Human Rights Commission.

Australian Senate 2019. *Question on Notice No. 109: Portfolio Question Number: AE19/109 2018–19 Additional Estimates'. February 18, 2019* [Online], Canberra: Legal and Constitutional Affairs Committee, Home Affairs Portfolio. Available: www.aph.gov.au/api/qon/downloadestimatesquestions/EstimatesQuestion-CommitteeId6-EstimatesRoundId5-PortfolioId20-QuestionNumber109 [Accessed 20/07/2019].

Bocco, R 2009. UNRWA and the Palestinian refugees: A history within history, *Refugee Survey Quarterly*, 28(2–3): 229–252. doi.org/10.1093/rsq/hdq001

Bosswick, W 2000. Development of asylum policy in Germany, *Journal of Refugee Studies*, 13(1): 43–60. doi.org/10.1093/jrs/13.1.43

Brotman, S, & Lee, EOJ 2011. Exploring gender and sexuality through the lens of intersectionality: Sexual minority refugees in Canada, *Canadian Social Work Review/Revue canadienne de service social*, 28(1): 151–156.

Canetti, D, Galea, S, Hall, BJ, Johnson, RJ, Palmieri, PA, & Hobfoll, SE 2010. Exposure to prolonged socio-political conflict and the risk of PTSD and depression among Palestinians, *Psychiatry: Interpersonal and Biological Processes*, 73(3): 219–231. doi.org/10.1521/psyc.2010.73.3.219

Carrol, A, & Mendos, LR 2017. *International Lesbian, Gay, Bisexual, Trans and Intersex Association*, Geneva: ILGA.

Cook, L, & Sherrell, H 2018. *Social Services Legislation Amendment (Encouraging Self-Sufficiency for Newly Arrived Migrants) Bill 2018*, 45 ed., Canberra.

Cousins, S 2018. Rohingya threatened by infectious diseases, *The Lancet Infectious Diseases*, 18(6): 609–610. doi.org/10.1016/S1473-3099(18)30304-9

Davies, AA, Basten, A, & Frattini, C 2009. Migration: A social determinant of the health of migrants, *Eurohealth*, 16(1): 10–12.

DIBP 2018. *Immigration Detention and Community Statistics Summary*, Canberra: DIBP.

Doocy, S, Lyles, E, Roberton, T, Akhu-Zaheya, L, Oweis, A, & Burnham, G 2015. Prevalence and care-seeking for chronic diseases among Syrian refugees in Jordan, *BMC Public Health*, 15(1): 1097. doi.org/10.1186/s12889-015-2429-3

Dörschner, J, & Machts, F 2011. *The 1951 Convention Relating to the Status of Refugees and Its 1967 Protocol: A Commentary*, Oxford: Oxford University Press.

Edwards, A, & Van Waas, L 2014. Statelessness, in *The Oxford Handbook of Refugee and Forced Migration Studies*, Oxford: Oxford University Press.

Equaldex 2019. *Homosexual Activity* [Online]. Available: www.equaldex.com/ [Accessed 18/03/2019].

Erakat, N 2014. Palestinian refugees and the Syrian uprising: Filling the protection gap during secondary forced displacement, *International Journal of Refugee Law*, 26(4): 581–621. doi.org/10.1093/ijrl/eeu047

Fazel, M, & Silove, D 2006. Detention of refugees, *British Medical Journal Publishing Group*. doi.org/10.1136/bmj.332.7536.251

Fiddian-Qasmiyeh, E 2014. Gender and forced migration, in E Fiddian-Qasmiyeh, G Loescher, K Long, & N Sigona (eds.) *The Oxford Handbook of Refugee and Forced Migration Studies*, Oxford: Oxford University Press. doi.org/10.1093/oxfordhb/9780199652433.013.0010

Filges, T, Montgomery, E, & Kastrup, M 2018. The impact of detention on the health of asylum seekers: A systematic review, *Research on Social Work Practice*, 28(4): 399–414. doi.org/10.1177/1049731516630384

Goodwin-Gill, GS 2014. The international law of refugee protection, *The Oxford Handbook of Refugee and Forced Migration Studies* (pp. 36–47), Oxford: Oxford University Press.

Grigg-Saito, D, Och, S, Liang, S, Toof, R, & Silka, L 2008. Building on the strengths of a Cambodian refugee community through community-based outreach, *Health Promotion Practice*, 9(4): 415–425. doi.org/10.1177/1524839906292176

Harvey, C 2015. Time for reform? Refugees, asylum-seekers, and protection under international human rights law, *Refugee Survey Quarterly*, 34(1): 43–60. doi.org/10.1093/rsq/hdu018

Heenan, RC, Volkman, T, Stokes, S, Tosif, S, Graham, H, Smith, A, Tran, D, & Paxton, G 2019. 'I think we've had a health screen': New offshore screening, new refugee health guidelines, new Syrian and Iraqi cohorts: Recommendations, reality, results and review, *Journal of Paediatrics and Child Health*. doi.org/10.1111/jpc.14142

Holborn, L 1939. The league of nations and the refugee problem, *Annals of the American Academy of Political and Social Science*, 203, ArticleType: Research-article/Issue Title: Refugees/Full publication date: May, 1939, American Academy of Political and Social Science, 124–135. doi.org/10.1177/000271623920300115

Hollander, A-C 2013. Social inequalities in mental health and mortality among refugees and other immigrants to Sweden: Epidemiological studies of register data, *Global Health Action*, 6(1): 21059. doi.org/10.3402/gha.v6i0.21059

Ismail, MB, Rafei, R, Dabboussi, F, & Hamze, M 2018. Tuberculosis, war, and refugees: Spotlight on the Syrian humanitarian crisis, *PLoS Pathogens*, 14(6): e1007014. doi.org/10.1371/journal.ppat.1007014

Jansen, S 2013. Introduction: Fleeing homophobia, asylum claims related to sexual orientation and gender identity in Europe, in T Spijkerboer (ed.) *Fleeing Homophobia: Sexual Orientation, Gender Identity and Asylum*, London: Routledge.

Jordan, S, & Morrissey, C 2013. 'On what grounds?' LGBT asylum claims in Canada, *Forced Migration Review*, 42.

Karlsen, E 2016. Refugee resettlement to Australia: What are the facts?, *Research Paper Series*, 201–7, Canberra, ACT: Parliament of Australia.

Kidane, W 2006. An injury to the citizen, a pleasure to the state: A peculiar challenge to the enforcement of international refugee law, *Chicago-Kent Journal of International and Comparative Law*, 6(116).

Kimmerling, B 2009. *The Palestinian People: A History*, Cambridge, MA: Harvard University Press.

Loescher, G 2014. UNHCR and forced migration, *The Oxford Handbook of Refugee and Forced Migration Studies* (pp. 215–226), Oxford: Oxford University Press.

McAdam, J, & Chong, F 2014. *Refugees: Why Seeking Asylum Is Legal and Australia's Policies Are Not*, Sydney: UNSW Press.

McKay, FH, & Dunn, M 2015. Food security among asylum seekers in Melbourne, *Australia and New Zealand Journal of Public Health*, 39(4): 344–349. https://doi.org/10.1111/1753-6405.12368

McKay, FH, Hall, L, & Lippi, K 2017. Compassionate deterrence: A Howard government legacy, *Politics & Policy*, 45(2): 169–193. doi.org/10.1111/polp.12198

McKay, FH, Thomas, SL, & Blood, RW 2011. Any one of these boat people could be a terrorist for all we know! Media representations and public perceptions of 'boat people' arrivals in Australia, *Journalism: Theory, Practice and Criticism*, 12(5): 608–626. doi.org/10.1177/1464884911408219

O'Byrne, K 2013. Is there a need for better supervision of the refugee convention?, *Journal of Refugee Studies*, 26(3): 330–359. doi.org/10.1093/jrs/fet024

OHCHR 2019. *Opinions Adopted by the Working Group on Arbitrary Detention* [Online], Geneva. Available: www.ohchr.org/EN/Issues/Detention/Pages/OpinionsadoptedbytheWGAD.aspx [Accessed 19/06/2019].

Physicians for Human Rights 2013. *From Persecution to Prison: The Health Consequences of Detention for Asylum Seekers* [Online]. Available: https://phr.org/resources/from-persecution-to-prison/ [Accessed 22/03/2019].

Poutrus, PG 2014. Asylum in postwar Germany: Refugee admission policies and their practical implementation in the federal republic and the GDR between the late 1940s and the mid-1970s, *Journal of Contemporary History*, 49(1): 115–133. doi.org/10.1177/0022009413505667

Rehr, M, Shoaib, M, Ellithy, S, Okour, S, Ariti, C, Ait-Bouziad, I, van den Bosch, P, Deprade, A, Altarawneh, M, & Shafei, A 2018. Prevalence of non-communicable diseases and access to care among non-camp Syrian refugees in northern Jordan, *Conflict and Health*, 12(1): 33. doi.org/10.1186/s13031-018-0168-7

Rondinelli, AJ, Morris, MD, Rodwell, TC, Moser, KS, Paida, P, Popper, ST, & Brouwer, KC 2011. Under-and over-nutrition among refugees in San Diego County, California, *Journal of Immigrant and Minority Health*, 13(1): 161–168. doi.org/10.1007/s10903-010-9353-5

Sanggaran, J-P, & Zion, D 2016. Is Australia engaged in torturing asylum seekers? A cautionary tale for Europe, *Journal of Medical Ethics*, 42(7): 420–423. doi.org/10.1136/medethics-2015-103326

Saul, B 2012. Dark justice: Australia's indefinite detention of refugees on security grounds under international human rights law, *Melbourne Journal of International Law*, 13: 685.

Schultz, C 2019. A prospect of staying? Differentiated access to integration for asylum seekers in Germany, *Ethnic and Racial Studies*: 1–19. doi.org/10.1080/01419870.2019.1640376

Sethi, S, Jonsson, R, Skaff, R, & Tyler, F 2017. Community-based noncommunicable disease care for Syrian refugees in Lebanon, *Global Health: Science and Practice*, 5(3): 495–506. doi.org/10.9745/GHSP-D-17-00043

Shishehgar, S, Gholizadeh, L, DiGiacomo, M, Green, A, & Davidson, PM 2017. Health and socio-cultural experiences of refugee women: An integrative review, *Journal of Immigrant and Minority Health*, 19(4): 959–973. doi.org/10.1007/s10903-016-0379-1

Silove, D, Steel, Z, Mollica, RF, & Sultan, A 2001. Detention of asylum seekers: Assault on health, human rights, and social developments, *The Lancet*, 357(9266): 1436. doi.org/10.1016/S0140-6736(00)04575-X

Silove, D, Ventevogel, P, & Rees, S 2017. The contemporary refugee crisis: An overview of mental health challenges, *World Psychiatry*, 16(2): 130–139. doi.org/10.1002/wps.20438

Skran, C 1995. *Refugees in Inter-War Europe: The Emergence of a Regime*, Oxford: Oxford University Press. doi.org/10.1093/acprof:oso/9780198273929.001.0001

Sphere Association 2018. *The Sphere Handbook: Humanitarian Charter and Minimum Standards in Humanitarian Response*, Geneva, Switzerland: Sphere.

Takahashi, S 2002. Recourse to human rights treaty bodies for monitoring of the refugee convention, *Netherlands Quarterly of Human Rights*, 20(1): 53–74. doi.org/10.1177/016934410202000104

UNHCR 1951. *Convention Relating to the Status of Refugees*, Geneva: UNHCR.

UNHCR 2012. *Guidelines on International Protection No. 9: Claims to Refugee Status Based on Sexual Orientation and/or Gender Identity within the Context of Article 1A(2) of the 1951 Convention Relating to the Status of Refugees*, Geneva: UNHCR.

UNHCR 2017. *UNHCR chief Filippo Grandi Calls on Australia to End Harmful Practice of Offshore Processing* [Online]. Available: www.unhcr.org/uk/news/press/2017/7/597217484/unhcr-chief-filippo-grandi-calls-australia-end-harmful-practice-offshore.html [Accessed 16/03/2019].

UNHCR 2018a. *Germany* [Online], Geneva. Available: http://popstats.unhcr.org/en/asylum_seekers [Accessed 20/07/2019].

UNHCR 2018b. *Global trends: Forced displacement in 2017*, Geneva: United Nations High Commissioner for Refugees.

UNHCR 2018c. *UNHCR Condemns Forced Returns of Cameroon Asylum-Seekers from Nigeria* [Online]. Available: www.unhcr.org/en-lk/news/press/2018/2/5a731fcf4/unhcr-condemns-forced-returns-cameroon-asylum-seekers-nigeria.html [Accessed 16/03/2019].

UNHCR 2018d. *UNHCR Urges Family Unity at Southern US Border* [Online]. Available: www.unhcr.org/en-au/news/press/2018/6/5b27fea84/unhcr-urges-family-unity-southern-border.html [Accessed 16/03/2019].

UNHCR 2019. *Statelessness* [Online]. Available: www.unhcr.org/statelessness.html [Accessed 15/03/2019].

United Nations 2019. *Treaty Collection* [Online], Geneva. Available: https://treaties.un.org/ [Accessed 08/04/2019].

UNRWA 2007. *Report of the Commissioner-General of the United Nations Relief and Works Agency for Palestine Refugees in the Near East*, Geneva: United Nations.

UNRWA 2019. *UNRWA* [Online]. Available: www.unrwa.org/ [Accessed 14/03/2019].

Waterston, T, & Nasser, D 2017. Access to healthcare for children in Palestine, *BMJ Paediatrics Open*, 1(1). doi.org/10.1136/bmjpo-2017-000115

Weiss, P 1954. International protection of refugees, *American Journal of International Law*, 48(2): 193–221. doi.org/10.2307/2194371

White, E 2017. The legal status of Russian refugees, 1921–1936, *Comparativ*, 27(1): 18–32.

WHO 2003. *International Migration, Health and Human Rights*, Geneva: World Health Organization.

WHO 2016. *Health Conditions in the Occupied Palestinian Territory, Including East Jerusalem, and in the Occupied Syrian Golan Sixty-Ninth World Health Assembly*, Geneva: World Health Organization.

WHO 2019. *WHO in Emergencies* [Online]. Available: www.who.int/emergencies/en/ [Accessed 20/03/2019].

Willems, K, & Vernimmen, J 2018. The fundamental human right to education for refugees: Some legal remarks, *European Educational Research Journal*, 17(2): 219–232. doi.org/10.1177/1474904117709386

Woodhead, M 2015. Australian doctors face two years in jail for reporting asylum seekers' health, *BMJ: British Medical Journal* [Online], 350. doi.org/10.1136/bmj.h3008

8

HUMAN RIGHTS FOR PEOPLE WITH A DISABILITY

Joanne Watson, Kate Anderson, Patsie Frawley and Susan Balandin

Introduction

According to the World Report on Disability, 15 percent of the world's population has a disability, of whom approximately 80 percent are located in the Global South (WHO and World Bank 2011). People with disability are subjected to a range of oppressions and inequalities that include limited opportunities to engage with education and employment, the experience of violence and abuse, poor health care, discrimination, poverty, and limited freedom to express their sexuality. The Convention on the Rights of Persons with Disabilities (CRPD) adopted in 2006 was crucial in responding to the oppression and inequality experienced by people with disability. It is considered by some to be the most important international legislation of the twenty-first century for people with disability and represents a historical landmark in the disability rights movement globally.

Before the adoption of the CRPD, few human rights instruments specifically addressed the human rights of people with disability, those that did address these issues were not legally binding, and as such, had little impact beyond an advisory role. Recognising the need for a legally binding instrument to highlight and reinforce the rights of people with a disability, in 2001, the Office of the High Commissioner for Human Rights (OHCHR) commissioned a study focused on human rights and people with disability (Quinn et al. 2002). The findings of this study suggested that the existing instruments and mechanisms were not paying sufficient attention to the promotion and protection of the rights of people with disabilities, and that the absence of explicit legal protection represented a significant gap in equality for people with disabilities (UN 2002). The study concluded that existing human rights instruments were failing people with disability, reinforcing a need for a disability specific human rights treaty. Following the release of this report a strong advocacy movement, led by people with disability, their representatives, NGOs, and academics, drew attention to the need for a broad, legally binding instrument. The approach used during this early stage of the Convention's development reflected the collaborative and participatory spirit of the CRPD, driven by the now familiar slogan 'nothing about us without us'.

The CRPD is the first legally binding instrument to explicitly focus on how human rights apply to people with disability. This chapter will discuss the CRPD, changes in the understanding of disability, followed by a consideration of the process of formulation of the CRPD and its underlying principles. Finally, this chapter will explore some diverse responses to the Convention, illustrated in a case study on sexual and reproductive rights. The chapter concludes with a look forward in terms of disability rights.

Shaping new global understandings of disability

Disability has traditionally been viewed through a medical or scientific lens, as a problem of, and for, an individual. This view of disability is referred to as the medical model, and results in the categorisation of a person through medical terminology, treating them as patients, and can lead to practices such as segregation, sterilisation, and institutionalisation (Haegele and Hodge 2016). Disability is understood as existing inside the individual, originating from personal biological characteristics that are labelled in terms of impairment or deficiency – an intellectual, sensory, or physical deviation from the norm (Haegele and Hodge 2016). For example, the medical model would view a person's spinal injury or vision impairment as the primary reason for their disability, and the cause of any participation restrictions they experience. This focus on organic 'deficits' can also have a limiting effect on the way people with disability are viewed in society, meaning they are typically characterised by their impairment and not by other aspects of their personhood, a situation that may have a profound impact on self-perception (Roush and Sharby 2011). Such a model reinforces a public policy response that isolates and segregates an individual from mainstream community life and services. Practically, for a person with disability, this means that education is provided through segregated schools, employment options are restricted to segregated facilities (for example, through sheltered workshops), pathways to physical and virtual environments are inaccessible, and a person's right to participate in civil society is restricted. These unacceptable consequences of the medical model were summarised by the OHCHR (2010: 8):

> When disability is perceived in this way, society's responses are restricted to only one of two paths: individuals can be "fixed" through medicine or rehabilitation (medical approach); or they can be cared for, through charity or welfare programmes (charity approach). According to this old model, the lives of persons with disabilities are handed over to professionals who control such fundamental decisions as where they will go to school, what support they will receive and where they will live.

The process of challenging the medical frame of disability led to the emergence of the social model of disability, a phrase coined by Oliver (2004). Describing the social model, Oliver (2004) states, 'the idea underpinning the individual [medical] model was that of personal tragedy, while the idea underpinning the social model was that of externally imposed restriction' (20). The social model views disability as a socio–political construct, seeing disability as socially constructed by social systems that act as a barrier to inclusion and that oppress people who are impacted by these barriers. It makes a distinction between impairment and disability, making the increasingly accepted case that the experience of disability can be ameliorated through social change (Haegele and Hodge 2016). For example, under the social model, disability and participation restrictions result from society's inability to accommodate diversity rather than being directly caused by the impairments themselves. This framework has been advocated for by disability researchers and advocates since the 1970s, particularly in the UK and United States as the way to understanding disability. While the social model of disability has assisted with a number of political successes for people with disability, including leading to the adoption of the CRPD, there is concern that it is becoming increasingly outdated. The main criticism is that model itself is too narrow and does not take into consideration the interplay of individual and environmental factors (Shakespeare 2016).

Disability is a complex phenomenon. Shakespeare (2016) suggests that approaches and responses that are more sophisticated are needed, including medical and socio-political approaches. Many now advocate for an interactional model of disability that takes in the ecological experience of disability, where disability is seen as separate from impairment (Harpur 2012). Within the interactional model, disability is seen as resulting from the interaction between the person and their embodied impairment and a disabling society. This model does not ignore a person's impairment, viewing disablement as a product of both a person's body and society, but allows for disability to be seen as a barrier to participation of people with impairments that arises from an interaction of that impairment with discriminatory attitudes, policies, or institutional practices. At a policy level, a biopsychosocial framing of disability can be seen in the World Health Organisation's, WHO (2001) International Classification of Functioning, Disability and Health (ICFDH) which is now increasingly used across the fields of public health, allied health, and health promotion (Roush and Sharby 2011).

Making the Convention a reality

Disability has been largely absent from international human rights law, neither the Universal Declaration of Human Rights (UDHR), the International Covenant on Civil and Political Rights (ICCPR), or the International Covenant on Economic, Social and Cultural Rights (ICESCR) mention people with disability. Only the Convention on the Rights of the Child includes reference to 'mentally and physically disabled' and describes the obligations of states to children with disability. Until the adoption of the CRPD, the UN had sought to address the absence of disability within the human rights system in two ways. The first was by applying existing core human rights instruments to people with disability, and second, by developing a series of policy and programmatic documents specifically focused on the needs and rights of people with disability (Kayess and French 2008).

These approaches achieved little in the way of recognition of human rights for people with disability. Part of this is related to the human rights system as a whole being based on an 'abled bodied' norm, while people with disability have typically been seen to sit within charity or welfare framework (Kayess and French 2008). This is not to say that the UN had not made some attempts before the establishment of the CRPD to address the needs and the rights of people with disabilities. In 1971, the General Assembly adopted the Declaration on the Rights of Mentally Retarded Persons, and the Declaration on the Rights of Disabled Persons in 1975. These two Declarations, while not legally binding, were the first to situate people with disability in international human rights law, despite doing so within a scope defined by the individual model of disability (Quinn et al. 2002). There were attempts at this time to establish a specific human rights convention for people with disability, however, it was considered that the rights of persons with disability were addressed in other human rights instruments (Kayess and French 2008).

In 1982 the UN adopted the World Programme of Action concerning Disabled Persons (WPA), which established as one of its goals the equalisation of opportunities for people with disability. In shifting the discussion of disability away from an individual or medical approach, the WPA marked a focus on rights and equality (General Assembly 1993). This was followed by the appointment of a Special Rapporteur, and a report making it clear that disability is a human rights concern (Despouy 1993).

Calls for a Convention to bring together a number of Declarations and Standards relating to people with disabilities had been made by many countries for years. In 2001, Mexico sought to secure a mandate from the General Assembly to develop a human rights convention in relation to people with disability. This request from Mexico came while countries were investing in the Millennium Development Goals. By highlighting that despite being among some of the world's poorest, people with disability were not identified as a specific target group for action in the Millennium Development Goals, Mexico was able to point to the potential development of a specific human rights instrument to address this omission (Kayess and French 2008). Framing the need for a new convention within terms of social development, enabled countries who, until that point, showed little interest in the human rights of people with disability, to more easily support such a convention.

The committee created to discuss and then draft a Convention Related to Persons with Disability were advised by the General Assembly that their mandate was not to create new rights, but rather express existing rights in a way that addresses the needs of people with disabilities. The CRPD was adopted on 13 December 2006, the first human rights treaty endorsed in the twenty-first century, and opened for signature on 30 March 2007. Reflecting the significant support for the Convention, an unprecedented eighty-one countries signed the Convention on the first day. The CRDP, and an associated Optional Protocol (CRPD Optional Protocol), were entered into force on 3 May 2008; by mid-2019, there were 162 signatories (United Nations 2019).

The CRPD consists of fifty Articles and a preamble. Unlike many other Conventions, the CRPD is not divided into formal sections, however informally, there are six areas, and eight general principles (see Table 8.1).

The CRPD sets out the legal obligations of signatory nations to promote and protect the rights of people with disability. These obligations are transferred to human service organisations and staff, and need to be reflected in these organisations mission statements, policy, and procedural requirements. The CRPD provides a guiding framework for States Party to the CRPD to strengthen and develop legislation, policy and practice that 'promote, protect and ensure the full and equal enjoyment of all human rights and fundamental freedoms by all

TABLE 8.1 Eight general principles of the Convention of the Rights of Persons with Disability

1. Respect for inherent dignity, individual autonomy including the freedom to make one's own choices, and independence of persons;
2. Non-discrimination;
3. Full and effective participation and inclusion in society;
4. Respect for difference and acceptance of persons with disabilities as part of human diversity and humanity;
5. Equality of opportunity;
6. Accessibility;
7. Equality between men and women;
8. Respect for the evolving capacities of children with disabilities and respect for the right of children with disabilities to preserve their identities.

(Adapted from UN General Assembly 2006, Article 3 'General Principles') persons with disabilities, and to promote respect for their inherent dignity' found in Article 1 (UN General Assembly 2006). Articles 2 and 3 provide definitions and general principles surrounding communication, including Braille, sign language, plain language, non-verbal communication, reasonable accommodation, and universal design.

Articles 4 to 32 define the rights of persons with disabilities and the obligations of States Party to the Convention, many of these rights are similar to those found in other conventions. Rights that are specific to the CRPD include the rights to accessibility including to information technology, the rights to live independently and be included in the community (Article 19), to personal mobility (Article 20), habilitation and rehabilitation (Article 26), and to participation in political and public life, and cultural life, recreation and sport (Articles 29 and 30).

Articles 33 to 39 are concerned with reporting and monitoring procedures of the convention by national human rights institutions (Article 33) and Committee on the Rights of Persons with Disabilities (Article 34). Articles 40 to 50 govern ratification, entry into force, and amendment of the Convention.

While there is not definition of disability within the CRPD, it has played a key role in ushering in the social model as a way of understanding disability in contemporary society. The wording of the Convention promotes disability as an interaction between an impairment and the environment, rather than a medical problem housed solely within an individual. The OHCHR (2014: 24) describe this interaction, stating

> *Persons become disabled when they clash with an unwelcoming or inaccessible environment. Persons with disabilities do not require to be fixed before accessing an environment (society); it is instead the environment that needs to be uniformly open to all its members. It does so by dismantling attitudinal and environmental barriers so that everyone can actively participate and enjoy the full range of rights.*

Graham Innes (2010) highlighted the need for the practical implementation of the CRPD by drawing on a quote from French jurist, Rene Cassin. Cassin, during the drafting of the UDHR, said: 'it would be deceiving the peoples of the world to let them think that a legal provision was all that was required . . . when in fact an entire social structure had to be transformed'. Innes (2010) claims that one of the things that sets the CRPD apart from other human rights instruments is its practical nature and the useful implementation and reporting guidelines it provides for signatory nations to follow. This can be seen specifically in Article 9 on accessibility and Article 24 on education, that include detailed, practical agendas for implementing rights, opposed to simply proclaiming rights in principle.

The CRPD is built the Human Rights model of disability. This model has firm roots in the interactional model (described above), acknowledging that disability can be the product of individual impairment and socially constructed disabling barriers. However, it extends further by considering the consequence of such barriers for the human rights of people with a disability. Degener (2016), proposes that the human rights model provides a blue print for reform, noting that adopting this perspective has allowed the CRPD drafters to recognise the intersectional nature of humanity. This is illustrated in several provisions in the CRPD acknowledging overlapping and intersecting identities, such as women and children with disabilities (Degener 2016).

There is little argument that the CRPD has marked a 'paradigm shift' in attitudes and approaches to people with disability (Kayess and French 2008). It has sparked a new way of understanding disability, as an evolving concept that results from changing environmental factors. The CRPD has made way for a new narrative around disability that recognises that the notion of 'disability' is not rigid and can be adapted according to the society of which a person with a disability is a part.

Diverse responses to the Convention across the globe

Different nations have responded to the requirements of the CRPD in different ways. The drafters of the CRPD understood that, on a global scale, issues like poverty and economic status, rurality, geographic isolation, and the environmental and political stability of the country will impact how disability is understood and responded. Being a signatory to the CRPD brings responsibilities to report on progress. States Party to the CRPD report their progress to the UN Committee on the Rights of Persons with Disabilities. The Committee is a UN body of eighteen experts who meet twice each year to consider reports submitted by UN member states. Each state is required to submit information regarding national legislation, policy, and practice to meet the rights enshrined in the CRPD. A close examination of some of these documents and the broader World Report on Disability (2011) reveal diverse responses to the issue of disability rights across nations. For some countries, such as Mongolia (ratified in May 2019), legislation is currently limited to broad social security or pension legislation. For others such as South Africa (ratified November 2007), specific issues are addressed, such as access to education and employment (for example, South Africa's Employment Equity Bill). In some countries, laws that protect the rights of people with disability are incorporated within broad human rights or anti-discrimination legislation (for example, New Zealand's Human Rights Act 1993), while in others, disability discrimination is covered in legislation that addresses disability discrimination directly (for example, Australia's Disability Discrimination Act 1992).

In addition, many States Party to the CRPD have developed a National Response to Disability, sometimes referred to as a National Disability Strategy or Framework. Such strategies aim to assist nations to fulfil their obligations under the CRPD, by establishing frameworks to promote, protect and monitor its implementation as articulated in Article 33. This Article enables State Parties to translate the generalities of the Convention into a practical agenda for local reform.

Consideration of where the largest populations of people with disability live need to be taken into account when observing the integration of the CRDP into national law. Grech (2016) points to poverty in many of these countries as providing and containing to 'provide multiple conditions for the creation and maintenance of impairment' (26). The rising number of people with disability in the Global South can be attributed to hunger, malnutrition, inaccessible health care and rehabilitation, unsanitary living conditions, and violence and conflict (Grech 2016). In recent years there has been a focus on finding a place for disability in the development agenda and practice, resulting in the inclusion of a disability component in the Sustainable Development Goals (SDGs). However, despite this increased focus, concern remains that the everyday experiences of people with disability living in the Global South have little relevance to most human rights instruments including the CRPD. Meekosha and Soldatic (2011) argue that despite the Global South supporting the Convention, the struggles of people with disability in the Global North cannot be equated with the struggles in the South, and there needs to be critical engagement with the disability politics of the South. The case study provided below highlights an area where implementation experiences particular challenges, namely sexual and reproductive rights.

CASE STUDY: SEXUAL AND REPRODUCTIVE RIGHTS FOR PERSONS WITH DISABILITY

The CRPD is silent on sexuality rights per se, which some researchers and commentators have noted reflects the continuation of a protective and paternalistic regime in relation to sexuality and disability, in particular intellectual disability, that has seen people with a disability infantilised or regarded as asexual (Addlakha et al. 2017). Ruiz (2017) notes, 'the silence on affirmative sexual and reproductive rights [in the Convention] reinforces prejudices that equate disability with incompetence, incapacity, impotence, and asexuality' (Ruiz 2017: 94). The Articles that make reference to or that could be referred to regarding sexuality are Articles 23, which outlines the right to respect for home and family, which notes, 'States Parties shall take effective and appropriate measures to eliminate discrimination against persons with disabilities in all matters relating to marriage, family, parenthood and relationships, on an equal basis with others' and Article 25 relating to the right to health, noting in 25(a) that States Parties 'Provide persons with disabilities with the same range, quality and standard of free or affordable health care and programmes as provided to other persons, including in the area of sexual and reproductive health and population-based public health programmes'.

As noted by Schaaf (2011), these Articles reflect a framing of sexuality as biological in the Convention, being about reproduction and is heteronormative in its framing of sexuality in this context. For individuals with disabilities who seek to made decisions about their own sexual or reproductive health, the strength of the Convention might be in other Articles. This includes Article 12 which provides for Equal Recognition before the law, with the key assumption that everyone can make decisions with support (Watson 2016), and Article 22 which provides the right of respect for privacy, states that 'no person with disabilities, regardless of place of residence or living arrangements, shall be subjected to arbitrary or unlawful interference with his or her privacy'. For an individual living with disability, this means they have the right to conduct their sexual life in privacy and for their living environment to ensure this privacy. It also means they should not have to disclose their sexuality to anyone or be questioned about it as it is a private aspect of their life.

Looking forward to disability rights

There has been a profound paradigm shift over the past three decades relating to the lives of people with disability; the culmination of this shift can be seen in the creation of the CRPD. However, this shift has largely been driven and located in the Global North. Further critical engagement with the disability politics of the Global South are needed in order to ensure the rights enshrined in the CRPD can be achieved by all citizens.

In concluding this chapter, we give just two examples of how this agenda is being taken up. In 2013 and 2015, Jenkin and colleagues (2017, 2020, forthcoming) worked in Vanuatu and Papua New Guinea between 2013 and 2015, with Save the Children Vanuatu, Papua New Guinea and Australia and the Disabled Persons Organisation in each country, to answer, 'What are the human rights needs and priorities of children with disability in Vanuatu and

Papua New Guinea?'. They used an inclusive research design, enabling children with diverse disabilities to self report. Data were collected from eighty-nine children with disability (aged five to eighteen), across both countries. Jenkin and colleagues (2020, forthcoming) consider the important issue of how to imbed the change produced in short term funded projects at a variety of levels in order to ensure the social inclusion of the group continues beyond the life of the project. The project also left a legacy in terms of a website containing a set of resources for supporting the involvement of children with disability in research, consultation, policy and service development, monitoring, and evaluation (see www.voicesofchildrenwith disability.com/).

The second example is focussed on understanding and supporting the livelihoods of rural Indonesian villagers with disability. Liu and colleagues (2020, forthcoming) describe a collaborative and multi-methods participatory research project conducted in the context of the Indonesian Inclusive Village Model. Economic and social inclusion for rural Indonesian villagers with disability are dependent on participation in key deliberative mechanisms of the village and of wider social and economic programs. This participation is fundamentally linked to attitudes towards people with disability and constructions of disability. The process of participating in research, and in particular the public theatre performance by research participants that formed part of the research dissemination (see www.youtu.be/WunxVBxxHbk for a short video that was made on the process), was a mechanism to change the way disability is viewed, challenge exclusive social relations and open opportunities for discussion of economic participation for people with disability. In this context, villagers with disability came to be seen as valued community members with the desire and potential for equal roles in economic participation as well as village decision making about this. Kortschak (2019) discusses the creation of the theatre piece in more detail. In these two examples local NGOs of, and with, people with disabilities in the global south can be seen taking action to achieve their rights, drawing on the CRPD for legitimation of their work.

References

Addlakha, R, Price, J, & Heidari, S 2017. Disability and sexuality: Claiming sexual and reproductive rights, *Reproductive Health Matters*, 25(50): 4–9. https://doi.org/10.1080/09688080.2017.1336375

Degener, T 2016. Disability in a human rights context, *Laws*, 5(3): 35. doi.org/10.3390/laws5030035

Despouy, L 1993. *Human Rights and Disabled Persons*, Geneva: United Nations.

General Assembly 1993. *The Standard Rules on the Equalization of Opportunities for Persons with Disabilities*, Geneva: United Nations.

Grech, S 2016. Disability and development: Critical connections, gaps and contradictions, in *Disability in the Global South*, Switzerland: Springer. doi.org/10.1007/978-3-319-42488-0

Haegele, JA, & Hodge, S 2016. Disability discourse: Overview and critiques of the medical and social models, *Quest*, 68(2): 193–206. doi.org/10.1080/00336297.2016.1143849

Harpur, P 2012. Embracing the new disability rights paradigm: The importance of the Convention on the Rights of Persons with Disabilities, *Disability & Society*, 27(1): 1–14. doi.org/10.1080/0968759 9.2012.631794

Innes, G 2010. *National Disability Strategies as tools for Implementing the Convention on the Rights of Persons with Disabilities*, Centre for disability law and policy, University College Galway, Ireland: Delivered via video link.

Jenkin, E, Wilson, E, Campain, R, Murfitt, K, & Clarke, M 2020, forthcoming. Embedding change: Designing short term projects for sustainable effects, in BR Crisp and A Taket (eds.) *Sustaining Social Inclusion*, London: Routledge.

Jenkin, E, Wilson, E, Clarke, M, Campain, R, & Murfitt, K 2017. Listening to the voices of children: Understanding the human rights priorities of children with disability in Vanuatu and Papua New Guinea, *Disability and Society*, 32(3): 358–380. doi.org/10.1080/09687599.2017.1296348

Kayess, R, & French, P 2008. Out of darkness into light? Introducing the Convention on the Rights of Persons with Disabilities, *Human Rights Law Review*, 8(1): 1–34. doi.org/10.1093/hrlr/ngm044

Kortschak, I 2019. Radical theatre of the difabled, *The Theatre Times* [Online], Available: https://thethheatretimes.com/radical-theatre-of-the-difabled/ [Accessed 05/09/2019].

Liu, E, Wahyu, Y, Kortschak, I, Insriani, H, & Wilson, E 2020, forthcoming. Sustaining inclusion through work: Livelihoods experience of rural Indonesian villagers with disability, in BR Crisp and A Taket (eds.) *Sustaining Social Inclusion*, London: Routledge.

Meekosha, H, & Soldatic, K 2011. Human rights and the global south: The case of disability, *Third World Quarterly*, 32(8): 1383–1397. doi.org/10.1080/01436597.2011.614800

Office of the High Commissioner for Human Rights 2010. *Monitoring the Convention on the Rights of Persons with Disabilities: Guidance for Human Rights Monitors*, Professional Training Series No. 17, New York/Geneva: United Nations.

Office of the High Commissioner for Human Rights 2014. *The Convention on the Rights of Persons with Disabilities: Training Guide*, Professional Training Series No. 19, New York/Geneva: United Nations.

Oliver, M 2004. Chapter 2: The social model in action: If I had a hammer, in C Barnes & G Mercer (eds.) *Implementing the Social Model of Disability: Theory and Research* (pp. 18–31), Leeds: The Disability Press.

Quinn, G, Degener, T, & Bruce, A 2002. *Human Rights and Disability: The Current Use and Future Potential of United Nations Human Rights Instruments in the Context of Disability*, Geneva: United Nations Publications.

Quinn, G, Degener, T, Bruce, A, Burke, C, Castellino, J, Kenna, P, Kilkelly, U, & Quinlivan, S 2002. *The Current Use and Future Potential of United Nations Human Rights Instruments in the Context of Disability*, Geneva: United Nations.

Roush, SE, & Sharby, N 2011. Disability reconsidered: The paradox of physical therapy, *Physical Therapy*, 91: 1715–1727. doi.org/10.2522/ptj.20100389

Ruiz, J 2017. The Committee on the Rights of Persons with Disabilities and Its Take on Sexuality, *Reproductive Health Matters*, 25: 92–103. doi.org/10.1080/09688080.2017.1332449

Schaaf, M 2011. Negotiating Sexuality in the Convention on the Rights of Persons with Disabilities, *International Journal on Human Rights*, (14): 113.

Shakespeare, T 2016. Chapter 13: The social model of disability, in L. Davis (ed.) *The Disability Studies Reader*, 5th edn, New York: Taylor & Francis.

UN General Assembly 2006. *Convention on the Rights of Persons with Disabilities*, Geneva, Switzerland: United Nations.

United Nations 2002. *Human Rights and Disability: The Current Use and Future Potential of United Nations Human Rights Instruments in the Context of Disability*, Geneva, Switzerland: United Nations.

United Nations 2019. *Treaty Collection* [Online], Geneva. Available: https://treaties.un.org/ [Accessed 08/04/2019].

Watson, J 2016. Assumptions of decision-making capacity: The role supporter attitudes play in the realisation of article 12 for people with severe or profound intellectual disability, *Laws*, 5: 6. doi.org/10.3390/laws5010006

World Health Organization 2001. *International Classification of Functioning, Disability and Health: ICF*, Geneva, Switzerland: World Health Organization.

World Health Organization 2011. *World Report on Disability 2011*, Geneva: World Health Organization.

9

ELIMINATION OF RACIAL DISCRIMINATION

Fiona H. McKay and Ann Taket

Introduction

The principle that all humans have equal rights, including the right to dignity and the right to equal treatment without discrimination, is a cornerstone of international human rights. This notion, that everyone is equal under the law means that governments should grant the same rights, responsibilities, and privileges to all citizens. In reality, however, not everyone is treated equally. Across the globe, people have been discriminated against because of the colour of their skin, their religion, or their nationality for centuries.

While the word 'race' did not appear in the Covenant of the League of Nations, signed in 1919, the language of racism and paternalism were present in the work of the League, with the mandate system giving western countries legal control over the 'colonies' (Keane and Waughray 2017). Many countries at the beginning of the twentieth century had discriminatory immigration policies and policies of segregation in place; however, after the conclusion of the Second World War, where the effects of overt racism and discrimination had terrible consequences, such policies became intolerable. Through the creation of the United Nations (UN), global powers sought to eliminate racist language by creating a system that endorsed equality. This was first articulated in Article 1(3) of the 1945 UN Charter, that the UN was created to achieve international cooperation in promoting and encouraging respect for human rights for all 'without distinction as to race'. The UN General Assembly, reiterated this when it adopted a resolution during its first session declaring that it is 'in the higher interests of humanity to put an immediate end to religious and so-called racial persecution and discrimination' (UN 2007). The non-discriminatory approach of the UN was reinforced in Article 2 of the 1948 Universal Declaration of Human Rights (UDHR), where it was declared that everyone is entitled to the same rights and freedoms 'without distinction of any kind, such as race, colour, sex, language, religion, political or other opinion, national or social origin, property, birth or other status'.

This chapter focuses on discrimination based on race, colour, or ethnicity, racism, racial discrimination and the related issues of xenophobia and intolerance. Although current understandings of 'race' are as a social construct rather than a fact of biology, racism as a social problem is real (Smedley and Smedley 2005). Racism affects a large number of people every day in both small and large ways and with considerable impacts on physical and mental health. The impact of racism can prevent an individual from seeking or receiving health care, employment, housing, and education. The impacts of racism and discrimination can last for generations.

There has been increased focus on the impact of racism and discrimination on health outcomes. A recent review found that racism and discrimination have significant negative effects on health outcomes, with researchers suggesting that racism and discrimination are determents of health (Paradies et al. 2015). A range of studies has shown the experience of discrimination can cause considerable distress (Bailey et al. 2017), can have an impact on cardiovascular health (Calvin et al. 2003), pregnancy and birth outcomes (Dominguez et al. 2008), and poor mental health (Berger and Sarnyai 2015). Other research has shown that health inequalities affect minority groups who suffer from lower life expectancy, lower access to health services and a higher burden of disease (Berger and Sarnyai 2015).

From the vast literature on racism and health outcomes are three clear findings. The first is the direct impact of racism or discrimination on health; this can include poor mental or physical health as a result of vilification, harassment, or assault (Hemmings and Evans 2018). The second is the impact of poor health care or mistreatment on health (Hall et al. 2015). The third area is related to systematic discrimination that results in socioeconomic differences and can lead to poor housing and working conditions, lower wages, and lower education (Williams and Williams-Morris 2000).

Race based discrimination

Race is not a biological or genetic construct, but rather an ideology that has been used to justify the domination of one identifiable group of people by another (Miller and Garran 2017). For a racist group to translate racial bias and prejudice into racial discrimination, it must be politically, socially, and economically dominant (LeMelle and Shepherd 1971). The idea that one group is superior to another, based on biology, has supported a number of oppressive regimes and activities over centuries, including genocide, slavery, and colonialism, resulting in extensive death and torture (Fredrickson 2015).

Racism scholars regularly draw a line from current racism to religious intolerance in Europe during the fifteenth and sixteenth centuries. For example, in Spain during the fifteenth century, Jews who converted to Christianity as a result of religious violence were discriminated against based on notions of 'impure blood' (Fredrickson 2015). These race-based distinctions were used by Spanish and Portuguese colonial rulers during the 'discovery' of Latin America, when they introduced a complex hierarchical caste system focused on 'blood purity'. Those most negatively impacted by this classification system were the local Indigenous population and the slaves imported from Africa who were situated at the base of the hierarchy, while the European colonists placed themselves at the top (Miller and Garran 2017). The systematic categorisation and enslavement created the economic underpinning for later colonisation, legitimising the racially oppressive social structures put in place by colonial powers (Waldrep 2008). The structures employed by European colonial powers during this period endure throughout the world: colonial powers continue to be wealthier than their colonies, an inequality that can exist even when a country has gained independence (Finlay 2017).

In the eighteenth and nineteenth centuries, these ideas spread to the United States, where dissatisfaction after the conclusion of the Civil War lead to the creation of the Ku Klux Klan, who went on to terrorise and intimidate Black Americans with the plan to re-establish white supremacy (Waldrep 2008), and to Europe where the theory of Social Darwinism became popular, leading to colonial domination over the African continent (Mlambo 2006). These colonial influences continued into the twentieth century, with the racial hatred demonstrated by the Nazi regime, the institutional racism of apartheid in South Africa, and the ethnically motivated genocides in Rwanda and Bosnia (Valentino 2005). Today, we see the impact of intergenerational racism and discrimination in Indigenous populations all over the world, and poor health outcomes for many minorities. Even at the household level, colonialism is still present; domestic staff in western countries are often from former colonies, while it is unusual for the reverse to occur (Miller and Garran 2017).

There are many examples across the world of racism and acts of discrimination. In the following section, racism and discrimination in four countries (Australia, the United States, South Africa, and Indonesia) are discussed in order to give a historical perspective from four different geographical, social and cultural settings, before the chapter moves on to consider the International Convention on the Elimination of All Forms of Racial Discrimination, and then considers aspects of how racial discrimination has been tackled using the Convention and relation provisions, revisiting the same four countries as examples. As will be seen, the development of racism and discrimination in the different settings is intimately bound with the historical development of Western imperialism, colonialism, and neocapitalism.

Australia

Australia was settled primarily as a penal colony during the late eighteenth and early nineteenth centuries, with convict transportation, mostly from Britain, central to Australia's migration patterns. Vital to the development of relationships with the first peoples of Australia was the use of the doctrine of 'terra nullius', a principle in international law that was used to justify settlement, neglecting the first peoples' use of, and relationship to, the land, which would suggest that invasion and conquest was the more appropriate description (Reynolds 1989). With the discovery of gold, many free settlers made their way to Australia. The gold rushes transformed Australia; from 1851 to 1871 the population quadrupled, from 430,000 to 1.7 million (Department of Labor and Immigration 1975; Ozdowski 1984). This increase in population resulted in public concern regarding the security of Australia's borders, with Australia's Asian neighbours, particularly China, identified as the largest potential threat to Australia (Jupp 2002). Attracted by the prospect of gold, Australia's Chinese population increased in the mid-1800s, igniting the fear that Australia would be invaded by the 'hordes from the north' (McMaster 2002: 73). Responding to these fears were the anti-Chinese immigration policies of the 1850s. These policies, similar to those already operating in Canada and the United States, excluded all non-Europeans from settlement in Australia with the primary objective of creating a 'totally homogeneous white and British society' (Jupp 2002: 9).

One of the first federal laws passed by Australia when it became a nation in 1901 was the Immigration Restriction Act, forming the basis of the 'White Australia Policy'. This Act, modelled on a similar South African immigration act, included a number of restrictions on who could enter, stay, and move around freely. Most impacted were Chinese and Pacific Islanders, but the Act also prevented other potential immigrants who were 'undesirable' by virtue of their ethnicity from entering Australia. The Act remained in force until a relaxation of the policy in the 1960s and its abolition in 1972, resulting in changes in the Australian population, from one of predominantly British and then Western European character, toward a population that is more multicultural.

Despite a long and large presence in Australia, Asian-Australians, Muslims, and Aboriginal and Torres Strait Islander people have long been identified as outside of what it means to be Australian (Dunn et al. 2007). There is a large amount of research showing that intolerance of these groups is sustained through core stereotypes. For example, stereotypes that have been found applied to Aboriginal and Torres Strait Islander people include a supposed welfare dependency, drunkenness, and failure to assimilate or integrate into the 'Australian way of life' (Markwick et al. 2019).

Australia has recently seen an increase in migration from Muslim countries. While the building of mosques and prayer houses, Islamic schools, and increased access to Halal food are a clear indication of an increasing Muslim presence in Australia, not all Muslim Australians have a positive experience (Akbarzadeh 2016). Anti-Muslim sentiments have been identified, with discrimination against Muslims said to be increasingly normalised, made respectable, and presented as a precaution against violent extremism (Poynting and Briskman 2018). Despite some hugely successful Muslim Australians, including those in business, in the media, in sport, and through all areas of the community, international events and the failure of political leaders to defend multiculturalism or to separate ideas of Islamic terrorism from every day Muslim Australia have proven increasingly damaging to the relationship of many Australians with the Muslim community (Akbarzadeh 2016). Increased racism and discrimination in the immediate post-9/11 period made it more difficult for Muslim Australians to integrate into Australian society, resulting in increased isolation, leading to poor mental health and wellbeing (Kalek et al. 2010).

United States

Racism has existed in the United States for centuries, reflected in social and economic inequalities across different population groups (Miller and Garran 2017). Dehumanisation and racial segregation over the past three centuries have resulted in the enslavement of African Americans, the slaughter and dispossession of American Indians and Mexicans, and the exclusion and imprisonment of immigrants during periods of war (Bonilla-Silva 2015).

The United States gained independence from European colonisers in the eighteenth century. However, while the Declaration of Independence declaimed that all men were created equal, white or European American men were the key beneficiaries of the legal or social provision of privileges and rights during the founding of the United States. These privileges and rights were denied to others particularly those who had been purchased from Africa and sold on to the Americans as a form of indentured labour, and the Native Americans who were systematically murdered and removed from their lands (Bailey et al. 2017). During this period, European settlers built a prospering economy on the labour of many thousands of enslaved African people and their descendants, while at the same time, upholding the universal rights of 'man' (Bailey et al. 2017). As a way to hold these two contradictory ideas, the colonists established categories identifying Black and Native American populations as less than human, and as somehow intellectually and morally inferior (and therefore subordinate), while white peoples of European heritage were categorised as of a higher class and seen to be of higher intelligence (Omi and Winant 2014). Further entrenching these divisions were access to education, freedom of movement, voting rights, access to citizenship, and land ownership from a period extending from the seventeenth century to the 1960s, all only available to European Americans (Bailey et al. 2017).

The United States passed civil rights laws in the 1960s. These laws were designed to open voting, and to go part of the way to deal with the discriminatory laws and segregation practices prevalent in the southern states. Discrimination at the time was widespread and included legalisation and the enforcement of slavery, the Jim Crow laws enacted in the 1870s (legalising racial discrimination and minimising the social gains attained by the newly freed Black population in the period after the US Civil War), the forcible removal of Indigenous people from their lands, and the forcible transfer of Indigenous children from their families as a way to separate them from their culture (Hammonds 2009).

While no longer legal, there are a number of examples of institutionalised racism present in the United States. For example, the ongoing intergenerational effects of the Social Security Act of 1935, which, while creating an important system of employment-based aged pensions and unemployment compensation, the Act also excluded agricultural workers and domestic servants – occupations largely held by Black men and women (Omi and Winant 2014). The War on Drugs and tough-on-crime policies introduced by President Nixon in the 1970s, are additional examples. While the 'war' does not ever mention race, the penalties for some drugs, those more likely used by Black Americans, are harsher than those for other drugs used by white Americans, leading to disproportionate incarceration rates (Hinton 2016).

South Africa

Archaeological sites reveal that modern humanity and its predecessors have lived in the southern part of Africa for more than 100,000 years, and there is evidence of multiple political and material cultures preceding European colonisation and settlement (Delius and Hay 2009; Ndlovu and Smith 2019). The arrival of the Dutch East India Company in Cape Town in 1652 was followed by the British and the French who each established a footprint in southern Africa, with widespread conflict with first peoples occurring from the 1770s onwards. Following the second Boer War, in 1910, the Union of South Africa was created out of the British controlled colonies of Cape, Natal, Transvaal, and Free State, bringing together the various European settlers and controlled by them. Black opposition to the exclusion of Black people from power led to the foundation of the African National Congress (ANC), originally the South African Native National congress in 1912 (Dubow 2000).

In 1948, the National Party came to power with the ideology of apartheid, an even more authoritarian approach than the previous segregationist policies. In 1961, South Africa was declared a republic after the National Party government won a whites-only referendum, resulting in the enforcement of residential segregation and legislation encapsulating a concern with 'racial purity' (South African Government 2019). The government devised a policy of separate development, and the African population was divided into artificial ethnic 'nations', each with its own 'homeland'. Forced removals from areas defined as 'white' affected over 3 million people, and the homelands faced acute poverty and associated mortality and morbidity, along with environmental degradation (Fabricius and de Wet 2002).

The ANC adopted its Programme of Action against white domination in 1949, calling for protests, strikes, and demonstrations. During the early 1950s mass mobilisation continued to support non-violent resistance to the pass laws that restricted where they were allowed to travel. At the Congress of the People in Soweto in 1955, the Freedom Charter was created, enunciating the principles of the struggle, binding the movement to a culture of human rights and non-racialism. Soon the larger organisations, including the ANC and the Pan-Africanist Congress (PAC), were banned. Matters came to a head at Sharpeville in March 1960 when 69 PAC anti-pass demonstrators were killed. A state of emergency was imposed, and detention without trial was introduced (Marschall 2008).

Indonesia

Indonesia was formed from the former Dutch East Indies (the nationalised colonies of the Dutch East India Company), with the term *Indonesia* coming into use for the geographical location after 1880. In the early twentieth century, local intellectuals began developing the concept of Indonesia as a nation-state, setting the stage for an independence movement (Elson 2008). Following occupation by the Japanese in the Second World War and their surrender in 1945, Indonesian nationalists declared independence and Indonesian sovereignty was formally recognised after four years of struggle in 1949. The introduction of the Republic of Indonesia Citizenship Certificate reproduced the colonial racism that divided the population of the Dutch East Indies into three racial categories: the Europeans (highest status), the Foreign Orientals (Chinese, Indian, and Arab) in the middle, and the Inlanders (the natives or first peoples) at the lower end (Lan 2012).

The Constitution was adopted in 1945 by the new Republican government, and established the religious foundation of the state in language acceptable to both Christians and Muslims, and set out a provision for freedom of religion (Bouwman 2018). Despite this consultative consultation, concerns among Christians, and their potential to be treated as second-class citizens persisted, with theologians and missionaries actively participating in the debates shaping the final constitution. The constitution went through several further iterations in the following years, what was of particular concern to the missionaries was the right to evangelise. The final version of the constitution stops short of this, but incorporates text from Article 18 from the UDHR, truncating the language to limit its scope, and eventually reading that 'everyone is entitled to freedom of religion, conscience, and thought' (Bouwman 2018: 264). A separate provision covered the nature of the state and religious freedom.

The International Convention on the Elimination of All Forms of Racial Discrimination

Traditionally, international human rights instruments and the protections they offer have been developed to ensure individuals are protected from state interference. This has changed in recent decades, with the general understanding that while there are some cases where discrimination occurs at the state level, discrimination can also be perpetrated by private, non-state actors. The International Convention on the Elimination of All Forms of Racial Discrimination goes part of the way to addressing both non-state and state discrimination.

The discussions that lead to the development of a specific body of rules and regulations regarding racial discrimination began after a number of anti-Semitic incidents, first occurring in Germany and then spreading all over the world, in the late 1950s and early 1960s (Keane 2006). These anti-Semitic displays included swastika painting and other overt displays of racial and religious prejudice and lead the UN to adopt a resolution condemning these manifestations of prejudice as contradicting the UDHR (Schwelb 1966). Eventually, the UN General Assembly made the decision to split religious and racial discrimination into two separate resolutions, resulting in two separate decelerations, and then conventions, that would deal with the issues of racial and religious prejudice separately (Keane and Waughray 2017). This decisions to split racial and religious discrimination was largely political, with some countries viewing racial discrimination more serious than religious discrimination, resulting in the drafting of the non-binding Declaration on racial discrimination and then the following Convention receiving priority (Lerner 2014). Since this time, a Declaration on the Elimination of All Forms of Intolerance and of Discrimination Based on Religion or Belief has been adopted by the UN, but political sensitivities around religion have meant that it has not been drafted into a legally binding document.

The Declaration on the Elimination of All Forms of Racial Discrimination was adopted in 1963. This Declaration contained no definition of racial discrimination but did go as far as to declare that discrimination on the basis of race, colour, or ethnicity was an 'offence to human dignity'. This Declaration was followed, in 1965, by the preparation and acceptance of the International Convention on the Elimination of All Forms of Racial Discrimination (ICERD). In drafting the ICERD there were some discussions about the inclusion of a specific Article on anti-Semitism. Give that anti-Semitism was the catalyst for the creation of the Convention, and that only two decades had passed since the Holocaust and the loss of one third of the global population of people of Jewish faith and background, some countries, specifically the United States, Austria, and Poland, supported the inclusion of a specific example of such discrimination (Schwelb 1966). However, the Article did not enjoy broad enough support, with many countries fearing that to include a specific example of one type of racism would exclude or minimise others (Keane and Waughray 2017). In the end, a specific mention of anti-Semitism was not included in the ICERD.

While the so-called swastika epidemic was one of the key drivers for the development of the ICERD, the swift drafting of first the Declaration and then the Convention was largely a result of countries in Asia and Africa pushing back against colonialism and apartheid, and drawing direct links between colonialism, apartheid, and racism (van Boven 2000). This is particularly evident in Article 3 of the ICERD. Article 3 condemns apartheid and racial segregation and obliges parties to 'prevent, prohibit and eradicate' these practices in territories under their jurisdiction. While this Article was specifically directed at the apartheid occurring in South Africa, the Committee on the Elimination of Racial Discrimination (CERD), in General Recommendation 19, highlight the importance of prohibiting all forms of racial segregation in all countries, and eliminating the consequences of past acts of segregation. Article 3, with its specific mention of one example of racism was included as apartheid 'was the official policy of a State Member of the UN'. This Article has been strengthened by the recognition of apartheid as a crime against humanity.

The ICERD has 181 states parties and four signatories; only twelve countries have taken no action on this Convention (at mid-2019). However, only fifty-eight countries have made a declaration under Article 14 (discussed below) allowing the CERD to receive complaints from individuals; the countries that have not made such a declaration include China, India, Indonesia, Israel, the United States, and the UK.

The ICERD commits its members to the elimination of racial discrimination and the promotion of understanding among all races. The ICERD provides a definition of 'racial discrimination' found in Article 1:

> any distinction, exclusion, restriction or preference based on race, colour, descent, or national or ethnic origin which has the purpose or effect of nullifying or impairing the recognition, enjoyment or exercise, on an equal footing, of human rights and

fundamental freedoms in the political, economic, social, cultural or any other field of public life.

The treaty makes no comment or provides no definition of race, but rather provides protections against racial discrimination. In practice, this means that individuals who self-identify as experiencing racial discrimination under one (or more) of the five categories can seek protection. Importantly, this definition does not contain any specific examples, allowing the treaty to fulfil its intent to eliminate all forms of racial discrimination, and exist as a living document that can change over time (Keane and Waughray 2017).

Articles 2, 5, and 6 are concerned with the prevention of discrimination. Article 2 condemns racial discrimination and obliges parties to 'undertake to pursue by all appropriate means and without delay a policy of eliminating racial discrimination in all its forms'. Article 2 also obliges parties to promote understanding among all races through eliminating racial discrimination against its own citizens, terminating any support to parties who discriminate against any person or organisation, creating or amending laws to prevent discrimination, and actively supporting organisations who seek to eliminate discrimination. Article 5 expands on these ideas by requiring states to guarantee the right of everyone to equality before the law regardless of 'race, colour, or national or ethnic origin', including equality in courts and tribunals (reiterated in Article 6), providing security and freedom from violence, and ensuring right of access to any place or service used by the general public.

Article 4 seeks to address the issue of hate speech. It condemns propaganda and organisations that attempt to justify discrimination or are based on the idea of racial superiority. Specifically, it obliges parties to criminalise hate speech (speech that is intended to demonise or brutalise, or the use of derogatory language), hate crimes (a crime motivated by prejudice), as well as funding racist activities. This Article also seeks to prohibit and criminalise membership in organisations that promote and incite racial discrimination. Article 4 has been controversial, particularly around the perceived limits this Article puts on freedoms of speech, association, or assembly. The CERD regards this article as central to the operation of the ICERD, reinforcing this point in General Recommendation 15 by highlighting this Article as mandatory, and that States Parties are expected to both enact legislation to prevent organised violence based on ethnic origin, and to enforce it. A number of States Parties to the ICERD have expressed reservations on this Article. Specifically, the United States does not accept the obligation to restrict any individual freedom of speech, expression, or association, citing the Constitution and laws of the United States as above the obligations included in the ICERD. Many other countries have reservations to this Article, citing they will address any breaches within their own existing criminal law (United Nations 2019). Table 9.1 shows the positions of Australia, the United States, South Africa, and Indonesia in relation to the ICERD.

On the flip side of Article 4, is Article 7, obliging States Party to the ICERD to adopt measures that combat racial prejudice and encourage understanding and tolerance between different racial, ethnic, and national groups. This Article specifically suggests that these activities could be conducted through education and the promotion of a range of cultural activities to encourage understanding, tolerance, and friendship.

The remaining Articles provide the opportunity for complaints mechanism and for monitoring. Articles 11 through 13 of the Convention establish a dispute resolution mechanism between parties, and Article 22 allows unresolved complaints to be referred to the International Court of Justice.

TABLE 9.1 Positions of selected countries on ICERD

Australia: Ratified 30 September 1975
Declarations re article 14; Made
Reservations and declarations on ICERD
"The Government of Australia . . . declares that Australia is not at present in a position specifically
 to treat as offences all the matters covered by article 4 (a) of the Convention. Acts of the kind
 there mentioned are punishable only to the extent provided by the existing criminal law dealing
 with such matters as the maintenance of public order, public mischief, assault, riot, criminal libel,
 conspiracy and attempts. It is the intention of the Australian Government, at the first suitable
 moment, to seek from Parliament legislation specifically implementing the terms of article 4 (a)."

Indonesia Accession 25 Jun 1999
Declarations re article 14: Not made
Reservations and declarations on ICERD
"The Government of the Republic of Indonesia does not consider itself bound by the provision of
 Article 22 and takes the position that disputes relating to the interpretation and application of the
 [Convention] which cannot be settled through the channel provided for in the said article, may be
 referred to the International Court of Justice only with the consent of all the parties to the dispute."

South Africa Ratified 10 Dec 1998
Declarations re article 14: Made
Reservations and declarations on ICERD
None

USA Ratified 21 Oct 1994
Declarations re article 14: Not made
Reservations and declarations on ICERD
Upon signature:
"The Constitution of the United States contains provisions for the protection of individual rights,
 such as the right of free speech, and nothing in the Convention shall be deemed to require or
 to authorize legislation or other action by the United States of America incompatible with the
 provisions of the Constitution of the United States of America."
Upon ratification:
"I. The Senate's advice and consent is subject to the following reservations:
 (1) That the Constitution and laws of the United States contain extensive protections of individual
   freedom of speech, expression and association. Accordingly, the United States does not accept
   any obligation under this Convention, in particular under articles 4 and 7, to restrict those
   rights, through the adoption of legislation or any other measures, to the extent that they are
   protected by the Constitution and laws of the United States.
 (2) That the Constitution and laws of the United States establish extensive protections against
   discrimination, reaching significant areas of non-governmental activity. Individual privacy and
   freedom from governmental interference in private conduct, however, are also recognized as
   among the fundamental values which shape our free and democratic society. The United States
   understands that the identification of the rights protected under the Convention by reference in
   article 1 to fields of 'public life' reflects a similar distinction between spheres of public conduct
   that are customarily the subject of governmental regulation, and spheres of private conduct that
   are not. To the extent, however, that the Convention calls for a broader regulation of private
   conduct, the United States does not accept any obligation under this Convention to enact
   legislation or take other measures under paragraph (1) of article 2, subparagraphs (1) (c) and (d)
   of article 2, article 3 and article 5 with respect to private conduct except as mandated by the
   Constitution and laws of the United States.

(*Continued*)

TABLE 9.1 (Continued)

---

(3) That with reference to article 22 of the Convention, before any dispute to which the United States is a party may be submitted to the jurisdiction of the International Court of Justice under this article, the specific consent of the United States is required in each case.

II. The Senate's advice and consent is subject to the following understanding, which shall apply to the obligations of the United States under this Convention:

That the United States understands that this Convention shall be implemented by the Federal Government to the extent that it exercises jurisdiction over the matters covered therein, and otherwise by the state and local governments. To the extent that state and local governments exercise jurisdiction over such matters, the Federal Government shall, as necessary, take appropriate measures to ensure the fulfilment of this Convention.

III. The Senate's advice and consent is subject to the following declaration:

That the United States declares that the provisions of the Convention are not self-executing."

In addition to the CERD as a mechanism to resolve discrimination issues, the Working Group of Experts on People of African Descent, was established in 2002 by the Commission on Human Rights resolution 2002/68 (as a Special Procedure). The mandate was subsequently renewed by the Commission on Human Rights and the Human Rights Council in its resolutions (CHR 2003/30, 2008/HRC/RES/9/14, 2011/HRC/RES/18/28, 2014/HRC/RES/27/25 and A/HRC/RES/36/23). The last of these, passed in 2017, extended mandate of the group for a further three years. The main task of the Working Group is to investigate the problems of racial discrimination faced by people of African descent, and to propose measures to address these problems.

Monitoring

While states hold the responsibility for implementing international human rights, their effective implementation can only be achieved with an efficient monitoring and enforcement system. The CERD, established by Article 8 of the ICERD, is a body of 18 human rights experts, elected for four-year terms, who monitor the implementation of the ICERD. All States Party to the ICERD are required to submit reports to the Committee to provide an update on the activities related to the ICERD. The first report is due within a year of the Convention entering into effect for that state, and then reports are due every two years. However, the committee can request a report earlier if they have concerns about a specific country.

In addition to the regular reporting procedure, three other mechanisms have been established under the CERD. The first is the early-warning procedure, where the Committee works to prevent existing situations from escalating into conflicts and allows for urgent procedures to be enacted in respond to problems requiring immediate attention. The second is the examination of interstate complaints, where states can request the Committee investigate the activities of another state. The final mechanism is the process allowing for individual complaints, in which individuals or groups who claim to be victim of a violation of any of the Articles in the ICERD can petition to have their case heard.

Tackling racial discrimination

This section examines some of the overall issues that emerge from the operation of the CERD, before looking in particular at the four example countries introduced earlier in the chapter, including material drawn from the latest deliberations of the CERD for each country. The last annual report of the CERD (2018) lists forty-six countries with monitoring reports more than ten years overdue and a further seventeen countries with monitoring reports more than five years overdue. The chairs conclude of the CERD (1), that 'while progress has been made to address racial discrimination, major and multifaceted challenges remain in the struggle towards its elimination, including the inability or unwillingness to call racial discrimination by its shameful name'. At the time of adoption of the present report, CERD had registered, since 1984, sixty-two complaints concerning fifteen states brought under Article 14. Of those, two complaints were discontinued and nineteen were declared. The Committee adopted final decisions on the merits of thirty-five complaints, and declared and found violations of the Convention in nineteen of them. Six complaints were pending consideration.

Australia

Australia, like Canada, New Zealand, and the United States, has relied on large-scale immigration for population growth, and as a result, Australia has a large multicultural and ethnically diverse population. At the end of the Second World War, with concerns about low population growth, war-related causalities, and the myth of an invasion from Asian countries to the north, the Australian government launched a large-scale immigration program. Initially, Australia sought only those of British heritage, but when numbers failed to meet expectations, immigration was opened up to the thousands of people who were displaced by the war and living in camps across Europe (Jupp 2002). The entry of Europeans, including many thousands of Italians and Greeks, changed the Australian population from predominantly British, to what became multicultural Australia. Since this time, hundreds of thousands of people have migrated to Australia in response to government sponsored programs, family reunion, calls for skilled labour, and humanitarian crisis. By mid-2016, one in three Australians were born overseas, and almost half of the population had at least one overseas-born parent (ABS 2018). While eventually each new migrant group is accepted into Australia, upon their arrival, they can be subject to othering, discrimination, and racism (Poynting and Briskman 2018), making it difficult to find belonging in the community (Babacan 2010).

Australia has a number of laws that forbid racial and other forms of discrimination and protect freedom of religion, however, racism very much exists in Australia (Forrest et al. 2016). Contemporary racism in Australia, including intolerance towards specific cultural groups, is seen by researchers as being linked to past notions of what it means to be Australian and to Australian national identity (Dunn et al. 2004).

A Referendum in 1967 regarding the rights of Aboriginal and Torres Strait Islander people resulted in over 90 percent of Australians agreeing that Aboriginal and Torres Strait Islander people should be recognised as equal under Australian law. Since this time, legal reforms have re-established Aboriginal Land Rights under Australian law, allowing Aboriginal and Torres Strait Islander people to hold native title on important land. A large amount of work investigating the impact of historical policies such as the removal of mixed ethnicity Aboriginal and Torres Strait Islander children from their parents (called the Stolen Generations) resulted in a bipartisan Parliamentary apology to Aboriginal and Torres Strait Islander people in 2008. However, health indicators for Aboriginal and Torres Strait Islander people show health disparities between Aboriginal and Torres Strait Islander people and other groups within Australia.

CASE STUDY: CLOSE THE GAP

Australian Aboriginal and Torres Strait Islanders experience lower life expectancy and quality of life compared to other Australians. In response, the Australian government has implemented the Closing the Gap campaign, a strategy developed to address some of the issues that disproportionately affect Aboriginal and Torres Strait Islander Australians. In 2019, the life expectancy gap between an Aboriginal and Torres Strait Islander and non-Aboriginal and Torres Strait Islander was around 8 years, while this gap has decreased since the Closing the Gap program started in 2008, improvements in the past four years have been minimal. There are also gaps in relationship to child mortality, early years education, children's literacy and numeracy, school attendance and completion, employment, and life expectancy. While there have been some positive changes, more initiatives focusing on partnerships supported by community knowledge and wisdom will be needed to drive further change.

Find out more about Close the Gap here: https://closingthegap.pmc.gov.au/

Multiculturalism has been an important enabler for the integration of new Australians from all over the world, as religious beliefs and freedoms are protected by law, and sit alongside efforts to counter racism and discrimination (Akbarzadeh 2016). Legislation, including the Racial Discrimination Act (1975), the Commonwealth Racial Hatred Act (1995), and the Human Rights and Equal Opportunity Commission Act (1986), have outlawed racial discrimination in the public sphere in Australia. Together this anti-discrimination legislation prevents discrimination in the workplace, when purchasing or renting a house or other goods or services, when accessing public facilities (for example, libraries, pools, or places of worship), or when joining a trade union. However, there are some exceptions to this legislation. For example, the laws protect free speech by allowing exemptions if they are done 'reasonably and in good faith', and include artistic work or performance, a publication, discussion, or debate on a matter of public interest, or a fair and accurate report on a matter of public interest (for example, an accurate media report of an act of racial incitement or racially offensive conduct). However, a recent survey found that almost 20 percent of Australians had experienced religious or race based discrimination in the previous twelve months, suggesting that Australia still has a long way to go to be an accepting and tolerant nation (Markus 2018).

CASE STUDY: SECTION 18C OF THE RACIAL DISCRIMINATION ACT 1975

Section 18C of the Racial Discrimination Act 1975, deals with offensive behaviour 'because of race, colour or national or ethnic origin' and makes it unlawful to do an act otherwise than in private if 'the act is reasonably likely, in all the circumstances, to offend, insult, humiliate or intimidate another person or a group of people'. Introduced in 1975, and seeking to make racial discrimination unlawful, the Act has been controversial and subject to considerable debate around the potential of the Act to interfere with freedom of speech and political communication. Section 18C is seen as controversial by some, because it includes a statement that 'offending' or 'insulting' a person constitutes an offense, with the suggestion by some that if freedom of speech is only the freedom to say things about uncontroversial topics, or to say nice or inoffensive things, then it is not really freedom (Finlay 2017). However, others see this as an important inclusion in this Act, as the context surrounding speech that could be discriminatory is what makes it offensive or insulting, and not the terms themselves (Sorial 2017).

For an interesting discussion and implications of 18C in the media, see the *Eatock v Bolt* case from 2011 (Gelber and McNamara 2013).

The most recent report of the CERD (2017b) on Australia's periodic reports under the Convention provides comments on a number of positive legislative, institutional, and policy measures, but registers its continued concern about the decision not to adopt a federal human rights act, as recommended by the national human rights consultation of 2009, arguing that scrutiny by a Parliamentary Joint Committee on Human Rights of existing legislation and draft bills is insufficient to ensure compatibility. The Committee further raises concerns that protection against racial discrimination is not guaranteed by the Constitution and notes that section 25 and 51 (xxvi) in themselves raise issues of racial discrimination. The Committee also express concern that Australia continues to maintain a reservation on Article 4(a) of the Convention (see Table 9.1), which negatively impacts 'the sanctioning of racial hatred and redress for victims, within the context of the persistence in the State Party of racially motivated acts against Indigenous peoples, people of African descent, and Africans, South Asians, refugees, asylum seekers and migrants' (CERD 2017b: 2). It goes on to note the rise of racism in Australia. In relation to Indigenous Australians in particular, the Committee concludes that: 'despite statements by the State Party that it rejects the principle of *terra nullius*, grounded in the "discovery discourse", the State Party continues to conduct its relations with Indigenous peoples, in a manner that is not reconcilable with their rights to self-determination and to own and control their lands and natural resources' (CERD 2017b: 4). In response to the often overt racism in Australia, the Human Rights Commission has released a guide to assist Australians to discuss racism, seeking to encourage individuals, communities, and workplaces to have meaningful and productive conversations about racism (Human Rights Commission 2019).

United States

Racial politics remains a major phenomenon in the United States, and racism continues to be reflected in socioeconomic inequality in employment, housing, education, lending, and government. While the views held by average Americans have changed significantly over the past several decades, and many Americans would strive to present themselves as non-racist or as egalitarian, commonly held implicit biases toward historically marginalised groups suggest that racist attitudes may be unconscious (Konrad 2018). The election of Barack Obama, the first person of colour elected as president, was seen by some as a sign that the United States had moved on from a racist past (Ng and Stamper 2018). However, researchers suggest that many people voted for President Donald Trump in retaliation to the presidency of Obama, suggesting racist resentment and anti-immigration sentiment in voters (Hooghe and Dassonneville 2018). Since the election of President Trump, the United States has seen continued high levels of racism and bigotry, including the rise of the 'alt-right' movement, and increased awareness of race-based discrimination.

Alt-right groups, the term used for a range of white nationalist coalitions that seek segregation, expulsion, and/or subjection of minorities (Cole 2018), have been more active since the election of President Trump. For example, in August 2017, hundreds of self-styled white nationalists joined Klansmen (Ku Klux Klan), militia members, and affiliates of various white power organisations in Charlottesville, Virginia, for a rally to 'defend white heritage' (Atkinson 2018). While this rally was met with concern and disbelief by a large proportion of mainstream America, and resulted in the groups going back to ground, they have not totally disappeared. Alt-right and white supremacist groups continue to be active on the internet, and acts of terrorism attributed to these groups increased in the six months after the incident (Atkinson 2018).

Discrimination directed at Black Americans continues to be a problem in parts of the United States. In April 2018, two men, were arrested in a Starbucks store in Philadelphia while they waited for a friend to join them. A witness at the time of the arrests said that the men asked staff if they could use the bathroom to which an employee said it was reserved for paying customers and were instructed by staff to leave. When they did not comply, the store manager called the police, claiming that the men were trespassing, leading to their arrests. They were released without charge. The video of the arrest and the conduct of the Starbucks staff led the CEO of Starbucks to issue an apology, referring to the arrests as 'reprehensible' and promising to take steps to prevent future incidents. In response, Starbucks closed their stores and corporate offices for a day so that all staff could take part in racial-bias training.

Finally, there is the response to increased police brutality against mostly young Black men. The activist movement, Black Lives Matter, was created in response to the increasing number of Black men who were dying in police custody, and campaigns against violence and systemic racism toward Black people. In 2013, the movement began with the use of #BlackLivesMatter on social media after the acquittal of George Zimmerman in the shooting death of African-American teen Trayvon Martin the preceding February (Carney 2016). The campaign was reignited in 2014 following the deaths of Michael Brown, resulting in protests and unrest in Ferguson, and Eric Garner in New York City. Since these protests, participants in the movement have demonstrated against the deaths of numerous other Black Americans by police actions or while in police custody. The movement has been controversial, with some stating that the police are the real victims, with others trying to counter the hashtag with their own, saying #AllLivesMatter (Carney 2016).

The CERD, under its early warning and urgent action procedure has recently considered the situation in the United States and calls upon:

> the Government of the United States, including the high-level politicians and public officials, not only to unequivocally and unconditionally reject and condemn the racist hate speech and racist crimes in Charlottesville and throughout the country, but also to actively contribute to the promotion of understanding, tolerance and diversity between ethnic groups, and acknowledge their contribution to the history and diversity of the United States

recommending that:

> the Government of the United States identify and take concrete measures to address the root causes of the proliferation of such racist manifestations, and thoroughly investigate the phenomenon of

racial discrimination targeting in particular people of African descent, ethnic or ethno-religious minorities and migrants.

(CERD 2018: 7)

There are some counters to this long history of racism in the United States, particularly the policies of affirmative action or positive discrimination. Affirmative action describes the measures that aim to create equality and overcome past discrimination. Affirmative action policies have been controversial, as by design, they favour one group over another, in order to compensate for past wrongs. Despite such concerns, the number of minorities in work and education as a result of these programs has increased (Miller 2017).

South Africa

The International Day for the Elimination of Racial Discrimination is observed every year on 21 March. It is held on this day to commemorate police opening fire on a peaceful demonstration against the apartheid pass laws in the town of Sharpeville, South Africa, in 1960, killing sixty-nine demonstrators. The protestors had burned the 'pass books' they were required to carry, which restricted them from going into certain areas as a part of the apartheid regime. Apartheid, an Afrikaans word meaning separateness, was an official regime of the South African government that systematically institutionalised racism through white supremacy. It existed in South Africa from 1948 until 1994. During apartheid, the majority Black South Africans were separated from the minority white South Africans in public facilities and social events, and in housing and employment opportunities.

Like many countries that existed under colonial rule, a hierarchical stratification system in South Africa that saw the Dutch and then British colonial powers at the top, with an ethnically diverse enslaved population at the base, existed for centuries. However, the effect of an official apartheid in the twentieth century was that individuals could not marry across racial lines, and millions of people were forced to move out of their homes and into segregated neighbourhoods, with some Black South Africans losing their nationality in the process (Clark et al. 2016).

International criticism was levelled at the regime in South Africa by many nations who were concerned by the systematic discrimination and violence, and in 1966, the UN condemned 'the policies of apartheid practised by the Government of South Africa as a crime against humanity' (Clark et al. 2016). This was followed in 1977 by a mandatory embargo for all UN member states for the trade of arms to South Africa. During this time, internal resistance began to build, and South Africa entered a period of civil war, with the white ruling powers increasingly using military force to implement its policies. As South Africa became increasingly ungovernable, much of the rest of world began to impose additional sanctions, boycotts (in the economic, political, and sporting realms), and general condemnation. In response to this international pressure and the disintegration of life in South Africa, the government of South Africa announced in 1990 that that they would renounce the policy of apartheid, and released Nelson Mandela from prison after being held for almost thirty years as a political prisoner; in 1994 he became the first president of the new South Africa (Wilson 2001).

South Africa ratified the ICERD in 1998, declaring its agreement to be bound by Article 14, and made no reservations or declaration on the ICERD; it is the only one of the four countries considered as examples who made no reservation or declaration (see Table 9.1). CERD (2016) considered the combined fourth to eighth periodic reports from South Africa and published its concluding observations in 2016. This is the most recent consideration by CERD of South Africa. While this report identifies positive aspects in South Africa's adoption of a number of different legislative and policy measures, it notes a number of concerns and makes recommendations. One concern regards the statistics based on the use of classifications from the former apartheid era, without measurement of the disaggregated data specified in Article 1(1) of the ICERD. A second concern is the lack of provision of adequate financial resources to the South African national human rights institution (NHRI). While commending the work of the Truth and Reconciliation Commission, CERD expressed concern regarding lack of full implementation of its recommendations particularly in terms of prosecuting perpetrators and providing adequate reparations to victims (CERD 2017a). The response by the South African government demonstrates the provision of an increased budget to the NHRI and discusses the work underway to 'create a single umbrella body, under which all the institutions supporting democracy would be managed, thereby allowing for added efficiency and the optimal use of resources' (CERD 2017a: 5). The government's report also discusses the different educational campaigns to address the causes of prejudices and to promote respect for diversity as well as criminal justice responses to hate crime and hate speech. The report acknowledges that the eradication of all forms of racism and racial discrimination in South Africa is a work in progress but says that it is confident on being able to report of positive progress when they submit their next periodic review in 2020.

Indonesia

Indonesia's combined fourth to sixth periodic reports to CERD have been overdue since 2010. Indonesia submitted the first to third periodic reports in a single document which was submitted six years late and considered by CERD in 2007. The committee's concluding observations, while welcoming the initiation of dialogue with the State and identifying some positive aspects, presents a long list of concerns including the status and treatment of Indigenous peoples and their rights to self-determination and self-identification, and points to the threads posed by oil palm plantations (CERD 2007). Concerns were also raised about the rights of non-citizens and internally displaced persons, due to natural disasters as well as conflicts. CERD also takes issue with the government of Indonesia's statement that there is no racial discrimination in Indonesia, direct or indirect, and points out internal contradictions in their report (CERD 2007).

Indonesia is home to an estimated 50 to 70 million Indigenous peoples, with the government recognising 1,128 ethnic groups (IWGIA 2019). Despite laws that recognise the rights of Indigenous peoples (and Indonesia's vote in favour of the United Nations Declaration on the Rights of Indigenous Peoples), according to IWGIA (2019) 'government officials argue that the concept of Indigenous peoples is not applicable, since almost all Indonesians (with the exception of the Chinese) are Indigenous and have the same rights. As a result, the government has rejected calls for the specific needs of groups that identify themselves as Indigenous.' Indigenous peoples face violence and criminalisation, often linking to exploitation of lands for infrastructure projects and dams. These issues remain pressing concerns in Indonesia to the current day. The position of Indonesians of Chinese heritage remains of concern. According to Lan (2012), the Indonesian Constitution did not succeed in removing the colonial racism that created the category of Foreign Orientals, maintaining this through the Republic of Indonesia Citizenship Certificate. While this certificate has ostensibly been abolished, it is still used within many parts of the Indonesian bureaucracy. In April 2019, as presidential elections were about to commence, Nnoko-Mewanu (2019) reported on the damage and threats posed by the palm oil industry to the land rights of Indigenous peoples, and identified that neither of the two presidential candidates has any plan for protection of Indigenous rights. While in February 2019, a group of UN human rights experts called for 'prompt and impartial investigations must be carried out into numerous cases of alleged killings, unlawful arrests, and cruel, inhuman and degrading treatment of Indigenous Papuans by the Indonesian police and military in West Papua and Papua provinces' (OHCHR 2019).

Dealing with racism and discrimination in the twentieth century

The legacies of colonialism and western imperialism remain dominant and continue to negatively impact the lives of many people all over the world. Addressing the impact of the long history of domination by one group over others remains to be comprehensively accomplished, with many individuals, communities, workplaces, and organisations continuing to ignore the impacts of racism. Intersectionality, not only in the demographic sense, but also in terms of the integration of measures to eliminate discrimination with other instruments of the UN, including the Declaration on the Rights of Indigenous Peoples, the mandates of several other Special Rapporteurs, including Special Rapporteur on the situation of human rights defenders, Special Rapporteur on torture and cruel, inhuman or degrading treatment or punishment, and the Special Rapporteur on contemporary forms of racism, racial discrimination, xenophobia and related intolerance, will be necessary in the fight against ongoing discrimination. As seen in the discussion on racism in the United States in this chapter, global movements and migration also have an impact on the way that some communities respond to the presence and arrival of other groups. While many countries have come a long way since the introduction of the ICERD, there remains a long way to go to address the discrimination experienced by many.

References

ABS 2018. *3415.0: Migrant Data Matrices, 2018* [Online], Canberra. Available: www.abs.gov.au/AUSSTATS/abs@.nsf/Latestproducts/3415.0Main%20Features42018?opendocument&tabname=Summary&prodno=3415.0&issue=2018&num=&view= [Accessed 07/05/2019].

Akbarzadeh, S 2016. The Muslim question in Australia: Islamophobia and Muslim alienation, *Journal of Muslim Minority Affairs*, 36(3): 323–333. doi.org/10.1080/13602004.2016.1212493

Atkinson, DC 2018. Charlottesville and the alt-right: A turning point?, *Politics, Groups, and Identities*, 6(2): 309–315. doi.org/10.1080/21565503.2018.1454330

Babacan, H 2010. Immigration, nation state and belonging, in *Migration, Belonging and the Nation State*, Newcastle upon Tyne: Cambridge Scholars Publishing in association with GSE Research.

Bailey, ZD, Krieger, N, Agénor, M, Graves, J, Linos, N, & Bassett, MT 2017. Structural racism and health inequities in the USA: Evidence and interventions, *The Lancet*, 389(10077): 1453–1463. doi.org/10.1016/S0140-6736(17)30569-X

Berger, M, & Sarnyai, Z 2015. 'More than skin deep': Stress neurobiology and mental health consequences of racial discrimination, *Stress*, 18(1): 1–10. doi.org/10.3109/10253890.2014.989204

Bonilla-Silva, E 2015. *The Structure of Racism in Color-Blind, 'Post-Racial' America*, Los Angeles, CA: Sage Publications. doi.org/10.1177/0002764215586826

Bouwman, B 2018. From religious freedom to social justice: The human rights engagement of the ecumenical movement from the 1940s to the 1970s, *Journal of Global History*, 13(2): 252–273. doi. org/10.1017/S1740022818000074

Calvin, R, Winters, K, Wyatt, SB, Williams, DR, Henderson, FC, & Walker, ER 2003. Racism and cardiovascular disease in African Americans, *The American Journal of the Medical Sciences*, 325(6): 315–331. doi.org/10.1097/00000441-200306000-00003

Carney, N 2016. All lives matter, but so does race: Black lives matter and the evolving role of social media, *Humanity & Society*, 40(2): 180–199. doi.org/10.1177/0160597616643868

CERD 2007. Concluding observations, *CERD/C/IDN/CO/3*, Geneva: Committee on the Elimination of Racial Discrimination.

CERD 2016. Concluding observations on the combined fourth to eighth periodic reports of South Africa, *CERD/C/ZAF/CO/4–8*, Geneva: Committee for the Elimination of Racial Discrimination.

CERD 2017a. Addendum: Information received from South Africa on follow-up to the concluding observations, *CERD/C/ZAF/CO/4–8/Add.1*, Geneva: Committee on the Elimination of Racial Discrimination.

CERD 2017b. *Concluding Observations on the Eighteenth to Twentieth Periodic Reports of Australia*, Geneva: International Convention on the Elimination of All Forms of Racial Discrimination.

CERD 2018. *Report of the Committee on the Elimination of Racial Discrimination*, New York/United Nations: Official Records of the UN General Assembly, Seventy-Third Session, Supplement No. 18. A/73/18.

Clark, NL, Worger, WH, Clark, NL, & Worger, WH 2016. *South Africa: The Rise and Fall of Apartheid*, New York: Routledge.

Cole, M 2018. *Trump, the Alt-Right and Public Pedagogies of Hate and for Fascism: What Is to Be Done?*, Routledge. doi.org/10.4324/9780429467141

Delius, P, & Hay, M 2009. *Mpumalanga: An Illustrated History* [Online], Johannesburg: Highveld Press. Available: www.mpumalanga.gov.za/mpumalangabook/history.html [Accessed 04/06/2019].

Department of Labor and Immigration 1975. *1788–1975 Australia and Immigration*, Canberra: Australian Government Publishing Service.

Dominguez, TP, Dunkel-Schetter, C, Glynn, LM, Hobel, C, & Sandman, CA 2008. Racial differences in birth outcomes: The role of general, pregnancy, and racism stress, *Health Psychology*, 27(2): 194. doi.org/10.1037/0278-6133.27.2.194

Dubow, S 2000. *The African National Congress*, Stroud, UK: Sutton Publishing.

Dunn, KM, Forrest, J, Burnley, I, & McDonald, A 2004. Constructing racism in Australia, *Australian Journal of Social Issues*, 39(4): 409–430. doi.org/10.1002/j.1839-4655.2004.tb01191.x

Dunn, KM, Klocker, N, & Salabay, T 2007. Contemporary racism and Islamaphobia in Australia: Racializing religion, *Ethnicities*, 7(4): 564–589. doi.org/10.1177/1468796807084017

Elson, RE 2008. *The Idea of Indonesia: A History*, Cambridge: Cambridge University Press.

Fabricius, C, & de Wet, C 2002. The influence of forced removals and land restitution, in *Conservation and Mobile Indigenous Peoples: Displacement, Forced Settlement, and Sustainable Development* (Vol. 10, p. 142), Oxford: Berghahn Books.

Finlay, L 2017. The continuing fight against 18C where to from here?, *Policy: A Journal of Public Policy and Ideas*, 33(2): 32.

Forrest, J, Elias, A, & Paradies, Y 2016. Perspectives on the geography of intolerance: Racist attitudes and experience of racism in Melbourne, Australia, *Geoforum*, 70: 51–59. doi.org/10.1016/j. geoforum.2016.02.005

Fredrickson, GM 2015. *Racism: A Short History*, Princeton: Princeton University Press. doi.org/10.1515/9781400873678

Gelber, K, & McNamara, L 2013. Freedom of speech and racial vilification in Australia: 'The Bolt case' in public discourse, *Australian Journal of Political Science*, 48(4): 470–484. doi.org/10.1080/10361146. 2013.842540

Hall, WJ, Chapman, MV, Lee, KM, Merino, YM, Thomas, TW, Payne, BK, Eng, E, Day, SH, & Coyne-Beasley, T 2015. Implicit racial/ethnic bias among health care professionals and its influence on health care outcomes: A systematic review, *American Journal of Public Health*, 105(12): e60–e76. doi.org/10.2105/AJPH.2015.302903

Hammonds, E 2009. *The Nature of Difference: Sciences of Race in the United States from Jefferson to Genomics*, Cambridge: The MIT Press.

Hemmings, C, & Evans, AM 2018. Identifying and treating race-based trauma in counseling, *Journal of Multicultural Counseling and Development*, 46(1): 20–39. doi.org/10.1002/jmcd.12090

Hinton, E 2016. *From the War on Poverty to the War on Crime*, Cambridge: Harvard University Press. doi.org/10.4159/9780674969223

Hooghe, M, & Dassonneville, R 2018. Explaining the Trump vote: The effect of racist resentment and anti-immigrant sentiments, *PS: Political Science & Politics*, 51(3): 528–534. doi.org/10.1017/S1049096518000367

Human Rights Commission 2019. *Let's Talk Race: A Guide on How to Conduct a Conversation about Racism* [Online], Sydney. Available: www.humanrights.gov.au/sites/default/files/document/publication/ahrc_racism_conversation_guide_2019.pdf [Accessed 09/08/2019].

IWGIA 2019. *Indigenous Peoples in Indonesia* [Online], Denmark: International Work Group for Indigenous Affairs. Available: www.iwgia.org/en/indonesia [Accessed 18/07/2019].

Jupp, J 2002. *From White Australia to Woomera*, Melbourne: Cambridge University Press. doi.org/10.1017/CBO9781139195034

Kalek, S, Mak, AS, & Khawaja, NG 2010. Intergroup relations and Muslims' mental health in Western societies: Australia as a case study, *Journal of Muslim Mental Health*, 5(2): 160–193. doi.org/10.1080/15564908.2010.487722

Keane, D 2006. Addressing the aggravated meeting points of race and religion, *Race, Religion, Gender & Class*, 6: 367.

Keane, D, & Waughray, A 2017. *Fifty Years of the International Convention on the Elimination of All Forms of Racial Discrimination: A Living Instrument*, Oxford: Oxford University Press. doi.org/10.7228/manchester/9781784993047.001.0001

Konrad, AM 2018. Denial of racism and the Trump presidency, *Equality, Diversity and Inclusion: An International Journal*, 37(1): 14–30. doi.org/10.1108/EDI-07-2017-0155

Lan, TJ 2012. Contesting the post-colonial legal construction of Chinese Indonesians as 'foreign subjects', *Asian Ethnicity*, 13(4): 373–387. doi.org/10.1080/14631369.2012.710075

LeMelle, TJ, & Shepherd Jr, GW 1971. Race in the future of international relations, *Journal of International Affairs*: 302–314.

Lerner, N 2014. *The UN Convention on the Elimination of All Forms of Racial Discrimination: Reprint Revised by Natan Lerner*, Martinus Nijhoff Publishers. doi.org/10.1163/9789004279926

Markus, A 2018. *The Scanlon Foundation Surveys 2018* [Online], Melbourne: Monash University.

Markwick, A, Ansari, Z, Clinch, D, & McNeil, J 2019. Experiences of racism among Aboriginal and Torres Strait Islander adults living in the Australian state of Victoria: A cross-sectional population-based study, *BMC Public Health*, 19(1): 309. doi.org/10.1186/s12889-019-6614-7

Marschall, S 2008. Pointing to the dead: Victims, martyrs and public memory in South Africa, *South African Historical Journal*, 60(1): 103–123. doi.org/10.1080/02582470802287745

McMaster, D 2002. *Asylum Seekers: Australia's Response to Refugees*, Melbourne, Victoria: Melbourne University Press.

Miller, C 2017. The persistent effect of temporary affirmative action, *American Economic Journal: Applied Economics*, 9(3): 152–190. doi.org/10.1257/app.20160121

Miller, J, & Garran, AM 2017. *Racism in the United States: Implications for the Helping Professions*, Springer Publishing Company. doi.org/10.1891/9780826148858

Mlambo, AS 2006. Western social sciences and Africa: The domination and marginalisation of a continent, *African Sociological Review*, 10(1): 161–179.

Ndlovu, N, & Smith, B 2019. The past is a divided country: Transforming archaeology in South Africa, *African Archaeological Review*: 1–18.

Ng, ES, & Stamper, CL 2018. A Trump presidency and the prospect for equality and diversity, *Equality, Diversity and Inclusion: An International Journal*, 37(1): 2–13. doi.org/10.1108/EDI-12-2017-0282

Nnoko-Mewanu, J 2019. *Whoever Wins Indonesia's Presidential Election, Indigenous People Will Lose* [Online], Washington: Foreign Policy. Available: https://foreignpolicy.com/2019/04/16/whoever-wins-indonesias-presidential-election-indigenous-people-will-lose/ [Accessed 18/07/2019].

OHCHR 2019. *Indonesia: UN Experts Condemn Racism and Police Violence against Papuans, and Use of Snake against Arrested Boy* [Online], Geneva: The Office of the High Commissioner for Human Rights. Available: www.ohchr.org/EN/NewsEvents/Pages/DisplayNews.aspx?NewsID=24187&LangID=E [Accessed 18/07/2019].

Omi, M, & Winant, H 2014. *Racial Formation in the United States*, New York: Routledge.

Ozdowski, S 1984. *The Australian Migration Law: A Time for a Change? Multicultural Australian Papers*, Richmond: Clearing House on Migration Issues.

Paradies, Y, Ben, J, Denson, N, Elias, A, Priest, N, Pieterse, A, Gupta, A, Kelaher, M, & Gee, G 2015. Racism as a determinant of health: A systematic review and meta-analysis, *PLoS One*, 10(9): e0138511. doi.org/10.1371/journal.pone.0138511

Poynting, S, & Briskman, L 2018. Islamophobia in Australia: From far-right deplorables to respectable liberals, *Social Sciences*, 7(11): 213. doi.org/10.3390/socsci7110213

Reynolds, H 1989. *Dispossession: Black Australians and White Invaders*, Sydney: Allen & Unwin Sydney.

Schwelb, E 1966. The international convention on the elimination of all forms of racial discrimination, *International & Comparative Law Quarterly*, 15(4): 996–1068. doi.org/10.1093/iclqaj/15.4.996

Smedley, A, & Smedley, BD 2005. Race as biology is fiction, racism as a social problem is real: Anthropological and historical perspectives on the social construction of race, *American Psychologist*, 60(1): 16–26. doi: 10.1037/0003-066X.60.1.16

Sorial, S 2017. What does it mean to offend, insult, humiliate and intimidate: Section 18C of the Racial Discrimination Act 1975 (Cth) and the problem of harm, *Australian Journal of Legal Philosophy*, 42: 165.

South African Government 2019. *History* [Online], Pretoria: South African Government. Available: www.gov.za/about-sa/history [Accessed 18/07/2019].

UN 2007. *The Struggle against Apartheid: Lessons for Today's World* [Online]. Available: https://unchronicle.un.org/article/struggle-against-apartheid-lessons-today-s-world [Accessed 21/05/2019].

United Nations 2019. *Treaty Collection* [Online], Geneva. Available: https://treaties.un.org/ [Accessed 08/04/2019].

Valentino, BA 2005. *Final Solutions: Mass Killing and Genocide in the 20th Century*, New York: Cornell University Press.

van Boven, T 2000. The petition system under the international convention on the elimination of all forms of racial discrimination, *Max Planck Yearbook of United Nations Law Online*, 4(1): 271–287. doi.org/10.1163/187574100X00106

Waldrep, C 2008. *African Americans Confront Lynching: Strategies of Resistance from the Civil War to the Civil Rights Era*, Plymouth: Rowman & Littlefield Publishers.

Williams, DR, & Williams-Morris, R 2000. Racism and mental health: The African American experience, *Ethnicity & Health*, 5(3–4): 243–268. doi.org/10.1080/713667453

Wilson, RA 2001. *The Politics of Truth and Reconciliation in South Africa: Legitimizing the Post-Apartheid State*, Cambridge: Cambridge University Press. doi.org/10.1017/CBO9780511522291

10

MONITORING HUMAN RIGHTS

Fiona H. McKay and Ann Taket

Introduction

There are a range of different mechanisms that can be employed to monitor the promotion, protection, and fulfilment of human rights. This chapter will focus on the range of proactive activities and actions undertaken by institutions and government bodies to promote and protect human rights. It will include a discussion of the role of the United Nations (UN) Universal Periodic Review system in encouraging states to meet obligations, the role of regional and country level courts in monitoring and responding to breaches through courts, commissions, and ombudsmen. This chapter does not seek to present a comprehensive overview of all human rights monitoring activities, but instead will present an overview of current activities, and examples of monitoring at global, regional and national level.

Universal Periodic Review system

The Universal Periodic Review (UPR) is a mechanism of the UN Human Rights Council. The UPR, first introduced in Chapter 2, allows for the periodic examination of the human rights performance of all 193 UN member states (OHCHR 2019). The UPR aims is to increase transparency and credibility of global human rights, and their implementation by the UN (Gaer 2007). Part of the appeal of this system is that all states are reviewed by their peers in a non-selective, universal, and transparent manner (Abebe 2009). Forty-two states are reviewed each year during three sessions of a Working Group of the Human Rights Council, with each country benchmarked against the Charter of the UN, the Universal Declaration of Human Rights (UDHR), other human rights instruments to which a state is party, and any voluntary pledges or commitments made. The UPR is the first international human rights mechanism to address all countries and all human rights.

The Working Group is formed by forty-seven members of the Human Rights Council, the process of the UPR Working Group consists of three steps (OHCHR 2019). First, the country under review offers an assessment of its own human rights record. Second, other UN member states peer-review the country under review and make recommendations for improvement, this assessment is conducted through a dialogue. Finally, based on this dialogue, the UPR Working Group submits an 'Outcome Report' to the plenary of the Human Rights Council for adoption by a formal decision. A group of three states (the troika), is drawn from the members of the Human Rights Council to facilitate the UPR Working Group, who then receive questions raised by states ahead of the review, this is followed by the creation of a report prepared by the state under review. The troika drafts the Outcome Report, reflecting the proceedings of the review, with the full involvement of the State concerned and the cooperation of the Office of the High Commissioner for Human Rights (OHCHR). States can then indicate if they accept or reject the recommendations (Dominguez-Redondo 2012).

NGOs can play a significant role in the UPR process (Moss 2010). NGO submissions are published on the OHCHR website and become a part of a central reference on the human rights situation for the country concerned, providing a valuable opportunity for advocacy. NGO reports can include specific recommendations, which may then be picked up in the review sessions. Moss (2010) analysed the proceedings of the second session of the UPR in which sixteen states were reviewed, finding that 745 factual statements, observations, or recommendations by NGOs were included in the summaries of 'other stakeholder information'. Of these 523, or 70 percent, correspond to recommendations made by member states to the states under review, and 199 of those were accepted by the relevant state under review (Moss 2010).

In responding to breaches of human rights, states and other interested bodies have long employed a naming and shaming approach, often influenced by strategic ties between countries. While countries are more likely to condemn their friends and allies less harshly in order to maintain relationships, these ties can provide a key leverage point when dealing with human rights problems. Research investigating the operations and effectiveness of the UPR have found that states will give less severe commentary to their allies overall, but when they do offer criticism, their recommendations are more likely to be accepted, compared to similar recommendations from other countries (Terman and Voeten 2018).

The NGO, UPR Info, works to report on the outcomes of the UPR process, including the adoption and action by countries of their recommendations. In 2014, UPR Info released a report detailing the concrete and immediate results of the promises made in the first cycle of the UPR (Info UPR 2014). This report shows that 48 percent of UPR recommendations triggered action by the mid-term (2.5 years after the review), with most of the action taken by countries in Eastern Europe and the least in Asia. During the review, states are able to accept or note the recommendations. Recommendations that were accepted were more likely to have progressed (with 55 percent of accepted recommendations triggering action by mid-term), while noted recommendations are less likely to be actioned at mid-term (19 percent of noted recommendations triggered action) (Info UPR 2014). Issues such as women's rights, the adoption of international instruments, and children's rights had the highest number of recommendations that triggered action, but the issues with the highest percentage of implementation within the issue categories were HIV/AIDS, human trafficking, and the rights of people with disability (Info UPR 2014). Actions that were least likely to be implemented were related to freedom of movement, right to land, and the death penalty.

In their 2016 follow up to this report, UPR Info address the successes and challenges of the UPR system, drawing on approximately 57,000 recommendations addressed to 193 states reviewed over two cycles of the UPR (Info UPR 2016). They point to several human rights successes, such as Fiji removing the death penalty from the military code, the criminalisation of marital rape in the Republic of Korea, and China reducing the number of crimes that carry the death penalty. However, as pointed out by UPR Info, the UPR cannot compel states to make changes, for example, Switzerland recommended that Australia in its first review 'not detain migrants other than in exceptional cases, limit this detention to six months and bring detention conditions into line with international standards in the field of human rights'. The recommendation was noted, and Switzerland reiterated the recommendation in the second cycle, adding 'as previously recommended'. A number of Australian NGOs attended these sessions, making similar submissions on the issue of the detention of asylum seekers, however, despite these calls from other nations and NGOs, the Australian government largely ignored calls for changes to the policy relating to people seeking asylum (OHCHR 2019).

MONITORING HUMAN RIGHTS USING SDGDATA. HUMANRIGHTS.DK

The Sustainable Development Goals (SDGs) and human rights are closely interrelated. More than 92 percent of SDG targets reflect specific provision of international human rights and labour standards (Hassler 2019). The Danish Institute for Human Rights has produced an online SDG-Human rights data explorer (https://sdgdata.humanrights. dk/en/explorer) which allows for the exploration of human rights recommendations and their connection to the 2030 Agenda. The database can be browsed by the SDG goals and associated targets, country or region, different groups of rights-holders and different human rights mechanisms (treaty body, special procedure, or UPR). Future linkages to other data from the SDG indicator framework (https://unstats.un.org/sdgs) and Human Rights Measurement Initiative (https://humanrightsmeasurement.org) are also planned (Hassler 2019, personal communication).

As an example of the use of this database, this case study examines Indigenous peoples as a group of rights holders and looks at the recommendations made to two countries Argentina (Table 10.1) and the Russian Federation (Table 10.2) in the second and third cycles of the UPR.

The second UPR cycle finished in 2012 for Argentina. Thirteen recommendations were made and ten of these (77 percent) were accepted; recommendations covered seven of the seventeen SDGs and thirteen different countries were involved in making the recommendations. The third cycle for Argentina finished in 2017, a far higher number of recommendations were made in relation to Indigenous peoples (twenty-eight in total); twenty-four of these were accepted (86 percent). Recommendations covered six of the seventeen SDGs (4 SDG that had also been covered in the second cycle), and twenty-seven different countries were involved in making the recommendations.

TABLE 10.1 Argentina – Recommendations regarding Indigenous People in UPR cycles 2 and 3

	Cycle 2 (2012)	Cycle 3 (2017)
Number of recommendations	13	28
Recommendations accepted	10	24
Recommendations noted *	3	4
SDG goals affected	1 No poverty 2 Zero hunger 4 Quality education 5 Gender equality 10 Reduced inequalities 11 Sustainable cities and communities 16 Peace, justice and strong institutions	1 No poverty 2 Zero hunger 4 Gender equality 6 Clean water and sanitation 10 Reduced inequalities 16 Peace, justice, and strong institutions
Countries making recommendations	Algeria Oman Austria Pakistan Bolivia Peru Brazil South Africa Greece Spain Iraq Trinidad and Mexico Tobago	Algeria Iraq Austria Madagascar Bolivia Maldives Brazil Namibia Canada Norway Columbia Paraguay Czechia Peru Ecuador Republic of Korea Estonia Senegal France Sierra Leone Germany South Africa Honduras State of Palestine India Venezuela Iran

* Noted: this is used on the database where the recommendation was not accepted by the country.

Turning to the Russian Federation, the second UPR cycle finished in 2013. Ten recommendations were made, and five of these (50 percent) were accepted. Recommendations covered six of the seventeen SDGs (four of which were the same as in Argentina), and seven different countries were involved in making the recommendations. The third cycle for the Russian Federation finished in 2018, a similar number of recommendations were made in relation to Indigenous peoples (nine in total), and four of these were accepted (44 percent); recommendations covered four of the seventeen SDGs (two were the same as in the second cycle), and ten different countries were involved in making the recommendations.

The responses made by countries to recommendations classified as 'noted' on the database reveal the contested nature of interactions within the UPR cycles. See Table 10.3, which gives these for the recommendations noted in cycle 3 for the Russian Federation. The details of the responses are not recorded on the database.

TABLE 10.2 Russian Federation – Recommendations regarding Indigenous People in UPR cycles 2 and 3

	Cycle 2 (2013)	Cycle 3 (2018)
Number of recommendations	10	9
Recommendations accepted	5	4
Recommendations noted*	5	4
Status of recommendation ns		1**
SDG goals affected	1 No poverty	1 No poverty
	2 Zero hunger	2 Zero hunger
	4 Quality education	11 Sustainable cities and communities
	10 Reduced inequalities	12 Responsible production and consumption
	16 Peace, justice, and strong institutions	
	17 Partnerships for the goals	
Countries making recommendations	Bolivia	Bolivia
	Denmark	Estonia
	Estonia	Honduras
	Hungary	Hungary
	Mexico	Madagascar
	Namibia	Nicaragua
	Paraguay	Norway
		Paraguay
		South Africa
		Venezuela

* Noted: this is used on the database where the recommendation was not accepted by the country.
** The Russian Federation's response on this recommendation (https://lib.ohchr.org/HRBodies/UPR/Documents/Session30/RU/A_HRC_39_13_Add.1_RussianFederation_Annex_E.docx, p. 37) was 'Partially accepted: The legislation of the Russian Federation already provides for adequate protection of indigenous peoples' rights. Russia continues to make efforts to improve the relevant legislation and expand the safeguard system.' Such responses are not currently recorded on the system

TABLE 10.3 Responses on 'noted' recommendations in the UPR third cycle, Russian Federation

Recommendation	Response
Ratify the International Labour Organization (ILO) Indigenous and Tribal Peoples Convention, 1989 (No. 169) and Domestic Workers Convention, 2011 (No. 189)	The examination of the provisions of ILO Convention No. 169 has revealed that current legislation concerning small indigenous peoples in the Russian Federation is not only more comprehensive than the Convention but that it is also subject to constant amendment in line with circumstances on the ground and emerging challenges.
	As far as ILO Convention No. 189 is concerned, the Russian authorities note that national legislation adequately protects all categories of workers, including those working at home. Chapter 49 of the Labour Code of the Russian Federation addresses the specific situation of home workers.

(Continued)

TABLE 10.3 (Continued)

Recommendation	Response
Formally endorse the United Nations Declaration on the Rights of Indigenous Peoples and implement its principles in national legislation	The state policy of Russia on small indigenous peoples is aimed at ensuring those peoples' sustainable development and is based on provisions of national legislation that are, to a large degree, identical to the provisions of the United Nations Declaration or, in some respect, significantly surpass this document.
Accede to international human rights instruments to which the country is not yet a party, particularly the International Convention on the Rights of All Migrant Workers and Members of Their Families, the ILO Indigenous and Tribal Peoples Convention, 1989 (No. 169) and the 1954 Convention relating to the Status of Stateless Persons	See above two responses As for the 1954 Convention related to the status of stateless persons, there is no objective need at present for accession to it, since the domestic law contains no provisions diminishing the legal status of stateless persons compared to the provisions of this international treaty.
Improve the precarious situation of indigenous peoples	A comprehensive system of safeguards for indigenous peoples' rights has already been established in the Russian Federation.

Sources: Russian Federation A–HRC–39–13_Add.1_RussianFederation_Annex_E

Hassler, A. (2019) *Making the link between human rights and the 2030 Agenda*, The Danish Institute for Human Rights, available at: https://sdgdata.humanrights.dk/en/node/252884

Regional human rights monitoring

Regional human rights regimes are independent, human rights sub-regimes that are nested within the international human rights framework, but that sit outside of national human rights regimes (see Chapter 3). There are three key regional human rights instruments; the African Charter on Human and Peoples' Rights, the American Convention on Human Rights, and the European Convention on Human Rights that will be discussed here. These were introduced along with other regional systems in Chapter 4. While each of these regimes shares some similarities, they vary widely in their approach to human rights and their record of human rights protection.

The African Charter on Human and Peoples' Rights

The African Charter on Human and Peoples' Rights (the Banjul Charter), first introduced in Chapter 3, sets out the rights and obligations relating to human rights for fifty-three African states. Oversight and interpretation of the Charter is the task of the African Commission on Human and Peoples' Rights, established in November 1987 in Addis Ababa, Ethiopia, and is now headquartered in Banjul, The Gambia. The Commission is a quasi-judicial body that is responsible for the protection and promotion of rights, and the interpretation of the provisions of the Charter. The Commission can investigate and research relevant issues and can organise a wide range of meetings and symposia on issues of human rights. The Commission can receive communications from individuals as well as states, with the preference for any problem to be solved through a local remedy.

On receipt of communications from individuals or organisations (other than states), the Commissioners vote on whether the communication should be considered, the decision being with the majority. Once it is decided that a communication is to be considered, the relevant state concerned is notified and, if after deliberation it appears that there are serious or massive violations of rights involved, the Commission will report this to the Assembly of Heads of State and Government who may request the Commission to undertake an in-depth study; in cases of emergency the Chairperson of the Assembly may request a study.

As of 13 March 2019, 229 decisions in relation to communications have been documented on the Commission's website, covering the period 1988 to 2018. They relate to forty-four of the fifty-five countries in the African Union (AU). The two articles most closely connected to the right to health (Articles 16 and 18) are involved in twenty-eight of these decisions and involve sixteen countries. The majority of the communications related to the consequences of armed conflict within or between states and arrest, detention and torture, others involve systematic discrimination against particular national or ethnic groups.

The Charter did not establish a human rights court to apply or to enforce the rights provided by the Charter. At the time, there was little support for a human rights court, with some claiming that such a mechanism was 'alien' to an African concept of justice (Ssenyonjo 2012). While others suggest that some African states were not prepared to accept judicial scrutiny for human rights violations. A protocol to the Charter was adopted in 1998 allowing for the creation of an African Court on Human and Peoples' Rights, however, only nine of the thirty States Party to the Protocol recognise the Court to receive cases from NGOs and individuals (Evans and Murray 2008). In 2004, the African Court of Justice and Human Rights was founded through a merger of the African Court on Human and Peoples' Rights and the Court of Justice of the African Union. Of the fifty-three member states of the AU, thirty have recognised the court, but only seven member states allow NGOs and individuals to file cases.

While the gains made by the OAU/AU over the past few decades are positive and allow for a recognition of human rights in Africa, the attainment of human rights in the region is far from complete (Amnesty International 2018). Recent brutal and deadly clashes with protesters in Khartoum, Sudan have resulted in the AU suspending Sudan's membership and threatening the leadership with sanctions for failing to hand over power to a civilian-led government. Making matters more complicated, the military shut down the internet, thereby slowing the flow of information to and from Sudan (HRW 2019a). The people of Nigeria experienced violence related to the 2019 election, with Boko Haram increasingly playing a role the general instability. Similarly, in Cameroon, hundreds of people who support the opposition party have been arrested, with the government attempting to limit political dissent (HRW 2019a).

As of 2019, the court has received 202 cases, of which fifty-two have been finalised, four transferred, and 146 pending. Cases cover the following states: Benin, Burkina Faso, Côte d'Ivoire, Gabon, Ghana, Kenya, Libya, Malawi, Mali, Morocco, Nigeria, Rwanda, Senegal, South Africa, and Tanzania. Perhaps the most successful case relates to freedom of speech. In March 2014, the Court delivered a far-reaching decision on a case concerning the rights of journalists to practice their vocation free from intimidation or the fear of death. The court, in its first ruling on such matters, held that the failure of a government to diligently seek and bring to account the persons responsible for the assassination of a journalist, intimidates the media, stifles free expression, violates the human rights of journalists, and endangers truth. The journalist in question was Norbert Zongo, publisher and former editor of *l'Indépendant* in Burkina Faso, who was killed in December 1998 (Baker 2018).

At the time of his death, Zongo was working on a story about how a driver and domestic employee of the brother of the Prime Minister of Burkina Faso was tortured and killed for allegedly stealing money from his employer (Frère and Englebert 2015). A presidential commission later concluded that Zongo's killing was politically motivated, triggered by his journalistic investigation into the killing. While five members of Burkina Faso's presidential guards were implicated in the killing, only one was ever charged – charges that were subsequently dropped (Baker 2018). All efforts by Zongo's family and their lawyers to seek accountability for his killing were thwarted.

In 2011, Zongo's widow, instructed lawyers to make a final attempt at justice through the African Court. Almost two years after the case was originally filed and almost 15 years after Norbert was killed, his family finally had the opportunity to put their appeal for justice before a court not controlled by the government of Burkina Faso. Burkina Faso argued that its government could not be held responsible for failing to find the killers. However, in its judgment, the African Court decided that what Burkina Faso did was in effect a cover-up, which violated the African Charter on Human and Peoples' Rights, that the case was not properly investigated in Burkina Faso, and that the court action was too slow (Baker 2018).

American Convention on Human Rights

American Convention on Human Rights, introduced in Chapter 3, is an international human rights instrument for most of Latin America and parts of the Caribbean. There are two bodies responsible for overseeing compliance with the Convention: The Inter-American Commission on Human Rights (IACHR) and the Inter-American Court of Human Rights.

The Commission

The Commission is responsible for examining human rights of countries party to the American Convention. Those presenting petitions to the Commission must satisfy a number of conditions. First the petitioner must have exhausted all avenues open for remedying the situation in the country concerned, or, it must be shown that this has been tried, and failed due to lack of adequate due process, denial of access to remedies, or undue delay in decision. Once domestic remedies are exhausted, the petition must be presented within six months of the final decision in the domestic proceedings. If domestic remedies have not been exhausted, the petition must be presented within a reasonable time after the occurrence of the events complained about. The petition must also fulfil other minimal formal requirements which are set out in the Convention and the rules of procedure of the Commission.

When the Commission receives a petition that meets, in principle, all requirements, a number is assigned to the petition and its processing as a case begins. This decision to open a case does not prejudge the Commission's eventual decision on the admissibility or the merits of the case. Once a case is opened, the pertinent parts of the petition are sent to the government with a request for relevant information. During the processing of the case, each party is asked to comment on the responses of the other party. The Commission also may undertake its own investigations, which may include visits, and requests for specific information from parties involved. The Commission may also hold a hearing during the processing of the case, in which both parties are present. In almost every case, the Commission will also offer to assist the parties in negotiating a friendly settlement if they wish.

When the Commission decides that it has sufficient information, the processing of a case is completed. The Commission then prepares a report which includes its conclusions while also generally provides recommendations to the state concerned. This report is not public. The Commission gives the state a period to resolve the situation and to comply with the recommendations of the Commission. Upon the expiration of this period granted to the state, the Commission has two options. The Commission may prepare a second report, which is generally like the initial report and which also usually contains conclusions and recommendations. In this case, the state is again given a period to resolve the situation and to comply with the recommendations of the Commission, if such recommendations are made. At the end of this second period granted to the state, the Commission will usually publish its report, although the Convention does allow the Commission to decide otherwise.

Rather than preparing a second report for publication, the Commission may decide to take the case to the Inter-American Court. This must be done within three months of the date of transmission of the initial report to the state concerned. The initial report of the Commission will be attached to the application to the Court. The Commission will appear in all proceedings before the Court. The decision as to whether a case should be submitted to the Court or published is made according to the Commission's judgment about what is in the best interests of human rights.

The recommendations made by the Commission can be wide-ranging, including directions for the provision of services, resources and compensation to individuals affected, and well as recommendations regarding the policy and laws of the country against which the case is found. Recommendations are binding on member states, but enforcement lies with the state itself. Monitoring therefore is an important part of efforts to ensure full compliance with recommendations. The Commission follows up in detail the response of the member state to recommendations, publishing details of progress or lack of it in its annual reports and on their website.

A priority challenge identified by the Commission is to protect the right of children and adolescents to live free of violence and discrimination. During 2016, the Commission (2016) focused in particular on the workings of national child rights protection systems, the results of this examination were published in 2017 (IACHR 2017a). The report notes the gains made by states in establishing systems adapted to the obligations stemming from the Convention on the Rights of the Child, but identifies major challenges remaining and makes recommendations to meet these.

Finally, in direct relation to health, the Commission expressed its concern for the serious conditions in which the persons deprived of liberty find themselves: in facilities that are insufficient and inadequate; with serious overcrowding; with no access to drinkable water; with food inadequate in quantity and quality; with no access to health and sanitary services, education, and rehabilitation services (IACHR 2011). In 2016 the Commission noted the actions taken in a number of states to address this problem through focussing on reducing pretrial detention, and a project financed by Spain investigated measures aimed at reducing the use of pretrial detention throughout the region (IACHR 2016, 2017b) and resulted in the publication of a practical guide to reduce pretrial detention (IACHR 2017c).

The Court

The Inter-American Court of Human Rights, the judicial arm of the Convention, sits in San José, Costa Rica. The Court rules on whether a state has breached human rights against the Convention, not if an individual has. According to its Statute, the Court is an autonomous judicial institution, whose purpose is the interpretation and application of the American Convention on Human Rights. The Court consists of seven judges, elected in an individual capacity by secret ballot from candidates suggested by the States Party to the Convention. Judges serve for six years and may be re-elected only once; judges whose terms have expired continue to deal with those cases they have begun to hear.

Three different functions of the Court can be distinguished: adjudicatory, advisory, and the power to adopt provisional measures. In relation to adjudication, the cases before the Court are started by an application presented either by the Commission or by a state. The Court's judgments are final and not subject to appeal, but if within ninety days of the notification of the judgment there is disagreement regarding the sense or scope of the judgment, the Court can issue an interpretation of the judgment upon request of any of the parties involved. In 2017 the average duration of the proceedings in cases was 24.7 months, duration being calculated from the date the case is submitted to the Court to the date that the Court hands down judgment on reparations (IACHR 2018). Eighteen new cases were submitted for consideration in 2017, and as of December 2017, thirty-five cases were pending a decision by the Court (Inter-American Court of Human Rights 2018). The Court monitors compliance with judgments.

The advisory function involves the Court responding to consultations made by the member states of the Organization of American States (OAS), or the bodies of the OAS. This advisory competence strengthens the capacity of the organisation to solve matters that arise from the application of the Convention, since it allows the bodies of the OAS to consult the Court about relevant matters. Finally, the Court may adopt such provisional measures as considered necessary in cases of extreme gravity and urgency and when necessary in order to avoid irreparable damage to people, both in cases being processed before the Court and in matters that have not yet been submitted to it, upon request of the Commission. The resolutions that form the provisional measures are supervised by the Court.

Given how long the court has been in operation, there are a number of notable cases, and a significant body of law that has evolved from cased heard (Pasqualucci 2012). For example, the discrimination case of a Chilean judge who lost custody of her three daughters in 2004, after the Supreme Court of Chile ruled that allowing them to stay with their mother would leave them in a 'situation of risk' and turn them into 'objects of social discrimination'. The case, *Atala Riffo and Daughters v Chile*, was an LGBT-rights child custody case, which reviewed a Chilean court ruling from 2005, that awarded custody to a father because of the mother's sexual orientation (Celorio 2011). This was the first case the Inter-American Court took regarding LGBT rights (Paúl 2014). Atala Riffo separated from her husband in 2001, and originally reached a settlement and retained custody of the children. When it became know that she was a lesbian in 2002, her ex-husband sued for custody, with the case eventually heard by the Supreme Court of Chile (Celorio 2011). That court awarded the husband custody, saying that the relationship put the development of her children at risk. In 2008, the Inter-American Commission ruled that the case was admissible to the Court, as it concerned Article 24 of the American Convention on Human Rights concerning equal protection. In

2010, the Court ruled that sexual orientation was a was part of an individual's private life, and that in Atala Riffo had been discriminated against in the custody case in ways incompatible with the American Convention (Paúl 2014).

A more recent example relates to freedom of the press. The case of *Marcel Granier and other (Radio Caracas Television, RCTV) v. Venezuela*, relates to a Venezuelan television station RCTV that transmitted news coverage and opinion programs which were often critical to the then government of President Hugo Chavez (Global Freedom of Expression 2019). Following political turmoil in Venezuela between 2001 and 2002, Venezuelan government officials maintained that RCTV supported the coup against President Chávez, only covering the followers of the coup, but not the protests in favour of Chávez. RCTV's license to operate its news station was scheduled to end in 2007. After Chavez was reinstated as Venezuela's President in 2002, he criticised RCTV declaring that the station supported the coup, terrorism, and the destabilization of the Venezuelan government (Martínez 2016). The main issue before the Court was whether the Venezuelan government had violated RCTV's representatives right to freedom of expression under Article 13 of the American Convention of Human Rights. The Court considered that the decision to not renew RCTV's license was taken before it expired and that the decision to not renew came directly from the Executive branch (the President) and was a violation of freedom of speech (Martínez 2016).

The European Convention on Human Rights

The European Convention on Human Rights is an international treaty governing the human rights and political freedoms of people in Europe (see Chapter 3). The European Convention allowed for the establishment of the European Court of Human Rights (through Article 19), an international court that hears allegations of breaches of one or more of the human rights provisions concerning civil and political rights set out in the Convention and its protocols; the Court is located in Strasbourg, France. Both individuals and groups can lodge applications against a state to the Court. States that are judged to be in violation of the Convention are bound by the judgment and are obliged to execute it.

National laws in Europe have been overturned on the grounds that they contravene the European Convention on Human Rights (Neuwahl and Rosas 1995). The Court's jurisdiction in relation to health is limited, since the Convention on Human Rights does not contain a specific article on the right to health or the right to health care. An analysis of the cases dealt with by the court over the period 1959 to 2018 (European Court of Human Rights 2019) is summarised in Table 10.4; as this shows, the articles most often involved are those relating to timely access to justice (right to a fair trial, length of proceedings), followed by protection of property and right to liberty and security. The number of applications pending before the Court at the end of 2018 is around 56,000 (European Court of Human Rights 2019). Almost 72 percent of the pending cases concern six countries: Russia, Romania, Ukraine, Turkey, Italy, and Azerbaijan.

The Court has published two recent reports on case-law in relation to health-related issues and bioethics (European Court of Human Rights 2015, 2016). The first of these discusses the range of health-related cases brought before the court. It explains that health-related cases brought before the Court have most frequently been argued under Articles 2 (right to life), 3 (right to freedom from torture and inhuman or degrading treatment or

TABLE 10.4 Outcome of judgments and types of violation found by European Court of Human Rights, 1959–2018

Total number of judgments	*21,651*
Percentage of judgments finding at least one violation	84%
Percentage of judgments finding no violation	8%
Percentage of friendly settlements/Striking out judgments	5%
Percentage of other judgments (just satisfaction, revision judgments, preliminary objections, and lack of jurisdiction)	3%
Percentage of judgments with violation in respect of:	
Length of proceedings	27%
Right to a fair trial	23%
Right to liberty and security	17%
Protection of property	15%
Right to an effective remedy	12%
Inhuman or degrading treatment	10%
Right to respect for private and family life	6%
Freedom of expression	4%
Lack of effective investigation	4%
Non enforcement	2%
Right to life	2%
Prohibition of discrimination	1%
Freedom of assembly and association	1%
Prohibition of torture	1%
Other articles of the Convention	3%

Source: compiled from European Court of Human Rights 2019, pp. 178–179

punishment), 8 (respect for family and private life), and 14 (right to be free of discrimination) of the Convention (European Court of Human Rights 2015). The examples of cases given illustrate the potential of cases brought in terms of supporting access to health care for groups like prisoners and supporting action on health risks in the environment, such as traffic and other noise, as well as pollution.

The European Court of Human Rights has delivered over 16,000 judgments since its creation in 1959 (Council of Europe 2019b). Part of the strength of the Court is said to be that the Court interprets the Convention, rather than being bound by the intention of the drafters, allowing it to progressively incorporate any changing European social and legal developments (Helfer 1993). This evolving interpretation of the Court and the Convention has allowed a number of issues to be progressed and to make human rights issues more even across Europe.

In 2011, the Court heard a case relating to freedom of conscience and religion (Article 9). This case, *Bayatyan v Armenia*, concerned the conviction of a conscientious objector. When joining the Council of Europe in 2001, Armenia had agreed to introduce civilian service as an alternative to compulsory military service and to pardon all conscientious objectors sentenced to imprisonment. However, Bayatyan, a Jehovah's Witness, was imprisoned when he refused to perform military service (Council of Europe 2019b). The judge ruled that he was illegally imprisoned, and that Armenia was required to provide him with a civil option. This first ruling on a conscientious objection opens the way for others in similar positions to avoid military service and seek instead alternative civilian service (Muzny 2012).

In 1999 the Court heard a case related to the prohibition of torture (Article 3). This case, *Selmouni v France*, centred on a complaint of assault while in police custody in 1991. According to the Court, the acts of physical and mental violence inflicted on the applicant had caused 'severe' pain and been of a serious and cruel nature, and importantly caused problems that were not present when Selmouni was detained (Council of Europe 2019b). In its decision, the Court also made it clear that there was no requirement for intent to find that torture had occurred, but rather, if a state could not explain how the injuries occurred, then injury could be considered torture (Harper 2009).

Finally, a good example of the evolution of the Court since its creation is the case of *S. and Marper v United Kingdom* from 2008. This case was concerned with the right to privacy (Article 8) and focused on the retention by the authorities of fingerprints and DNA samples taken from the applicants during criminal proceedings against them, which did not result in their conviction (Council of Europe 2019b). The judges returned a unanimous verdict that Article 8 had been breached and the applicants were awarded a cash settlement. The United Kingdom were advised that they were to restrict the use of DNA profiles and establish a time-frame for removing this information from databases (Deray 2011).

National human rights monitoring

Many countries have their own human rights bodies to ensure that human rights are protected, and laws and regulations are adhered to. National human rights institutions (NHRI) are organisations that work to protect, promote, and monitor human rights at the country level. OHCHR encourages country level human rights bodies and instruments, measuring such organisations against an international benchmark; the Paris Principles (see Chapter 4). As of the end of 2018 there were 122 countries that have their own NHRI; seventy-nine were fully compliant with the Paris Principles, and a further thirty-three were partially compliant. Three of these countries are discussed here; Australia, Azerbaijan, and Ireland.

Australia

The Australian Human Rights Commission is an accredited NHRI. The current system for the protection of human rights in Australia is reliant on international, Commonwealth and state laws, and institutional arrangements. Australia has ratified all the main UN human rights treaties and Australia's record on human rights is generally regarded as comparatively good, with some important exceptions: Indigenous rights; treatment of refugees and asylum seekers and people with disabilities, and provision of mental health services. See for example, the documentation for the 2015 Universal Periodic Review for Australia, the latest UPR at time of writing. Australia also receives criticism for its lack of comprehensive national human rights laws, and lack of attention to full range of economic and social rights including health care and housing (Lynch 2009; Mapulanga-Hulston and Harpur 2009).

The first policy of the first federal Parliament of Australia was the White Australia Policy, since this time the Australian Government has violated the human rights of Aboriginal and Torres Strait Islander people in many ways including through the restriction of movement. Until 1967 Aboriginal and Torres Strait Islander people were not allowed access to public places such as pubs, swimming pools and public transport. Aboriginal and Torres Strait Islander people experienced widespread discrimination and inequalities. Much of this discrimination was through laws set up to prevent Aboriginal and Torres Strait Islander people from participating in society as equals. These laws, practices and attitudes have had economic, social, psychological, and political consequences that are still witnessed today. In 2017, the published *Report of the Special Rapporteur on the rights of Indigenous peoples on her visit to Australia A/HRC/36/46/ Add.2* observes that the policies of the government do not duly respect the rights to self-determination and effective participation; contribute to the failure to deliver on the targets in the areas of health, education and employment; and fuel the escalating and critical incarceration and child removal rates of Aboriginal and Torres Strait Islanders. The report concludes that a comprehensive revision of those policies needs to be a national priority, and the consequences and prevalence of intergenerational trauma and racism must be acknowledged and addressed.

The UN system has helped to effect positive change in Australia. One example is the Human Rights Committee's (as the monitoring committee for the ICCPR is called) adverse opinion in the Toonen case concerning the criminal laws relating to homosexuality in Tasmania. This resulted from a 1991 communication made by an individual, Toonen, arguing that the laws violated his rights as a homosexual man. The challenged provisions of the Tasmanian legislation were said to violate the articles of the ICCPR in three respects: The first of these was that the legislation made no distinction between sexual activity in public and in private and thus brought private activity into the public domain. Second, the legislation distinguished between individuals in the exercise of their right to privacy on the basis of sexual activity, sexual orientation, and sexual identity, thus discriminating in its effects. Third, the legislation did not outlaw homosexual activity between consenting homosexual women in private, outlawing only some forms of consenting heterosexual activity between adult men and women in private, again showing discrimination.

Toonen's communication was lodged in 1991, and the Committee reported its views in 1994 (United Nations Human Rights Committee Views on Communication, No. 488/1992, adopted 31 March 1994). Australia summarised its response to this in its third report to the Human Rights Committee (CCPR/C/AUS/98/3: 4–5, paras 12–14), where it reported that:

12 *Sections 122 (a) and (c) and 123 of the 1924 Criminal Code of Tasmania made homosexual sexual activity a criminal offence in Tasmania. The author of communication 488/1992 alleged that these provisions were discriminatory under the terms of Articles 2.1, 17 and 26 of the Covenant.*

13 *The Human Rights Committee declared the communication admissible on 5 November 1992 and published its final views on 31 March 1994. It found that sections 122 (a) and (c) and 123 of the Tasmanian code were an Arbitrary interference with privacy and placed Australia in breach of article 17.*

14 *In response to the Committee's views, the Federal Attorney-General held discussions with the Tasmanian Premier and Attorney-General. The Tasmanian Government's position was that no action would be taken in response to the Committee's findings. Accordingly, the Federal Government introduced legislation to provide protection for all Australians from arbitrary interferences with sexual privacy. The legislation, entitled the Human Rights (Sexual Conduct) Act, came into force on 19 December 1994.*

This laid the basis for further challenge to the Tasmanian Criminal code, this time in the Australian High Court. Eventually, in 1998 Tasmanian Anti-Discrimination Act passed into law, hailed by Croome (quoted in Bernardi 2001) as 'one of the best pieces of anti-discrimination legislation in the country'. A full discussion of the case can be found in Editors (1994) and Bernardi (2001).

Probably the most famous human rights case is the *Mabo v Queensland* case. This case, heard before the High Court, considered Eddie Mabo's claim that he had native title over his traditional lands in the Torres Strait (Simpson 1993). The Mabo decision altered the foundation of land law in Australia by overturning the doctrine of terra nullius (land belonging to no-one) on which British claims to possession of Australia were based. The High Court found that, on the assumption that Aboriginal and Torres Strait Islander people did have title to their traditional land, the Queensland law was discriminatory because it took away property rights from Aboriginal and Torres Strait Islander people, and not from anybody else (Hill 1995). The High Court later went on to consider whether, under Australian law, Aboriginal and Torres Strait Islander people did have title to their traditional land. This decision of the High Court was followed by the *Native Title Act 1993* (Cth). This Act attempted to codify the implications of the decision, providing a legislative framework under which Australia's Aboriginal and Torres Strait Islander people could seek recognition of their native title rights. By 2018, Native Title covered approximately 35 percent of Australia's land mass (AIATSIS 2018).

More recently in relation to Native Title legislation is the case of the Carmichael coal mine in central Queensland. The proposed mine site sits on the land of the Wangan and Jagalingou people, who have rejected all applications for a permit for the mine, a requirement for any activity on land which is claimed under Native Title. In late August 2019, the Queensland Government extinguished the Native Title in order to make way for the mine, including over lands that are used for ceremonial purposed.

A final important case to be heard in Australia was that of *McBain v Victoria* (2000). This case centred on a Melbourne gynaecologist, Dr John McBain, who, under Victorian law, was prohibited from assisting Ms Lisa Meldrum, a single woman, to conceive using IVF treatment (Human Rights Commission 2009). At the time, assisted reproductive services were only available to married, heterosexual couples (Walker 2000). McBain challenged the Victorian law in the Federal Court and argued that it was inconsistent with the Sex Discrimination Act, which prohibits discrimination in the provision of goods and services on the grounds of sex or marital status. Justice Sundberg of the Federal Court agreed. The decision was unsuccessfully challenged in the High Court by the Australian Catholic Bishops Conference. As a result of this case, the Victorian Infertility Treatment Act of 1995 was amended to allow heterosexual couples in a de facto relationship access to assisted reproductive services (Walker 2000), the law was later amended to allow people in same-sex relationships to access assisted reproductive technologies (Fiske and Weston 2014).

Azerbaijan

The establishment of the role of the Commissioner for Human Rights gave the Republic of Azerbaijan for the first time an Ombudsman for whose job it was to consider and protect human rights. The Ombudsman is also the country's NHRI. The first Ombudsman, Elmira Süleymanova, was elected by the Parliament on 2 July 2002, and was reappointed in 2010 for a second term. Human rights in Azerbaijan are inscribed within the Constitution, adopted in 1995, and include the rights of minorities, property rights, equality rights, intellectual property rights, civil rights, the rights of the accused, the right to strike, social security, the right to vote, and freedom of speech, conscience and thought.

Azerbaijan gained independence in 1991 and admission to the UN in 1992. However, the first few years of an independent Azerbaijan were characterised by a series of coups, violence, corruption, and a weak economy. With the election of Prime Minister Ilham Aliyev in 2003, Azerbaijan has made a number of positive gains, including the establishment of a market economy, and political and social reform. However, despite having ratified of fifteen of the eighteen UN human rights treaties, and recently chairing the Council of Europe, in practice, human rights in Azerbaijan are not universal, with serious breaches of human rights regularly occurring (Knaus 2015).

While the Constitution of Azerbaijan includes a right to freedom of speech, this is rarely applied in practice. After several years of decline in press and media freedom, in 2014, media freedom deteriorated with the government campaigning to silence opposition and criticism, even while the country led the Committee of Ministers of the Council of Europe (May – November 2014). The most recent annual report of the Ombudsman includes concerns related to the unethical, non-professional, incompatible, or incomplete ways that some government ministers respond to journalists' questions (Commissioner for Human Rights (Ombudsman) of the Republic of Azerbaijan 2019). Azerbaijan has also been known to act with impunity and violence toward journalists, with ten journalists currently imprisoned in Azerbaijan (Council of Europe 2019a).

Despite Azerbaijan appearing to have much of the human rights machinery required for the protection and promotion of human rights at a national level, government interference, bribery, and corruption, have meant that the potential of the NHRI of Azerbaijan have not been realised. International observers have suggested that the most recent Presidential elections were not free or fair, and a large number of human rights defenders, journalists, and activists are imprisoned as a result of a lack of respect for human rights (HRW 2019b).

Ireland

Human rights in Ireland are protected under both the Irish Constitution and European provisions, with the Irish Human Rights and Equality Commission overseeing human rights. Human rights protected in the Irish constitution include equality before the law, a prohibition on titles of nobility, the right to life, person, good name, and property rights of every citizen, the right to liberty, protection against sex discrimination, inviolability of the home and private property, freedom of speech, religion, assembly, and association, education, the probation of the death penalty, the guarantee of due process under the law, and the probation against retroactive laws.

The protection and promotion of human rights and equality in Ireland are undertaken by the independent Irish Human Rights and Equality Commission, Ireland's NHRI. Established in 2014, the Commission has a mandate under the Irish Human Rights and Equality Commission Act 2014. Ireland has undergone massive changes over recent years, probably the most notable was the repeal of the eighth amendment of the Constitution, prohibiting abortion. In 2018 this amendment was repealed through a constitutional referendum, with 66.4 percent of the vote. In the lead up to this vote, the Commission advised the Government of the Republic of Ireland that it should engage in constitution reform, as a matter of healthcare policy, and that to do so would be in keeping with its obligations under international human rights law (Irish Human Rights and Equality Commission 2018). The Regulation of Termination of Pregnancy Bill passed in the Irish Parliament on 13 December 2018, and came into force in January 2019, allowing for termination of a pregnancy up to twelve weeks. Prior to the change in legislation, abortion was only permitted when there was a risk to the woman's life; in other cases abortion could lead to a sentence of fourteen years imprisonment (Taylor et al. 2019).

During 2017, the Commission represented thirty-three cases, including cases related to discrimination on the basis of disability, nationality, and gender. In one case, the Commission represented a family who were living in a house without basic facilities (including running water), while they waited for the local council to assess their application for another house. The family argued that by deferring their housing application, the decision negatively impacted the rights of their children, such as their right to bodily integrity, to dignity, to freedom from degrading conditions, to nurture and support within the family structure, and to education (Irish Human Rights and Equality Commission 2018). The decision was that the local council was required to reconsider the family's request for social housing. While in another case, members of a 'travelling community' were denied service at a local licenced premise. The group entered the premises, and when they attempted to order drinks, they were refused with staff claiming that only regulars were being served that night (Irish Human Rights and Equality Commission 2018). The case was settled, and the staff were required to undertake a course of equality training.

Ongoing monitoring

With increased mechanisms for the monitoring and enforcement of human rights at all levels, increased resourcing will be needed to keep up with demand. There are considerable time delays between the lodging of complaints and the rulings and decisions of the relevant bodies at the global, regional, and national levels. A further challenge is the volume of cases accumulating in the systems, as seen here, there are many more cases pending then there have been cases heard. Without greater attention paid to all levels of the human rights monitoring systems, further delays will accumulate, undermining the effective functioning of systems.

References

Abebe, AM 2009. Of shaming and bargaining: African states and the Universal Periodic Review of the United Nations Human Rights Council, *Human Rights Law Review*, 9(1): 1–35. doi.org/10.1093/hrlr/ngn043

AIATSIS 2018. *Native Title Newsletter* [Online], Canberra. Available: https://aiatsis.gov.au/sites/default/files/products/native_title_newsletter/1802_nativetitlenewsletter_final_web_0.pdf [Accessed 17/09/2019].

Amnesty International 2018. *Rights Today in Africa-2018* [Online], Kenya. Available: www.amnesty.org/en/latest/research/2018/12/rights-today-2018-africa/ [Accessed 17/09/2019].

Baker, C 2018. Burkinabè dictator-Novels and the Struggle against Impunity, *Research in African Literatures*, 49(3): 116–130. doi.org/10.2979/reseafrilite.49.3.08

Bernardi, G 2001. From conflict to convergence: The evolution of Tasmanian anti-discrimination law, *Australian Journal of Human Rights*, 7(1): 134–154. doi.org/10.1080/1323238X.2001.11911054

Celorio, RM 2011. The case of Karen Atala and daughters: Toward a better understanding of discrimination, equality, and the rights of women, *City University of New York Law Review*, 15: 335. doi.org/10.31641/clr150216

Commissioner for Human Rights (Ombudsman) of the Republic of Azerbaijan 2019. *Annual Report*, Baku: Commissioner for Human Rights (Ombudsman) of the Republic of Azerbaijan.

Council of Europe 2019a. *Democracy at Risk: Threats and Attacks against Media Freedom in Europe*, Annual Report, Strasbourg: Council of Europe.

Council of Europe 2019b. *The European Convention on Human Rights* [Online]. Available: www.coe.int/en/web/human-rights-convention/landmark-judgments [Accessed 17/09/2019].

Deray, ES 2011. The Double-Helix Double-Edged Sword: Comparing DNA retention policies of the United States and the United Kingdom, *Vanderbilt Journal of Transnational Law*, 44: 745.

Dominguez-Redondo, E 2012. The universal periodic review: Is there life beyond naming and shaming in human rights implementation?, *New Zealand Law Review*, 4: 673–706.

Editors 1994. Gay rights victory at UN-I, *Human Rights Defender*, 1. Available: www.austlii.edu.au/au/journals/HRD/1994/1.html [Accessed 03/08/2019].

European Court of Human Rights 2015. *Thematic Report: Health-Related Issues in the Case-Law of the European Court of Human Rights, Council of Europe*, Strasbourg: Council of Europe/European Court of Human Rights.

European Court of Human Rights 2016. *Research Report: Bioethics and the Case-Law of the Court*, Strasbourg: Council of Europe/European Court of Human Rights.

European Court of Human Rights 2019. *Annual Report 2018 of the European Court of Human Rights, Council of Europe*, Strasbourg: Registry of the European Court of Human Rights.

Evans, M, & Murray, R 2008. *The African Charter on Human and Peoples' Rights: The System in Practice 1986–2006*, Cambridge, UK, Cambridge University Press. doi.org/10.1017/CBO9780511493966

Fiske, E, & Weston, G 2014. Utilisation of ART in single women and lesbian couples since the 2010 change in Victorian legislation, *Australian and New Zealand Journal of Obstetrics and Gynaecology*, 54(5): 497–499. doi.org/10.1111/ajo.12260

Frère, M-S, & Englebert, P 2015. Briefing: Burkina Faso: The Fall of Blaise Compaoré, *African Affairs*, 114(455): 295–307. doi.org/10.1093/afraf/adv010

Gaer, FD 2007. A voice not an echo: Universal Periodic Review and the UN treaty body system, *Human Rights Law Review*, 7(1): 109–139. doi.org/10.1093/hrlr/ngl040

Global Freedom of Expression 2019. *Granier (Radio Caracas Television) v. Venezuela* [Online]. Available: https://globalfreedomofexpression.columbia.edu/cases/granier-v-venezuela/ [Accessed 17/09/2019].

Harper, J 2009. Defining torture: Bridging the gap between rhetoric and reality, *Santa Clara Law Review*, 49: 893.

Hassler, A. (2019) *Making the Link Between Human Rights and the 2030 Agenda* [Online], The Danish Institute for Human Rights. Available: https://sdgdata.humanrights.dk/en/node/252884 [Accessed 08/02/2020].

Helfer, LR 1993. Consensus, coherence and the European convention on human rights, *Cornell International Law Journal*, 26: 133.

Hill, RP 1995. Blackfellas and whitefellas: Aboriginal land rights, the Mabo decision, and the meaning of land, *Human Rights Quarterly*, 17: 303. doi.org/10.1353/hrq.1995.0017

HRW 2019a. *Africa* [Online], New York. Available: www.hrw.org/africa [Accessed 11/06/2019].

HRW 2019b. *Azerbaijan: Events of 2018* [Online]. Available: www.hrw.org/world-report/2019/country-chapters/azerbaijan [Accessed 17/06/2019].

Human Rights Commission 2009. *Human Rights 21: From the Bench: Landmark Human Rights Cases* [Online]. Available: www.humanrights.gov.au/our-work/human-rights-21-bench-landmark-human-rights-cases

IACHR 2011. *Annual Report of the Inter-American Commission on Human Rights 2010*, Washington: Inter-American Commission on Human Rights.

IACHR 2016. *Annual Report of the Inter-American Commission on Human Rights 2016*, Washington: Inter-American Commission on Human Rights.

IACHR 2017a. *Towards the Effective Fulfilment of Children's Rights: National Protection Systems*, Washington: Inter-American Commission on Human Rights/Organization of American States.

IACHR 2017b. *Report on Measures Aimed at Reducing the Use of Pretrial Detention in the Americas*, Washington: Inter-American Commission on Human Rights/Organization of American States.

IACHR 2017c. *Practical Guide to Reduce Pretrial*, Washington: Inter-American Commission on Human Rights/Organization of American States.

IACHR 2018. *Annual Report 2018* [Online]. Available: www.oas.org/en/iachr/docs/annual/2018/TOC.asp [Accessed 03/08/2019].

Info UPR 2014. *Beyond Promises: The Impact of the UPR on the Ground*, Geneva, Switzerland, UPR Info.

Info UPR 2016. *The Butterfly Effect: Spreading Good Practices of UPR Implementation*, Geneva, Switzerland, UPR Info.

Irish Human Rights and Equality Commission 2018. *Annual Report, 2017*, Dublin: Irish Human Rights and Equality Commission.

Knaus, G 2015. Europe and Azerbaijan: The end of shame, *Journal of Democracy*, 26(3): 5–18. doi.org/10.1353/jod.2015.0040

Lynch, P 2009. Australia, human rights and foreign policy, *Alternative Law Journal*, 34(4): 218–226. doi.org/10.1177/1037969X0903400401

Mapulanga-Hulston, JK, & Harpur, PD 2009. Examining Australia's compliance to the International Covenant on economic, social and cultural rights: Problems and potential, *Asia-Pacific Journal on Human Rights and the Law*, 10(1): 48–66. doi.org/10.1163/138819009X12589762582574

Martínez, MC 2016. Granier v. Venezuela, *American Journal of International Law*, 110(1): 109–115. doi.org/10.5305/amerjintelaw.110.1.0109

Moss, LC 2010. Opportunities for nongovernmental organization advocacy in the Universal Periodic Review process at the UN Human Rights Council, *Journal of Human Rights Practice*, 2(1): 122–150. doi.org/10.1093/jhuman/hup031

Muzny, P 2012. Bayatyan v Armenia: The grand chamber renders a grand judgment, *Human Rights Law Review*, 12(1): 135–147. doi.org/10.1093/hrlr/ngr050

Neuwahl, N, & Rosas, A (eds.) 1995. *The European Union and Human Rights*, The Hague: Kluwer Law International.

OHCHR 2019. *Universal Periodic Review* [Online]. Available: www.ohchr.org/en/hrbodies/upr/pages/uprmain.aspx [Accessed 12/06/2019].

Pasqualucci, JM 2012. *The Practice and Procedure of the Inter-American Court of Human Rights*, Cambridge: Cambridge University Press. doi.org/10.1017/CBO9780511843884

Paúl, Á 2014. Examining Atala-Riffo and Daughters v. Chile, the first inter-American case on sexual orientation, and some of its implications, *Inter-American and European Human Rights Journal*, 7: 54.

Simpson, G 1993. Mabo, international law, terra nullius and the stories of settlement: An unresolved jurisprudence, *Melbourne University Law Review*, 19: 195.

Ssenyonjo, M 2012. *The African Regional Human Rights System: 30 Years after the African Charter on Human and Peoples' Rights*, Leiden: Brill/Nijhoff. doi.org/10.1163/9789004218154_022

Taylor, M, Spillane, A, & Arulkumaran, S 2019. The Irish journey: Removing the shackles of abortion restrictions in Ireland, *Best Practice & Research Clinical Obstetrics & Gynaecology*. doi.org/10.1016/j.bpobgyn.2019.05.011

Terman, R, & Voeten, E 2018. The relational politics of shame: Evidence from the Universal Periodic Review, *The Review of International Organizations*, 13(1): 1–23. doi.org/10.1007/s11558-016-9264-x

Walker, KL 2000. Equal access to assisted reproductive services: The effect of McBain v Victoria, *Alternative Law Journal*, 25(6): 288–291. doi.org/10.1177/1037969X0002500606

11

RESPONDING TO BREACHES OF HUMAN RIGHTS

Fiona H. McKay and Ann Taket

Introduction

While the Universal Periodic Review (UPR) system, presented in Chapter 10, works to pro-mote human rights through capacity building, encouragement, and peer-pressure, there are times when a more direct approach needs to be taken to remedy serious breaches of human rights. This chapter focuses on the role of intergovernmental courts, such as the International Criminal Court and the ad hoc courts in addressing serious human rights breaches. This chapter also includes a short overview of the steps taken to achieve the current system of international courts.

Crimes committed during times of war have been prosecuted for centuries; researchers have found records of war courts from time of the ancient Greeks (Schabas 2011). More recent approaches to prosecuting human rights breaches in times of war can be found in the laws applied by Abraham Lincoln to the Union Army during the American Civil War, referred to as the Lieber Code. These laws describe inhumane conduct, and detail the pen-alties, including the death penalty, for pillage, rape, and abuse of prisoners (Meron 1998). Unlike current practices, justice taken against war crimes in these early examples occurred in national, not international, courts.

Current responses to war crimes have advanced through the adoption of a number of conventions and treaties. The Geneva Conventions are the standards of international law for humanitarian treatment in war. Proposed in 1864, these laws were concerned with the treat-ment of the sick and wounded, and the treatment of prisoners, and were complimented by other declarations concerned with how international wars should be conducted (Perrigo and Whitman 2010). Gustave Moynier, one of the founders of the International Committee of the Red Cross, was a long-time proponent of an international court to deal specifically with breaches of the humanitarian law outlined in the Geneva Conventions (Hall 1998). However, almost another century passed before states agreed to an international court. At the time, most states preferred to settle breaches of humanitarian law through publicity, diplomacy, and arbitration.

These initial discussions resulted in the Hague Conventions of 1899 and 1907. These Conventions are a series of treaties, drafted at the conclusion of two international peace conferences that represent the first real steps toward the creation of an international treaty for the laws of war and for war crimes. The Hague Conventions were intended to impose obligations on States, rather than creating criminal liability for individuals, and as the Conventions stop short of proposing any sanction for a violation, some acts are described as illegal but not as criminal (Schabas 2011).

At the conclusion of the First World War, and with many aspects of the Hague Convention violated, calls were made for states to be investigated for crimes committed during the war. However, with no system for the prosecution of international crimes, and with the United States in particular arguing that a state could not be charged with a crime that did not exist at the time it was committed, such calls went unheard. The United States was also concerned about the attribution of a breach of international conventions, and for crimes against the 'laws of humanity', including atrocities that occur within a state's borders, suggesting that these were a question of morality, not law (Schabas 2011). Other countries disagreed with this approach, and in the end a compromise was reached that saw the 'laws of humanity' dropped (Röhl 2014).

The First World War officially came to an end with the signing of the Treaty of Versailles. Among other things, the Treaty allowed for the creation, by the victors, of military tribunals to try soldiers and leaders accused of war crimes by Allied governments (Maogoto 2004). Germany protested the terms of the agreement, and instead proposed trying offenders in German courts, trials now referred to as the Leipzig War Crimes Trials. The number of soldiers accused was close to 1600 at the beginning of the trials, however, through negotiation this was reduced to a handful of soldiers who either escaped conviction, or received short terms, often the periods already served (Schabas 2011). These trials also dealt with the sinking of two hospital ships by German forces, the Dover Castle and the Llandovery Castle, however, the cases were ultimately unsuccessful, with one soldier pleading innocence as he was following orders, and another receiving a short jail term (Kramer 2006).

While these trials were regarded as a failure at the time, dissatisfaction at this lack of a mechanism to deal with war crimes lead to greater discussion about the importance of international law during and after the Second World War (Kramer 2006). With the conclusion of the Second World War and the clear evidence of atrocities that had been committed, the Allied forces were committed to prosecuting those responsible for war crimes. A UN body was created specifically to investigate and prosecute war crimes, consisting of the four main powers; the United Kingdom, France, the United States, and the Soviet Union, this laid the groundwork for the prosecutions at of Nazis at Nuremberg and the Japanese at Tokyo through the establishment of two Charters of the International Military Tribunal (IMT) (Schabas 2011).

Nuremberg Tribunal

The Nuremberg Tribunal had jurisdiction over four categories of offence (see Table 11.1): crimes against peace (including planning, initiating and waging wars of aggression or wars in violation of international treaties); war crimes (including any violation of the rules of war that were created through the Geneva Conventions and related documents); crimes against humanity (including extermination, deportation, and genocide); and the planning of any of the three above crimes, this meant that a person could be convicted of a crime against humanity even if they themselves did not put a person to death (Reginbogin et al. 2006). The trials garnered significant interest, due largely to the prosecution of prominent members

TABLE 11.1 Definitions used in international criminal tribunals

The term **Crimes against humanity** has existed for at least a century and refers to acts that are deliberately committed as part of a widespread or systematic attack or individual attack directed against any civilian or an identifiable part of a civilian population. The first prosecution for crimes against humanity took place at the Nuremberg trials, and such crimes have since been prosecuted by other international and domestic courts. The law of crimes against humanity has not been codified in international law, however, it is now considered customary international law. Unlike genocide, crimes against humanity do not need to target a specific group, but rather, the victim of the attack can be any civilian population, regardless of its affiliation or identity. It is also not necessary to prove that there is an overall specific intent; it is enough for there to be intent to commit any of the acts listed, with the exception of the act of persecution, which requires additional discriminatory intent.

Genocide is intentional action to destroy a people (usually defined as an ethnic, national, racial, or religious group) in whole or in part. The word 'genocide' was first coined by Polish lawyer Raphäel Lemkin in 1944 and consists of the Greek prefix *genos*, meaning race or tribe, and the Latin suffix *cide*, meaning killing. The UN Genocide Convention was established in 1948 and defines genocide as 'acts committed with intent to destroy, in whole or in part, a national, ethnic, racial or religious group.' The Genocide Convention has been ratified or acceded to by 149 states.

War crimes constitute a serious violation of the laws of war that gives rise to individual criminal responsibility. There is no one document that details all war crimes, but some can be found in the Hague and Geneva Conventions. Examples of war crimes include intentionally killing civilians or prisoners, torture or inhumane treatment, experimentation, destroying civilian property, taking hostages, rape, the use of child soldiers, pillaging, depriving a prisoner of war a trial, and intentionally attacking civilian populations.

See UN definitions for more information: www.un.org/en/genocideprevention

of the political, military, judicial, and economic leadership of Nazi Germany. Twenty-four Nazi leaders who planned, conducted, and participated in the Holocaust and other atrocities during the Second World War were indicted with major war crimes in trials over a twelve-month period. Nineteen defendants were convicted, and the death penalty was served in twelve cases, with the remaining five sentenced to lengthy prison terms. Trials of lesser war criminals were conducted at the US Nuremberg Military Tribunal, including the Doctors' and Judges' Trials.

While the Nuremberg trials were successful in seeing some of the worst criminals of the Holocaust receive justice, there are important criticisms of the Nuremberg trials that deserve brief exploration. The questions raised by some scholars surround the fairness of the justice provided. One objection to the Nuremberg trials surrounds the inclusion of the jurists from Allied nations who were not only involved in drafting the IMT Statute, but who also acted as prosecutors or judges, while no judge from a neutral nation was included (Burchard 2006). The second critique relates to the notion of retrospective justice, all of those prosecuted were tried for crimes which did not exist in law when they were committed (Schabas 2009). The final critique of the Nuremberg trials relates to notions of victor's justice. Victor's justice is the term used to describe a situation of injustice where a victorious entity applies 'justice' using different rules to judge themselves and the defeated party. The Nuremberg trials were focused only on prosecuting German nationals, ignoring the crimes committed by the Allied forces (Reginbogin et al. 2006). Despite these challenges, the Nuremberg trials initiated new ways of thinking about international law and the impact of law on individuals. Interestingly, the tribunal made it clear that following orders was not a reasonable defence against crimes against peace or humanity.

Nuremberg Code

After the completion of the main Nuremberg trials, the United States conducted twelve additional trials of representative Nazis from various sectors of the Third Reich, including law, finance, ministry, and manufacturing, before American Military Tribunals, also at Nuremberg (Shuster 1997). One of these trials, the Doctors' Trial, involved twenty-three defendants, accused of murder and torture in the conduct of medical experiments on concentration camp inmates. Sixteen were found guilty; seven were sentenced to death by hanging, and nine sentenced to terms of imprisonment. While the trials were ostensibly for murder, the judges were clear that these were 'no mere murder trial', because the defendants were physicians who had sworn to 'do no harm' and to abide by the Hippocratic Oath (Wunder 2000).

While the judges at Nuremberg made it clear that they understood Hippocratic ethics they also recognised that more was necessary to protect humans against unethical research. In response, the judges developed ten research principles centred not on the physician but on the participants in the research. These principles, the Nuremberg Code, included principles relating to consent, that the research should have some benefit to society, that the research should seek to minimise any pain or suffering of the participant, and that the participant should have the ability to withdraw from the research (Shuster 1997). While these principles have not been included in law, and have been updated and modernised several times, the concepts included in the Code have become important in the ethical conduct of medical research (Moreno et al. 2017).

Tokyo Tribunal

Two months after Germany surrendered and the war in Europe began to end, a number of Allied leaders met in Potsdam, Germany, to discuss peace settlements, but also to discuss the ongoing conflict in the Pacific. Despite calls for an end to the war, Japanese forces were committed to fighting and continued their takeover of territory in the region. At the Potsdam conference, leaders from the United States, the UK, and China drafted a declaration, the Potsdam Declaration, which defined the terms for Japan's surrender and outlined a number of warnings if the country failed to cease fighting. Despite the warnings, the war went on, and two nuclear weapons were dropped in August 1945, one on Hiroshima and one on Nagasaki, killing over 200,000 people, forcing Japan to surrender.

Before the surrender, the Allied forces had discussed plans for a military tribunal to address war crimes during the war in the Pacific. The International Military Tribunal for the Far East, known as the Tokyo trials, were convened in 1946 in Ichigaya, Tokyo. The trials were conducted to investigate crimes including conspiring to start a war, war crimes, and other crimes against humanity, for crimes relating to activities of the Second World War in the Far East. Unlike the Nuremberg trials, eleven countries (Australia, Canada, China, France, India, the Netherlands, New Zealand, the Philippines, the Soviet Union, the United Kingdom, and the United States) provided judges and prosecutors for the court, and the defence comprised Japanese and American lawyers. However, despite this varying representation of jurors, the Tokyo trials receive some of the same criticism as the Nuremberg trials, particularly though notions of victor's justice, and that once again, charges were made against actions that were not crimes when they were committed (Tanaka et al. 2011).

Twenty-eight Japanese military and political leaders were charged with a range of offenses including waging of an aggressive war, murder, and conventional war crimes committed against prisoners-of-war, civilian internees, and the inhabitants of occupied territories (Pritchard 1995). The defendants included former prime ministers, former foreign ministers, and former military commanders. Two defendants died during the proceedings, and one was ruled unfit to stand trial. All remaining defendants were found guilty of at least one count. Sentences ranged from seven years imprisonment to death (Tanaka et al. 2011).

In addition, 5700 lower-ranking personnel were charged with war crimes in separate trials convened all over the Asia Pacific. These charges included prisoner abuse, rape, sexual slavery, torture, ill-treatment of labourers, execution without trial, and inhumane medical experiments (Tanaka et al. 2011). Most of the defendants were found guilty of conventional war crimes, some were sentenced to death, but most were given prison terms (Wilson et al. 2017).

The ICTY and ICTR

Since the Nuremberg and Tokyo trials in the post-World War Two period, there have been a number of international criminal tribunals established to respond to atrocities committed during conflicts. Included among these ad hoc tribunals are the Extraordinary Chambers in the Courts of Cambodia, a national court established in partnership between the UN and the Government of Cambodia to investigate serious crimes committed during the Cambodian genocide, the Special Court for Sierra Leone, a national court established in partnership between the UN and the government of Sierra Leone, and the International Criminal Tribunal for the former Yugoslavia (ICTY) and International Criminal Tribunal for Rwanda (ICTR) which were both created by the UN Security Council. The final two courts will be discussed here as examples of more modern responses to serious crimes.

International Criminal Tribunal for the former Yugoslavia (ICTY)

The ICTY was established in 1993 in response to the Yugoslav Wars (1991–2001). The wars were characterised by ethnic conflicts, and wars of independence as states of the former Yugoslavia sought independence (Jansen 2005). Beginning in 1991, Croatian Serbs fought to prevent Croatia from seceding 'Greater Serbia' and attaining independence (MacDonald 2018). After several years of fighting, and 200,000 causalities, Croatia was successful in gaining independence (Obradović 2016). The following year, the new Republic of Bosnia and Herzegovina received international recognition. Similar to the experience in Croatia, in an attempt to protect Serb territories, Bosnian-Serb forces supported by Serbia, launched a war with the aim of establishing Serb control over parts of Bosnian territory (Rudolph 2001). The war in Bosnia was more protracted and deadlier than the Croatian experience. From the beginning of the war, Bosnian Serb forces carried out brutal policies of 'ethnic cleansing' including the forcible removal of Bosniak (the term used to describe Bosnians Muslim) and Croat populations from territories under Serb control (Bartrop 2016). This ethnic cleansing was designed to create ethnically distinct areas within the country. One half of Bosnia's pre-war population was forced to leave their homes by fleeing the country or seeking protection in areas of Bosnia dominated by their own ethnic group.

The ethnic cleansing culminated in the Srebrenica massacre of more than 8,000 Bosniak men and boys, and the deportation of more than 30,000 women and children in July 1995 (Bartrop 2016). The killings were perpetrated by units of the Bosnian Serb Army of Republika Srpska under the command of Ratko Mladić (Parks 2001). In April 1993 the UN declared the besieged enclave of Srebrenica a 'safe area' but provided only 600 lightly armed troops from the UN Protection Force 'UNPROFOR' to protect the area (ICTY 2001). Failure to demilitarise the armies surrounding Srebrenica, combined with a deteriorating humanitarian situation including a lack of food, water, and medical supplies, left of the area vulnerable to attack (Long 2006).

Realising that they could not be protected by the UN in Srebrenica, by the evening of 11 July 1995, approximately 20,000 to 25,000 Bosniak refugees, mostly women, children, and elderly, from Srebrenica made their way to Potočari, seeking protection within the UN Dutch battalion headquarters. Several thousand people had forced their way inside the compound itself, while the rest were spread throughout the neighbouring factories and fields. Over the following days, the refugees in the compound could see Bosnian Serb soldiers setting houses and haystacks on fire, and raping women. On 12 and 13 July 1995, the women, children, and elderly were bussed out of Potočari, under the control of the Bosnian Serb forces, to Bosnian Muslim held territory near Kladanj. Most people on the busses were unaware of where they were headed but left as they were desperate to get away from the horrors of Potočari (ICTY 2001).

Many of the women, children, and elderly, were able to reach safety, the men, however, were separated, and detained in Potočari. While some of these men were able to escape, forming the so-called column of men, many were executed in Potočari. The executions followed a pattern, the men were first taken to empty schools or warehouses, where they were detained for several hours, loaded onto buses or trucks and taken to another site, usually an isolated field, and then executed (Long 2006). Those who survived the initial round of shooting were individually shot with an extra round, although for some men, this occurred well after they had been initially shot leaving them to suffer (ICTY 2001). Their bodies were then bulldozed into mass graves (Parks 2001). Many of these executions were witnessed by UN troops, unable to do anything to prevent the killings.

Following the Srebrenica massacre, the North Atlantic Treaty Organization (NATO) launched a bombing campaign, which together with a ground offensive conducted by local troops, convinced the Bosnian Serb leadership to consider a negotiated settlement, the Dayton Agreement of December 1995. The Dayton Agreement brought an end to active combat and proposed the basic political structure of the present-day state (Cox 1999). A NATO-led peacekeeping force was immediately dispatched to the country to enforce the agreement. However, by the end of the war, more than 100,000 people had been killed, and millions displaced (Tabeau and Bijak 2005). Bosnia had endured what is routinely described as the worst atrocity in Europe since the Second World War (Bartrop 2016).

In response to the Srebrenica massacre (and other conflicts that involved the former Yugoslavia, now Serbia, Montenegro, and Croatia), many Bosnian Serb officials and soldiers have been convicted for their role in war crimes and crimes against humanity during the conflict, as well as for the genocide in Srebrenica. Several high-ranking Croat and Bosniak officials have also been convicted (Steinberg 2011).

Initially, those who were indicted were low level offenders, who played a comparatively minor role in the system of atrocities in Bosnia. These low-level indictments occurred firstly so that the court could show some success in its function, but also as it can be easier to prove the guilt of direct perpetrators than that of individuals who are the chief architects of systemic atrocities but who did not carry out atrocities themselves (Orentlicher 2010). Eventually these smaller offenders led to the prosecution of the leaders, charged with war crimes, crimes against humanity, and genocide; a total of 161 persons were indicted, with 90 found guilty and sentenced to imprisonment (ICTY 2019). Slobodan Milošević was the first sitting head of state indicted for war crimes, having been accused of war crimes in Bosnia, Croatia, and Kosovo, only to die of a heart attack while detained in his cell in The Hague (ICTY 2006).

The final case heard by the ICTY was that of Ratko Mladić. Mladić was the Bosnian Serb general, convicted of war crimes for crimes committed in Bosnia. On 24 July 1995, Mladić was indicted by the ICTY for genocide, crimes against humanity, and other war crimes, these charges were later expanded to include charges of war crimes for the attack on Srebrenica in July 1995 (ICTY 2017). In July 1996, the ICTY issued an international arrest warrant for Mladić, however, he evaded arrest until 2011, having been sheltered by Serbian and Bosnian Serb security forces and family. His capture was considered to be one of the preconditions for Serbia being awarded candidate status for European Union membership (Dragović-Soso 2012). On 22 November 2017, Mladić was sentenced to life in prison by the ICTY after being found guilty of 10 charges, one of genocide, five of crimes against humanity, and four of violations of the laws or customs of war. As the top military officer with command responsibility, Mladić was deemed by the ICTY to be responsible for both the siege of Sarajevo and the Srebrenica massacre (ICTY 2017). The ICTY formally ceased to exist on 31 December 2017, with any residual activities taken over by the Mechanism for International Criminal Tribunals.

International Criminal Tribunal for Rwanda (ICTR)

While the war in the Former Yugoslavia was still going, a large-scale conflict emerged in Rwanda. In response to violence in Rwanda, the UN Security Council, through Resolution 977 in November 1994, established the ICTR. The mandate of the ICTR was to judge people responsible for the Rwandan genocide, crimes against humanity, and violations of Common Article Three and Additional Protocol II of the Geneva Conventions (which deals with internal conflicts) in Rwanda, or by Rwandan citizens in nearby states, between 1 January and 31 December 1994. In addition, the court sort to foster national reconciliation between Hutu and Tutsi, and to strengthen the Rwandan legal system (Peskin 2005).

The Rwandan genocide refers to the mass slaughter of more than one million Rwandans, mostly Tutsis and politically moderate Hutus, by government-directed gangs of Hutu extremist soldiers and police, but also regular civilians who had been recruited and pressured to engage in the violence (Herr 2018). The war also featured widespread sexual violence against women, with some estimates suggesting that 500,000 women were raped during the war, with many thousands infected with HIV as a result (Donovan 2002). The duration of the Rwandan genocide is usually described as 100 days.

Tension between the Hutu and Tutsi developed over many decades but were particularly emphasised late in the nineteenth and early in the twentieth century as a result of German and then Belgian colonial rule in Rwanda, enabled by the mandate system of the League of Nations (Melvern 2006). The ethnic categorisation of Hutu and Tutsi were imposed, based largely on physical characteristics rather than ethnic background, as a way for colonial rulers to more effectively control the population. Under Belgium rule, all citizens of Rwanda carried an identity card that identified their ethnic group, a feature that would be exploited during the genocide (Caplan and Torpey 2001). Before the genocide, the Hutu were the majority population, but thanks to preferential treatment from Belgium colonial powers, the Tutsi minority had long dominated positions of power. By the time Rwanda gained independence in 1962, the situation had reversed, and the Hutus held power, forcing many Tutsi into exile in retaliation (LeBor 2006).

The genocide followed a civil war and decades of simmering tensions between Hutus and Tutsis but is generally agreed to have begun with the assignation of the Rwandan President, a Hutu, on 6 April 1994. A French Judge has blamed current president, Paul Kagame, at the time the head of the Tutsi rebel group, for the attack, while he in response blames Hutu extremists (Kosicki 2007). Either way, the death of President Habyarimana sparked immediate violence with a genocide targeting both Tutsis and moderate Hutus, including political leaders whose deaths created a political vacuum that was soon filled by Hutu extremists (Melvern 2006). For several months, thousands of Tutsi civilians, Hutu who looked like Tutsis, and Twa (an African Pygmy people) were shot, speared, clubbed, or hacked to pieces, with most of those killed, killed by hand (Herr 2018). Frequently the killers were people the victims knew personally, neighbours, colleagues, occasionally relatives through marriage. This devastation went on with little interference from the international community, despite both Belgium and UN troops being present in Rwanda at the time of the genocide.

The genocide was planned, and many say that the plans had been in motion for months, if not a year before killing actually began (Melvern 2006). While much of the killing during the Rwandan genocide was carried out by the radical Hutu groups, radio broadcasts were an integral part of the genocide, which encouraged Hutu civilians to kill their Tutsi neighbours (Yanagizawa-Drott 2014). This 'hate radio' was found to have incited violence, and those involved were found guilty of inciting genocide by the ICTR (Straus 2007).

By the time the ICTR completed its work, it had indicted ninety individuals, including high-ranking military and government officials, politicians, businessmen, and religious, militia, and media leaders, with sixty-two sentenced, and a further ten referred to national jurisdictions for trial. The main challenge during the initial period of the court was how to get the court to function under difficult conditions. The UN Security Council made the controversial decision to locate the seat of the Tribunal in Arusha, Tanzania, as no other location could service the needs of the international court, and it was decided that the for the trial to be just and fair, the proceedings needed be held in a neutral country (Møse 2005). Another controversial point was the ability to only to provide life in jail as the maximum sentence, many Rwandans regarded this insufficient, and as serving only to appease the conscience of the international community who did little to prevent the genocide (Cruvellier and Voss 2010).

Dissatisfied with the progress of the ICTR and the UN in general, and with the collapse of the government leaving Tutsi leaders with power, the Tutsi victors began to pursue their own efforts to render justice. Within the country, tens of thousands of Rwandans suspected of having taken part in the genocide were captured and jailed, with some tried at Gacaca courts. Gacaca courts are a form of community justice, designed to promote community healing, and allowed for cases to be heard much quicker than if they were heard in regular courts (Schabas 2005). At the same time, former leaders in exile were identified and international arrest warrants were prepared. However, before Rwandan courts could carry out these arrests, the ICTR informed Rwandan courts that the international court had precedence over national courts and that any person of interest to them would have to be sent to Tanzania, further infuriating the government and judiciary of Rwanda (Cruvellier and Voss 2010). This effectively established a two-tier system where those with the greatest responsibility for the genocide were tried at the ICTR while the remainder were left to national courts, meaning that those most responsible for genocide were put on trial with due process and, if convicted, the worst possible outcome was incarceration for life in prisons that met international standards. While lower-level perpetrators who were tried in Kigali were kept in custody in appalling conditions and subjected to the death penalty if found guilty (Rodman 2011).

Including convictions of those responsible for propaganda under the 'hate radio' case, a number of perpetrators of genocide and violence were found guilty. Jean-Paul Akayesu was found guilty of nine counts of genocide, and crimes against humanity including for the first-time rape as an activity of genocide, and former Rwandan Prime Minister Jean Kambanda became the first head of a government ever to be convicted of genocide by an international court. However, critics point to the number of high-profile acquittals, leaving many Rwandans doubting the ability of the ICTR to find justice. While others point to the discrepancy in indictments, with most indictments for crimes to be heard at the international court focused at Hutus and not to Tutsis who were also involved (Rodman 2011).

Despite these shortcomings, together with the ICTY, the ICTR has been credited with the establishment of a large body of international law. Importantly the successes and failures of these tribunals lead to the creation of the Permanent International Courts.

Permanent International Courts

The International Criminal Court (ICC) is a permanent court, that works as an intergovernmental organisation and sits in The Hague in the Netherlands. The ICC has the jurisdiction to prosecute individuals for the international crimes of genocide, crimes against humanity, war crimes, and crimes of aggression (Bassiouni 2012). The ICC is intended to complement existing national judicial systems (not to substitute for them) and operates when national courts are unwilling or unable to prosecute criminals, or when the UN Security Council or individual states refer situations to the Court.

While there had been calls for an international court after the Second World War, the Cold War interrupted this progress, and it was not until 1989 when, in response to a problem with drug trafficking, the Prime Minister of Trinidad and Tobago revived the idea of a permanent international criminal court (Schabas 2011). The progress of the court was again delayed, as while these discussions took place and a draft of the structure of the operation of the court was in progress, the Security Council had to establish the two ad hoc tribunals described above.

The ICC sits outside the UN, governed instead by a treaty, the Rome Statute, and is therefore only binding on States Party to that treaty (Bassiouni 2012). It is the first permanent, treaty based, international criminal court established to help end impunity for the perpetrators of the most serious crimes of concern to the international community. The ICC began functioning on 1 July 2002, the date that the Rome Statute entered into force, and cannot prosecute any crimes committed before this date (Schabas 2011). As of mid-2019, 122 states are party to the Rome Statute and therefore members of the ICC (United Nations 2019).

The United States is one of the key states opposed to the ICC. While the United States participated in negotiations leading up to the creation of the court (including playing key roles in the ad hoc international tribunals), in 1998 it was one of seven countries (including China, Iraq, Israel, Libya, Qatar, and Yemen) who voted against the Rome Statute (Scharf 1999). In 2000, President Bill Clinton signed the Rome Statute, but did not submit the treaty for ratification. In 2002, President George W. Bush sent a note to the UN Secretary General stating that the United States no longer intended to ratify the treaty and that it did not have any obligations toward it; however, the United States would not veto Security Council actions to refer cases to the ICC, with actions continuing to soften under President Obama. Under President Trump, the United States has been somewhat more hostile toward the ICC, imposing visa bans on ICC officials in March 2019 and stating that the United States will not cooperate with ICC investigations.

Other countries have withdrawn support from the ICC. In October 2016, after repeated claims that the court was biased against African states, Burundi, South Africa, and The Gambia announced their withdrawals from the Rome Statute; however, only Burundi acted on this withdrawal. The Philippines have also withdrawn from the Rome Statute, with the President of the Philippines, Rodrigo Duterte, claiming that the ICC was being used to attack weak states (Atienza 2019).

At mid-2019, the ICC has opened investigations in eleven situations, of which ten are in Africa: Burundi, Georgia, Central African Republic I and II, Mali, Cote d'Ivoire, Libya, Kenya, Sudan, Uganda, and Democratic Republic of Congo (ICC 2019). There are additionally preliminary examinations in eleven situations to determine whether they meet the legal criteria required to be investigated. These situations are in Afghanistan, Bangladesh, Colombia, Guinea, Iraq/the United Kingdom, Nigeria, Palestine, the Philippines, Ukraine, and Venezuela.

A few notable cases that have been decided by the ICC are worthy of further investigation here. There have been six cases from the Democratic Republic of Congo taken to the ICC. These cases relate to the war in Congo from 1998 until 2003, ultimately involving nine African countries, and resulting in the deaths of 5.4 million people, primarily through disease and starvation (Hawkins 2016). Arrest warrants have been made for six people involved: Thomas Lubanga Dyilo, Germain Katanga, Mathieu Ngudjolo Chui, Bosco Ntaganda, Callixte Mbarushimana, and Sylvestre Mudacumura for their involvement in war crimes and crimes against humanity, including conscripting, enlisting, and using child soldiers, committed in the context of armed conflict (ICC 2019). Several of these cases are ongoing, but by mid-2019, Lubanga and Katanga had been convicted and sentenced to fourteen and twelve years in prison, respectively; Chui was acquitted; and the case against Mbarushimana was dismissed. The case against Ntaganda is ongoing, and Mudacumura is considered a fugitive. As the ICC does not try individuals in their absence, this latter case will remain at the pretrial stage until he is captured (ICC 2019).

The ICC has an ongoing investigation into criminal acts committed in Darfur region of Sudan between 2003 and 2009–2010. Although Sudan is not a State Party to the Rome Statute, the situation in Darfur was referred to the ICC by the UN Security Council in 2005. Sudan's refusal to recognise the ICC has made finalising these cases more difficult (Du Plessis and Gevers 2005). So far, seven suspects have been indicted by the court accused of the crimes of genocide, crimes against humanity, and war crimes (ICC 2019). Of the seven suspects, one died before his case could be heard, and six remain at large, with the trials unable to continue until they have been arrested and brought to The Hague. The most famous, Omar al-Bashir, was the first sitting president to be indicted by the ICC. Both the Arab League and the African Union criticised the action, appealing to the UN Security Council to ask the ICC to freeze the indictment for twelve months (Ciampi 2008). Al-Bashir also travelled to a number of countries, all of which refused to arrest him and surrender him to the ICC upon arrival. After his recent defeat in the Sudanese national elections, al-Bashir was arrested and detained in a prison in Khartoum on a charge of inciting and killing protesters.

Responding to breaches of human rights into the future

Given the large number of ongoing and unresolved cases in front of the range of international courts, and the frequent disappointment with the role of the courts in brining perpetrators to justice, there is some concern about the role of these courts in the future. A general lack of resourcing and unprecedented demand further complicates and impinges on the impact of these courts. However, it is clear that when atrocities occur with no or little justice, they are repeated, and more people suffer. Some of the successes of the international system of justice has been truth telling, transparency, reparations, and documenting some of the most serious crimes, honouring the victims and shining a light on those involved. Holding people accountable for the crimes they commit, and ensuring justice through all levels of courts, is important in advancing and defending human rights.

References

Atienza, MEL 2019. The Philippines in 2018: Broken promises, growing impatience, *Asian Survey*, 59(1): 185–192. doi.org/10.1525/as.2019.59.1.185

Bartrop, PR 2016. *Bosnian Genocide: The Essential Reference Guide: The Essential Reference Guide*, Santa Barbara, CA: ABC-CLIO.

Bassiouni, MC 2012. *Introduction to International Criminal Law*, Brill Nijhoff. doi.org/10.1163/9789004231696

Burchard, C 2006. *The Nuremberg Trial and Its Impact on Germany*, Oxford: Oxford University Press. doi.org/10.1093/jicj/mql052

Caplan, J, & Torpey, J 2001. Identity cards, ethnic self-perception, and genocide in Rwanda, *Documenting Individual Identity: The Development of State Practices in the Modern World*, 345. doi.org/10.1515/9780691186856

Ciampi, A 2008. The proceedings against President Al Bashir and the prospects of their suspension under Article 16 ICC Statute, *Journal of International Criminal Justice*, 6(5): 885–897. doi.org/10.1093/jicj/mqn078

Cox, M 1999. The Dayton agreement in Bosnia and Herzegovina: A study of implementation strategies, *The British Year Book of International Law*, 69(1): 201. doi.org/10.1093/bybil/69.1.201

Cruvellier, T, & Voss, C 2010. *Court of Remorse: Inside the International Criminal Tribunal for Rwanda*, Madison, US: University of Wisconsin Press.

Donovan, P 2002. Rape and HIV/AIDS in Rwanda, *The Lancet*, 360: s17–s18. doi.org/10.1016/S0140-6736(02)11804-6

Dragović-Soso, J 2012. Apologising for Srebrenica: The declaration of the Serbian parliament, the European Union and the politics of compromise, *East European Politics*, 28(2): 163–179. doi.org/10.1080/21599165.2012.669731

Du Plessis, M, & Gevers, C 2005. Darfur goes to the international criminal court (perhaps), *African Security Studies*, 14(2): 23–34. doi.org/10.1080/10246029.2005.9627349

Hall, CK 1998. The first proposal for a permanent international criminal court, *International Review of the Red Cross Archive*, 38(322): 57–74. doi.org/10.1017/S0020860400090768

Hawkins, V 2016. *Stealth Conflicts: How the World's Worst Violence Is Ignored*, Abingdon, UK: Routledge. doi.org/10.4324/9781315242408

Herr, A 2018. *Rwandan Genocide: The Essential Reference Guide*, Santa Barbara, US: ABC-CLIO, LLC.

ICC 2019. *Situations under Investigation* [Online]. Available: www.icc-cpi.int/pages/situations.aspx [Accessed 04/06/2019].

ICTY 2001. *Case No. IT-98–33* [Online]. Available: www.icty.org/x/cases/krstic/tjug/en/krs-tj010802e.pdf

ICTY 2006. *Report to the President Death of Slobodan Milošević*, The Hague: ICTY.

ICTY 2017. *Mladić (IT-09–92)* [Online], The Hague: ICTY. Available: www.icty.org/case/mladic/4#custom5 [Accessed 21/07/2019].

ICTY 2019. *International Criminal Tribunal for the Former Yugoslavia* [Online]. Available: www.icty.org/en

Jansen, S 2005. National numbers in context: Maps and stats in representations of the post-Yugoslav wars, *Identities: Global Studies in Culture and Power*, 12(1): 45–68. doi.org/10.1080/10702890590914311

Kosicki, PH 2007. Sites of aggressor-victim memory: The Rwandan genocide, theory and practice, *International Journal of Sociology*, 37(1): 10–29. doi.org/10.2753/IJS0020-7659370101

Kramer, A 2006. The first wave of international war crimes trials: Istanbul and Leipzig, *European Review*, 14(4): 441–455. doi.org/10.1017/S1062798706000470

LeBor, A 2006. *'Complicity with Evil': The United Nations in the Age of Modern Genocide*, New Haven, CT: Yale University Press.

Long, L 2006. The Srebrenica massacre, *Forensic Examiner*, 15(2): 43.

MacDonald, DB 2018. Balkan holocausts? Serbian and Croatian victim-centred propaganda and the war in Yugoslavia. doi.org/10.7765/9781526137258

Maogoto, JN 2004. *War Crimes and Realpolitik: International Justice from World War I to the 21st Century*, Boulder, CO: Lynne Rienner Publishers.

Melvern, L 2006. *Conspiracy to Murder: The Rwandan Genocide*, New York: Verso.

Meron, T 1998. Francis Lieber's Code and principles of humanity, *Columbia Journal of Transnational Law*, 36: 269.

Moreno, JD, Schmidt, U, & Joffe, S 2017. The Nuremberg code 70 years later, *JAMA*, 318(9): 795–796. doi.org/10.1001/jama.2017.10265

Møse, E 2005. Main achievements of the ICTR, *Journal of International Criminal Justice*, 3(4): 920–943. doi.org/10.1093/jicj/mqi068

Obradović, S 2016. Don't forget to remember: Collective memory of the Yugoslav wars in present-day Serbia, *Peace and Conflict: Journal of Peace Psychology*, 22(1): 12. doi.org/10.1037/pac0000144

Orentlicher, DF 2010. *That Someone Guilty Be Punished: The Impact of the ICTY in Bosnia*, New York: Open Society Justice Initiative, International Center for Transitional Justice.

Parks, L 2001. Satellite views of Srebrenica: Tele-visuality and the politics of witnessing, *Social Identities*, 7(4): 585–611. doi.org/10.1080/13504630120107728

Perrigo, S, & Whitman, JR 2010. *The Geneva Conventions under Assault*, Chicago: Pluto Press.

Peskin, V 2005. Courting Rwanda: The promises and pitfalls of the ICTR Outreach Programme, *Journal of International Criminal Justice*, 3(4): 950–961. doi.org/10.1093/jicj/mqi072

Pritchard, RJ 1995. The international military tribunal for the Far East and its contemporary resonances, *Military Law Review*, 149(25).

Reginbogin, HR, Safferling, CJM, & Hippel, WR 2006. *The Nuremberg Trials: International Criminal Law since 1945: 60th Anniversary International Conference*, Nuremberg, Germany: K.G. Saur.

Rodman, KA 2011. International Criminal Tribunal for Rwanda (ICTR), in DK Chatterjee (ed.) *Encyclopedia of Global Justice*, Dordrecht: Springer Netherlands. doi.org/10.1007/978-1-4020-9160-5_718

Röhl, JC 2014. *Wilhelm II: Into the Abyss of War and Exile, 1900–1941*, Cambridge: Cambridge University Press. doi.org/10.1017/CBO9781139046275

Rudolph, C 2001. Constructing an atrocities regime: The politics of war crimes tribunals, *International Organization*, 55(3): 655–691. doi.org/10.1162/00208180152507588

Schabas, WA 2005. Genocide trials and gacaca courts, *Journal of International Criminal Justice*, 3(4): 879–895. doi.org/10.1093/jicj/mqi062

Schabas, WA 2009. Victor's justice: Selecting situations at the international criminal court, *The John Marshall Law Review*, 43: 535.

Schabas, WA 2011. *An Introduction to the International Criminal Court*, Cambridge: Cambridge University Press.

Scharf, MP 1999. The politics behind the US opposition to the international criminal court, *New England International and Comparative Law Annual*, 5(1).

Shuster, E 1997. Fifty years later: The significance of the Nuremberg code, *New England Journal of Medicine*, 337(20): 1436–1440. doi.org/10.1056/NEJM199711133372006

Steinberg, RH 2011. *Assessing the Legacy of the ICTY*, Leiden, Netherlands: The, Brill. doi.org/10.1163/ ej.9789004186248.i-318.8

Straus, S 2007. What is the relationship between hate radio and violence? Rethinking Rwanda's 'radio machete', *Politics & Society*, 35(4): 609–637. doi.org/10.1177/0032329207308181

Tabeau, E, & Bijak, J 2005. War-related deaths in the 1992–1995 armed conflicts in Bosnia and Herzegovina: A critique of previous estimates and recent results, *European Journal of Population/Revue européenne de Démographie*, 21(2–3): 187–215. doi.org/10.1007/s10680-005-6852-5

Tanaka, Y, McCormack, TL, & Simpson, G 2011. *Beyond Victor's Justice? The Tokyo War Crimes Trial Revisited*, Brill. doi.org/10.1163/ej.9789004203037.i-404

United Nations 2019. *Treaty Collection* [Online], Geneva. Available: https://treaties.un.org/ [Accessed 08/04/2019].

Wilson, S, Cribb, R, Trefalt, B, & Aszkielowicz, D 2017. *Japanese War Criminals: The Politics of Justice after the Second World War*, New York: Columbia University Press.

Wunder, M 2000. Medicine and conscience: The debate on medical ethics and research in Germany 50 years after Nuremberg, *Perspectives in Biology and Medicine*, 43(3): 373–381. doi.org/10.1353/ pbm.2000.0031

Yanagizawa-Drott, D 2014. Propaganda and conflict: Evidence from the Rwandan genocide, *The Quarterly Journal of Economics*, 129(4): 1947–1994. doi.org/10.1093/qje/qju020

12

ADVOCACY FOR HUMAN RIGHTS

Fiona H. McKay and Ann Taket

Introduction

Advocacy can take many forms, however, in general, advocacy encompasses actions that are taken to effect change for a specific cause. Human rights advocates work to promote and protect the human rights of particular groups or relating to specific issues, taking actions to support the positive advancement of those causes. Some of the activities that individuals or groups of advocates will employ to advance their cause include awareness raising, creating change, and movement building.

This chapter will present a range of approaches to advocating for human rights. This includes a discussion of human rights defenders, the role of non-government organisations (NGOs) in advocacy, including a number of examples of successful advocacy, and the range of activities that advocates might engage in. This chapter will conclude with an overview of some of the key steps involved in advocacy.

Human rights defenders

Human rights defenders are people who work to promote and protect human rights. The actions of human rights defenders can be taken individually or in groups, and can be taken by people who are engaging in human rights activism as part of their employment or as a volunteer (Landman 2006). Human rights defenders may include community leaders, lawyers, journalists, teachers, civil society actors, and concerned citizens. Given the nature of the work, the activities of human rights defenders can pose dangers to defenders. At times, human rights defenders can be the subject of reprisals, attacks, persecution, intimidation, or violence. Some countries prevent the actions of human rights defenders or ban or expel, human rights organisations from acting to promote and protect human rights (Nah et al. 2013).

Human rights defenders employ a range of methods to complete their work. These methods can include direct action or intervention, lobbying, or protesting. As more and more people around the world have access to the internet through smartphones, human rights defenders are increasingly turning to the digital technologies to engage their communities, and to spread their human rights messages (Hankey and Ó Clunaigh 2013). Digital technologies, particularly smart phones are accessible for most populations, meaning that more people have access to a mobile device than to justice or legal services (Zambrano and Seward 2012). While the use of the internet and other technology can allow human rights defenders to reach a wider population, they also come with risk by exposing the human rights defender's location, activities, and networks, and creating the potential for surveillance and interception. Attacks on human rights defenders have increased over the past few years (Global Witness 2018), as has the number of entrapments and networks being compromised through the use of computers, cameras, mobile phones, and the internet (Hankey and Ó Clunaigh 2013).

To address the concerns of those working as human rights defenders, in 1998, the UN General Assembly adopted the United Nations Declaration on Human Rights Defenders (Declaration on the Right and Responsibility of Individuals, Groups and Organs of Society to Promote and Protect Universally Recognized Human Rights and Fundamental Freedoms). This Declaration aims to provide support and protection to human rights defenders in the context of their work, and going beyond the defenders themselves, by outlining the role of every citizen in promoting and protecting the human rights of all. Under the Declaration, a human rights defender is anyone working alone, or as part of group or an institution, who is working for the promotion and protection of human rights (OHCHR 1998). This broad definition encompasses professional as well as non-professional human rights workers, volunteers, journalists, lawyers, and anyone else carrying out, even on an occasional basis, a human rights activity. The rights included under the Declaration include the right to seek protection, the right to conduct work as a human rights defender, the right to freedom of assembly, and of association, the right to develop and discuss new human rights ideas and to advocate for their acceptance, the right to criticise, or make complaints about, government bodies and agencies and to make proposals to improve their functioning, the right to provide legal assistance or other advice and assistance in defence of human rights, the right to attend public hearings, and the right to receive funds for the purpose of defending and promoting human rights (OHCHR 1998).

The mandate on the situation of human rights defenders was established in 2000 by the Commission on Human Rights (as a Special Procedure) to support implementation of the 1998 Declaration on human rights defenders. To operationalise the mandate, the President of the Human Rights Council appoints a UN Special Rapporteur on the situation of human rights defenders to seek, receive, examine, and respond to information on their situation; to establish cooperation and conduct dialogue with governments and other interested actors on the promotion and effective implementation of the Declaration; to recommend effective strategies to better protect human rights defenders and follow up on these recommendations; and to integrate a gender perspective throughout the work (OHCHR 2019a). The Special Rapporteur is required to provide an annual report to the Human Rights Council and the General Assembly (OHCHR 2019c). These annual reports describe the primary trends and concerns identified during the year and make recommendations for how these should be addressed. The reports are generally focused on major themes.

The report presented to the fortieth session of the Human Rights Council in 2019 focused on Women Human Rights Defenders. This report highlights the additional gendered risks and obstacles women human rights defenders face. For example, women can experience stigma for the same actions for which men are venerated, and women are often perceived not as agents of change but as vulnerable or victimized persons in need of protection by others, typically men (OHCHR 2019b). The report highlights the work of the thousands of women human rights defenders who work to promote and protect gender equality, Indigenous women who seek land and environmental rights, women in rural areas pressing for socioeconomic rights, girls campaigning on social issues, trans women speaking up against discrimination, lesbians calling for equality, migrant and refugee women advocating for their rights and security, homeless women demanding the right to housing and shelter, women fighting for justice for the disappeared, gender non-conforming persons resisting gender-based violence, women promoting choice and bodily autonomy, women expanding digital rights, women with disabilities fighting for independent living and women involved in peace processes (OHCHR 2019b).

The report to the UN General Assembly in 2016 highlighted the situation, and particularly the violence, surrounding the work of environmental human rights defenders (OHCHR 2016). Environmental human rights defenders are those, in their personal or professional capacity and in a peaceful manner, who strive to protect and promote human rights relating to the environment, including water, air, land, flora, and fauna. As the demand for natural resources grows, environmental concerns will play an increasingly important role in human rights activities. In many countries, activists and communities are seeking to prevent environmental harm and the promotion of alternatives to development. The report presented to the General Assembly details the almost 200 killings of environmental human rights defenders in 2015, linked to mining, hydroelectric dams and water rights, agribusiness, and logging, most of which occurred in Asia (OHCHR 2016). This is consistent with work from the NGO Global Witness, who work to protect human rights and the environment, finding that over 200 people were killed in 2017 through their work as environmental human rights defenders (Global Witness 2018). The perpetrators of this violence include governments, corporations, and investors, and are most linked to agribusiness.

There are a number of other ways that the work of human rights defenders is shared. For example, the Asian Forum for Human Rights and Development has been organising the Asian Regional Human Rights Defenders Forum for almost a decade. This forum provides a platform for human rights defenders to discuss work and advocacy efforts and share experiences and the challenges. Addressing the situation of human rights defenders across Asia, a recent report from the Forum reveals that 'violations have become more extreme, and the safe spaces in which human rights defenders can work have increasingly shrunk' (AFHRD 2019). The number of people killed or harmed as a result of their human rights work in this region increased throughout 2017–2018, with 164 cases of physical violence, 61 resulting in death. The majority of these cases occurred in the Philippines (48 per cent) and India (25 per cent). Concerningly, most of the perpetrators of these killings remain unknown, a reality which perpetuates impunity in the region (AFHRD 2019).

The situation of human rights defenders on the US–Mexico border is also becoming increasingly complex and dangerous. Since the election of President Trump, a humanitarian crisis, related to unlawful US asylum policies, has been worsening on the US–Mexico border. US authorities have turned away thousands of people requesting asylum at the border and are forcibly returning thousands more. According to Amnesty International (2019a), since 2018 the US government has executed an unlawful and politically motivated campaign of intimidation, threat, harassment, and criminal investigations against people who defend the human rights of migrants, refugees, and asylum seekers. Save the Children, a large NGO focused specifically on the human rights of children, have reported that children are being detained for longer than is legal, and are being separated from their families (Save the Children 2019). In addition to denying many people to their right to seek asylum, neither the US nor the Mexican government have provided adequate shelter, food, services, or legal assistance to those asylum seekers now stranded in the violent and dangerous border region of northern Mexico. As a result, NGOs and volunteers from communities of faith are trying to fill these service gaps. Among the human rights defenders targeted by US authorities are activists, lawyers, journalists, and volunteers (Amnesty International 2019c). US government departments have accused and investigated human rights defenders for alleged crimes including conspiracy, fraud, and the harbouring and smuggling of migrants and asylum seekers, as well as misdemeanour crimes related to the provision of humanitarian aid. These reports of intimidation and violence against human rights defenders are supported by recommendations from the 2009, 2013, and 2019 Universal Periodic Review of Mexico which highlight the dangers for human rights defenders, and other reports suggesting that Mexico has become one of the most dangerous countries for journalists (Tucker 2017).

NGOs in the global system

NGOs can play an important role in raising human rights issues within the global system. Many NGOs work to document human rights violations and call for action, both at a governmental and grass roots level, and by working with the Human Rights Council and the Universal Periodic Review system to report on issues at the country level. NGOs bring in a range of experts and community leaders, as well as the public, into human rights activities. There are a number of important NGOs who are key stakeholders in the global human rights system. In this section, a brief overview of some of the larger NGOs is given, as is some discussion of smaller, grass roots or single issue or group NGOs.

Amnesty International

The beginning of Amnesty International lay in an article by a British lawyer, Peter Benenson, published in the Observer newspaper, on 28 May 1961 (Power 1981). 'The Forgotten Prisoners' was written after Benenson learned about two Portuguese students who had been imprisoned for raising their wine glasses in a toast to freedom (although this account is refuted by some researchers, see Buchanan (2002) for example). The Forgotten Prisoners article highlighted the plight of those 'imprisoned, tortured or executed because his opinions or religion are unacceptable to his government' (Lake and Wong 2007), representing a violation, by governments, of Articles 18 and 19 of the Universal Declaration of Human Rights (UDHR). The publication of the article in the Observer, marked the launch of the 'Appeal for Amnesty, 1961', the aim of which was to mobilise public opinion, quickly, and widely (Power 1981). Soon after the launch, the leadership decided that the appeal would form the basis of a permanent organisation, Amnesty, with the first meeting taking place in London, with delegates from Belgium, the UK, France, Germany, Ireland, Switzerland, and the United States. At this meeting, it was decided to establish 'a permanent international movement in defence of freedom of opinion and religion'. The following year Amnesty International groups were started in Australia, Belgium, Denmark, Greece, Ireland, Norway, Sweden, and the United States. What started as a short appeal, soon became an international movement working to protect those imprisoned for non-violent expression of their views, harnessing research, community engagement, and campaigning. While Amnesty International had initially been concerned with Article 18, freedom of thought, conscious, and religion, and Article 19 freedom of expression, as the organisation became bigger and attracted more supporters, other human rights were included into their remit. In 2001, Amnesty International voted to transform its focus from mostly civil and political rights, to include a focus on economic, social, and cultural rights (Nelson and Dorsey 2008).

By the end of 2018, Amnesty International had grown into a global movement with more than seven million supporters, members, and activists in almost 160 countries and territories who campaign to end grave abuses of human rights. Amnesty's vision is 'for every person to enjoy all the rights enshrined in the Universal Declaration of Human Rights and other international human rights standards' (Amnesty International 2019a). The organisation is independent of any government, political ideology, economic interest, or religion and is funded mainly by membership and public donations. The main actions of Amnesty International, as a mass-membership organisation, are through the mobilization of their members through letter writing and direct lobbying.

Amnesty International had a number of early successes through actions of membership mobilisation. This included having a Serbian Archbishop Josyf Slipyj released from prison, the release of a number of political prisoners in Ghana, and the release of a trade unionist who was sentenced to 'hard labor' by an East German court (Power 1981). These successes were all the result of sustained letter writing campaigns followed by personal visits from members of Amnesty International. These initial successes allowed the organisation to grow and attract more support, and to branch out into other areas of human rights.

In the 1970s Amnesty International launched a campaign against torture, a campaign that eventually led to the adoption of the UN Convention against Torture, in 1987, now ratified by 166 countries (United Nations 2019). This was followed by efforts to abolish the death penalty. When Amnesty International began their work in 1961, only nine countries had abolished the death penalty, by 1977 when they began actively working on a campaign against the death penalty, 16 countries had removed the death penalty from their laws (Amnesty International 2019a). By the end of 2018, 106 countries had abolished the death penalty in law for all crimes and 142 countries had abolished the death penalty in law or practice, with China, Iran, Saudi Arabia, and Vietnam the main countries employing the death penalty for crimes (Amnesty International 2019b).

Amnesty International continues to work across a number of areas where human rights abuses are occurring. This includes working to ensure that anyone who is detained or imprisoned is given access to a fair trial with access to lawyers and fair judges, that they are not subject to torture, or to solitary confinement for prolonged periods. Through support of the UN Declaration on the Rights of Indigenous Peoples, Amnesty International works with Indigenous populations to develop laws that protect lands, cultures, and livelihoods. A large amount of recent work has focused on ensuring everyone has access to sexual and reproductive rights, including access to contraception, and working to eliminate discrimination against gay men, lesbian women and trans people (Amnesty International 2019a).

Human Rights Watch

Human Rights Watch began in 1978 (under the name Helsinki Watch) as a body to observe the Soviet Union's compliance with the Helsinki Accords, the agreements that would see greater communication and cooperation between Communist Eastern Europe and Western Europe. One if the key roles of Helsinki Watch was to provide advocacy for imprisoned monitors arrested by Soviet officials, but also to promote civil and political freedoms in Eastern Europe (HRW 2019c).

The Cold War and the resulting tensions between the United States and the Soviet Union led to the creation of the Americas Watch in 1981. The focus of the Americas Watch was to observe human rights abuses occurring in Central America, particularly through the interference of the United States. The establishment of other similar organisations rapidly increased through their classification as 'The Watch Committees' and eventually these committees joined, adopting the overarching title, Human Rights Watch (HRW 2019c). Human Rights Watch is now one of the world's leading independent organisations dedicated to defending and protecting human rights. It is an independent, non-governmental organisation, supported by contributions from private individuals and foundations worldwide, accepting no government funds, directly or indirectly.

Human Rights Watch opposes violations of the basic human rights found in the UDHR. The organisation works on the abolition of capital punishment and discrimination on the basis of sexual orientation, it works to promote freedom of religion, and freedom of the press, and the rights of women, children, refugees, and migrant workers, bringing a human rights perspective to issues including domestic violence, trafficking, rape as a war crime, and child soldiers (HRW 2019c). Human Rights Watch works by publicly pressuring governments and policy makers to curb human rights abuses. To progress these issues, Human Rights Watch publishes a number of reports on violations of international human rights.

Since its creation, Human Rights Watch has had a number of successes. It was one of six international NGOs in 1998 that founded the Coalition to Stop the Use of Child Soldiers (now called Child Soldiers International), a group that aimed to increase awareness of the plight of child soldiers through the use of photographs and other documentary artefacts (Druba 2002). The Coalition campaigned for the adoption of the Optional Protocol to the Convention on the Rights of the Child on the involvement of children in armed conflict (OPAC). This Protocol prevents the use of child soldiers in armed conflict and raises the age that a person can be recruited into the military to 18 years. By the middle of 2019, 168 states were party to this Protocol (United Nations 2019).

Another important area of work for Human Rights Watch has been on the International Campaign to Ban Landmines, a global coalition of civil society groups that successfully lobbied to introduce the Ottawa Treaty (the Convention on the Prohibition of the Use, Stockpiling, Production and Transfer of Anti-Personnel Mines and on their Destruction), to prohibit the use, production, stockpiling, and transfer of anti-personnel mines. By the middle of 2019, 164 states were party to this treaty. Those not party include China, Russia, and the United States (United Nations 2019).

CASE STUDY 1: PROTECTING THE RIGHTS OF LGBT PEOPLE – NGO ADVOCACY IN ACTION

In response to a global advocacy campaign led by Human Rights Watch, the UN General Assembly held a rare re-vote on a resolution protecting people from extrajudicial killings. The provision on sexual orientation was first added to the UN resolution on extrajudicial killings in 1999 at the insistence of the UN Special Rapporteur on Torture, whose findings evidenced the link between homophobia, perceived sexual orientation, and fatal hate crimes in a number of places around the world. During a November 2010 meeting of the UN committee that oversees decisions on human rights, that part of the resolution was removed. The initiative for the provision's removal was spearheaded, ostensibly for religious and cultural reasons, by some members of the Organisation of the Islamic Conference and of the United Nation's African Regional Group, including Uganda, South Africa, and Rwanda.

Human Rights Watch took a number of significant steps:

Boris Dittrich, Human Rights Watch's LGBT rights advocacy director, used a UN event he was co-organising to celebrate International Human Rights Day on 10 December as a catalyst to prompt a re-vote. UN Secretary General Ban Ki-moon and US Ambassador to the United Nations Susan Rice were invited, and both accepted. The Secretary General opened the session by calling for an end to laws that criminalise consenting homosexual conduct. Rice, during her keynote speech, announced that the United States sought to reopen the debate on the controversial amendment at a meeting of the UN General Assembly just eleven days later.

Human Rights Watch's South Africa director, Sipho Mthathi, increased pressure on the government in Pretoria, and encouraged South African LGBT rights groups to do the same. This was supported by Dittrich's appearance on South African television pointing out the contrast between the robust protections for the LGBT community in the South African constitution, and a vote in favour of an amendment that would remove protections for LGBT people.

Human Rights Watch contacted as many diplomats ahead of the reopened debate as possible. This outreach helped secure fresh support from many countries, including a block of seven countries in the Caribbean Community (Caricom). Meetings were held with UN mission diplomats from Colombia and Suriname, and LGBT human rights activists in these countries mobilised. Both of these countries changed their vote, as did South Africa.

During the final vote by the General Assembly, the UN Ambassador from Rwanda made a strong statement in favour of undoing the homophobic amendment. Together with cooperation from Argentina, Belgium, Brazil, France, the Netherlands, Norway and Gabon, these efforts led to an overwhelming majority of ninety-four countries in favour of restoring the resolution to ensure that LGBT people would continue to be protected.

(Extracted from Human Rights Watch. Restoring Protection for LGBT People against Extrajudicial Executions. www.hrw.org/en/news/2011/02/14/restoring-protection-lgbt-people-against-extrajudicial-executions, accessed June 2019)

Médecins Sans Frontières

Médecins Sans Frontières (MSF) (Doctors Without Borders in English) is an international medical humanitarian organisation created by doctors and journalists in France in 1971. MSF provides emergency medical assistance to populations in conflict zones and countries affected by epidemic diseases in more than seventy countries. One feature of the work of MSF is their emphasis on neutrality, impartiality, independence, and bearing witness, allowing MSF to explicitly preclude political, economic, or religious factors in decision making (MSF 2019b). By limiting the amount of funding received from governments, MSF is more able to speak openly about acts of war, aggression, corruption, and other issues that impact the human rights of those they work with.

Since its creation, MSF has expanded its role and reach and now provides medical assistance in both conflict and non-conflict settings, including treating HIV/AIDS, malnutrition, cholera, mental health, infectious diseases, and providing surgery. One of its key activities is the Campaign for Access to Essential Medicines, established in 1999 to increase the access to, and the development of, life-saving and life-prolonging medicines, diagnostic tests and vaccines for patients in MSF program and beyond (MSF 2019a).

MSF have a number of ongoing missions and activities. Recently, MSF have responded to the humanitarian needs of the Rohingya minority in Myanmar by providing sexual and reproductive health care, vaccination, and basic health care to thousands of Rohingya refugees. The Rohingya are a Muslim minority who have long been persecuted and denied rights in Myanmar, but recently have been the target of attacks of unprecedented scale by the government of Myanmar, a mostly Buddhist country, driving many thousands into neighbouring Bangladesh. As a result of the violence in northern Myanmar, in Rakhine state, at least 6,700 Rohingya were killed in the space of a month in late 2017, and over 600,000 have fled into Bangladesh (MSF 2018). These crimes are being investigated by the International Criminal Court, with the United States recently placing sanctions on some members of Myanmar's military over extrajudicial killings of Rohingya Muslims, barring them from entry to the United States.

CARE International

CARE (Cooperative for Assistance and Relief Everywhere) International is a large independent relief and development organisation, working in over ninety countries and benefiting over eighty million poor and marginalised people directly. CARE positions itself as a practical, hands-on organisation with thousands of programs around the world. CARE deal with a wide range of issues that keep people trapped in poverty, including HIV/AIDS, discrimination, lack of clean water, employment, substandard living conditions, and a range of other social determinants of health and issues of social justice. According to their organisational mission: 'We seek a world of hope, tolerance and social justice, where poverty has been overcome and people live in dignity and security' (CARE 2019). CARE has no political or religious affiliation.

CARE was founded in 1945 as a non-sectarian, impartial, and non-governmental organisation to provide food relief to those who were starving as a result of the Second World War. CARE's first activity was the provision of 'CARE packages', made of surplus army rations with enough food for a day's meal for ten people (called '10-in-ones'), including cigarettes, that were sent all across Europe (Henry 1999). When the army surplus food was exhausted, CARE began to make their own packages with the assistance of a nutritionist and without an allocation of cigarettes. As the need for CARE packages receded, the organisation shifted its work to a focus on supplementary feeding programs using surplus agricultural products, while at the same time responding to disasters, both natural and man-made (Henry 1999). After the Second World War, CARE began working more in the developing world, with missions in the Philippines, India, Pakistan, and Mexico. This work included providing non-food resources including tools for farming and other forms of employment (O'Keefe et al. 1991). CARE eventually phased out CARE packages, with the last of over 100 million packages delivered in 1967 (CARE International 2019a). Since this time, CARE has been involved in the creation of schools, nutrition centres, health education, and access to clean water and sanitation.

In recent years, CARE has moved to address the underlying causes of poverty, rather than to simply deal with its symptoms. CARE views poverty as the product of complex social processes that affect people's dignity and security as well as their material wellbeing and seeks to understand all the factors that make and keep people poor before choosing which ones to concentrate on in each individual project. CARE developed a number of microfinance programs as one way to address poverty. First trailed in 1991, in a village in southern Niger, CARE assisted a group of women to harness the practice of group savings and create a sustainable system of home-grown microfinance (CARE International 2019a). Since this initial group, hundreds of thousands of women-lead village savings and loan groups have been established, training members in group dynamics, governance, and in money management, a model that has been replicated by other NGOs (Allen 2006).

CARE conducts much of its work through an explicit human rights-based approach using six program principles: promote empowerment; work in partnership with others; ensure accountability and promote responsibility; address discrimination; promote the non-violent resolution of conflicts; and seek sustainable results. CARE makes their evaluations public, allowing for transparency and scrutiny of their projects and impact. They carried out a self-evaluation of the application of this rights-based approach in practice, examining sixteen projects from Bangladesh, Bolivia, Burundi, Cambodia, Guatemala, Honduras, India, Peru, Rwanda, Sierra Leone, Somalia, and Thailand (Picard 2005). For each project achievements against each of the six principles and at the local level were measured. Not all projects were equally successful, but analysis of their different experiences offers some useful findings which can serve as guidance for future work. One key finding was that client groups and partners reported that more time and support were needed than for a conventional project. Obtaining the support of key stakeholders was not always possible at the outset, and required persistence, advocacy, transparency, and negotiation. It was particularly important that any effort to raise awareness of rights and responsibilities relating to the problems facing marginalised groups include rights holders and duty bearers, both of whom are equally capable of transformation. Also identified was that attention needed to be paid to assessing, managing, and taking risk related to both staff and client groups.

This research found that a rights-based approach needs variety and flexibility in use of participatory methods at all different stages, for needs analysis, problem diagnosis, option generation and appraisal, and finally for decision-making (Picard 2005). Projects involved empowering marginalised groups were integral in understanding development and dignity as a basic human right. All projects took as their starting point the need to give voice to the most marginalised groups, whether or not the projects chose to invoke the language of rights. A few projects found that they needed to design processes to facilitate and mobilise community groups, while others demonstrated the importance of empowerment through solidarity. Without proper engagement and research into social, cultural, and economic differentiation, some social groups can be left out of a program, mirroring their social exclusion. The self-evaluation concluded that exemplary relationships with marginalised people bear characteristics of trust, friendship, and a 'journeying together'. One key finding in terms of promoting responsibility was that the process of dialogue between rights holders and duty bearers proved to be transforming for both groups. In most projects, this was accomplished by facilitating discussion and dialogue in an open and collaborative manner; while in others organised groups put pressure on responsible actors.

A more recent evaluations was of CARE's Gender Equality and Women's Empowerment Programme, a program that works with poor and vulnerable women and girls in some of the world's most fragile states: Burundi, the Democratic Republic of Congo, Mali, Myanmar, Niger, and Rwanda (CARE International 2019b). By the end of 2018, the program had worked with over one million women and girls, training more than 50,000 in leadership, and giving over 300,000 access to microfinance. The report indicates, that overall the program has been able to influence positive change in the perception and attitude to women's economic, political, and social empowerment; however, there remain areas of concern. For example, in Burundi, the percentage of women who state they are able to influence decisions has gone down since baseline, with the patriarchal system remaining strong in Niger. However, despite challenges in changing men's attitudes, women are reporting increased participation and social inclusion, and overall, women's sole decision-making has seen some progress. CARE's commitment to sharing these results, both positive and areas that need further attention, mean that other groups and NGOs can learn from existing work.

The International Network for Economic, Social and Cultural Rights (ESCR- Net)

The International Network for Economic, Social and Cultural Rights (ESCR- Net) is a decentralised collaborative initiative of more than 280 Members (ESCR-Net 2019). This structure aims to complement and strengthen, rather than replicate, the efforts of organisation's members working at the national or grassroots level through building bridges across regions, disciplines, and approaches. Through ESCR-Net, groups and individuals exchange information, develop a collective voice, amplify their actions, and develop new tools and strategies. As a network, ESCR-Net is not in itself an NGO, but rather a way for other smaller NGOs and groups to work together.

The substantive work of ESCR-Net is carried out through decentralised structures that are comprised of, and coordinated by, members based in different countries. These structures can take the form of a Working Group, Initiative, or Discussion Group, each providing a different way for organisations to work together on an issue of shared concern and enable joint action. ESCR-Net seeks to strengthen economic, social, and cultural rights by working with organisations and activists worldwide to facilitate mutual learning and strategy exchange; to develop new tools and resources; to engage in advocacy; and to provide information sharing and networking.

One of several current working groups is the Women and ESCR Working Group. This group is working to advancing women's rights related to land, housing, and natural resources and at the intersection of women and work, as well as supporting the wider network to operationalise an intersectional gender analysis and approach (ESCR-Net 2019). Part of

ESCR-Net's recent work has included lobbying the International Labour Organization (ILO) to adopt a convention on gender-based violence. In June 2019, the ILO adopted the Convention concerning the Elimination of Violence and Harassment in the World of Work. With this Convention, states will be able to adopt laws, policies, and other mechanisms that will assist in preventing violence and harassment at work (ILO 2019).

The International Service for Human Rights (ISHR)

The International Service for Human Rights (ISHR) is an international NGO that works by supporting human rights defenders, strengthening human rights systems, and leading and participating in coalitions for human rights change. The ISHR was created in 1984 with the objective of bridging the gap between the UN human rights system and the realities of the work of human rights defenders at the national level. It has enabled defenders to access the UN system and to effectively participate at the international level. Over time, ISHR's geographic reach has broadened to incorporate regional systems of protection.

One of ISHR's key achievements has been the adoption, by the UN, of the Declaration on the Right and Responsibility of Individuals, Groups and Organs of Society to Promote and Protect Universally Recognized Human Rights and Fundamental Freedoms (usually referred to as the Declaration on the Rights of Human Rights Defenders). This Declaration, adopted in 1998, works to protect those at risk for carrying out legitimate human rights activities. It is the first UN instrument that recognises the important work of human rights defenders, as well as the right and responsibility of all to protect human rights (OHCHR 1998).

The People's Health Movement

The People's Health Movement developed as a response to the failure to realise the goal of 'Health for All by the Year 2000' in the Alma Ata Declaration (PHM 2019). By the end of 2000 several international organisations, civil society movements, NGOs, and women's groups organised the first People's Health Assembly in Savar, Bangladesh. During this meeting, the People's Charter for Health was formulated and endorsed. The People's Health Movement rose from this Assembly as a body of health rights proponents who would demand Health for All Now across the globe; a worldwide citizens' movement committed to making the Alma Ata dream a reality.

The People's Health Movement plays a role in coordinating the production of the Global Health watch. The Global Health Watch works with the World Health Organization and other international and intergovernmental organisations to monitor their activities, and then report back in terms of the progress they are making on health (PHM 2019). These reports are then able to be used by a range of community groups and other NGOs to inform their activities.

Women's Global Network for Reproductive Rights

Women's Global Network for Reproductive Rights (WGNRR) is an NGO that works to promote and protect sexual and reproductive health, rights, and justice. Based in the Global South, WGNRR are a membership-driven organisation that works to realise the full sexual and reproductive health and rights of all people, with a particular focus on the most marginalised. Through their member activities, WGNRR work with their partners through a number of approaches (WGNRR 2019):

> Empowerment – Our members and allies are empowered and supported to take actions based on their own knowledge and experiences.
>
> Grassroots and community led – Our actions are informed and led by grassroots and community organisations and the people whose lives are affected by international agreements such as Human Rights treaties, ICPD and the MDGs.
>
> In partnership – We work globally, in partnership with members, SRHR activists and allies to strengthen its impact and work to achieve shared goals.

WGNRR advocates for sexual and reproductive health for all people. They have specific program areas around advocating for the recognition of young peoples' sexual and reproductive rights as human rights, addressing the cultural, social, economic, and political barriers that young people face in accessing their sexual and reproductive human rights (WGNRR 2019). They also work to increase access to contraception for the approximately 220 million women in low income countries who do not have access to contraception (WHO 2019b). The other main area of work for WGNRR is in advocating access to safe and legal abortions. According to the WHO, between 2010 and 2014, 56 million women access a either a safe or unsafe abortion, with around one in four pregnancies ending with abortion. Each year, it is estimated that around 25 million unsafe abortions are performed each year, with between 4.7% and 13.2% of all maternal deaths attributed to unsafe abortions (WHO 2019b). Most unsafe abortions are performed in low income countries.

JASS

JASS is a global women-led human rights network of activists, educators, and scholars across thirty-one countries. JASS works to ensure women leaders are confident, organised, louder, and safer as they take on critical human rights issues (JASS 2019). The organisation undertakes training of women grassroots leaders and activists across many countries. They also work with the UN Special Rapporteur on Human Rights Defenders to influence other international human rights organisations to better understand and promote gender, women's leadership, and collective protection strategies for human rights activists, especially feminist, LGBTIQ, Indigenous, environmental, and labour rights activists (JASS 2019).

JASS has a large body of work in Central and South America. In response to increased levels of violence in Mexico and other Central American, women's rights and freedoms are under threat and, with women human rights defenders facing serious dangers. Guatemala, Honduras, and Mexico report the most cases of violence against women, journalists, and activists (JASS 2019). In response, JASS is a founding member of the Mesoamerican Women Human Rights Defenders Initiative to facilitate dialogue, joint action, and capacity building through coordination with other organisations from El Salvador, Mexico, Guatemala, and the Central American Women's Fund. This work seeks to provide alternatives and to protect women human rights defenders, keeping them free from violence, enabling them to continue their human rights work.

How to advocate for human rights

So far, this chapter has provided examples of organisations that engage in human rights activities, overviews of the approaches that they take to their work, and some examples of where they have had success. While there are a number of ways that advocacy can occur, there are a commonalities in the approaches of these organisations to human rights advocacy, see Figure 12.1 for an overview of these steps (adapted from The Advocates for Human Rights (2019)).

The first step is to decide on the issue to be addressed. This may be through consideration of the biggest problems in the community, for particular population groups, or an issue that arouses particular passion. At this point, it is useful to ask what the ultimate human rights goal of the advocacy is, and to identify the possible outcomes of the advocacy.

The second step requires that you identify the related human rights. At this step, it is essential to be very clear on the human rights that are connected to the identified problem. This may include becoming aware and familiar with the UDHR, as well as any of the specific UN Declarations, Conventions, or Protocols related to the issue. At this step, becoming familiar with any related regional or state based human rights instruments would also be beneficial.

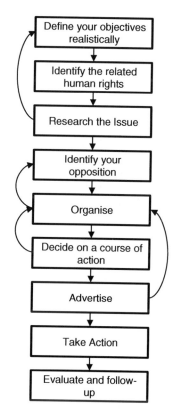

FIGURE 12.1   Steps for advocacy

Not all projects will require the need to invoke human rights legislation or frameworks, but a familiarity with the language is useful.

The third step allows for research into the issue. Before decisions are made on how to act, being informed on the issue is crucial. This could include reading the research published by reputable organisations, for example, Amnesty International and Human Rights Watch both produce comprehensive reports on a range of human rights abuses, and reading reports published by the range of UN human rights committees. Beyond this, at this stage engaging with the media, including social media will ensure the most up to date information on the issue. This step may lead back to the beginning and require a re-definition of the issue.

The next step is to identify the opposition. As part of researching the issue, identifying the individuals, groups, or policies that are in opposition on the issue will assist with the advocacy. At this stage, the opposition may be able to be met personally, allowing for, if possible, an exchange of ideas and possibly a compromise.

Following this is the organisation step. By working with an established group, the advocacy is more likely to be able to achieve greater accuracy in human rights reporting thanks to shared information and analysis, garner increased credibility with external actors such as UN officials or government diplomats and achieve higher concentration of international attention through complementary rather than competing advocacy efforts. Although the nature and structure of every network or coalition will differ, any coordinated advocacy strategy will benefit from open discussions to determine a common purpose, shared objectives, discussion of resources and strengths. Many civil society groups or individuals can make useful network partners, including grassroots organisations, national social justice organisations, universities, and journalists. This step may lead back to an identification of the opposition. It may not be clear until the organisation stage who the opposition is, this process will allow for a re-identification of any groups in opposition.

The next step is to decide on a course of action. It is this point where a human rights defender or advocate can begin to plan the most appropriate method for effecting change. Some approaches that can be considered include dialogue and awareness raising, raising awareness of rights and responsibilities, fostering dialogues to achieve a common understanding of problems, creating safe space for discussion of sensitive or taboo subjects, lobbying, or empowering. Deciding which course of action to take will depend greatly on the previous steps, and may require some re-consideration of the previous organise step, and of other areas of previous work and key stakeholders.

It is important that as many people as possible know about the human rights breach and the advocacy to resolve it, as such, the next step is to Advertise. Use all possible media to achieve this including newspapers, radio, television, along with social media and blogs. The more people know about the issue, the more likely that positive change will occur. If this step is not as effective as it needs to be, it may be worth returning to the organise step to ensure all key stakeholders are involved.

The next step is to carry out the actions as planned. While not all activities may go ahead exactly as planned, the only way to effect change is through action, making change happen takes time.

At the completion of the advocacy, and at periodical intervals, take time to think and talk about what happened through an evaluation of the program or activity. Were the goals and key objectives of the advocacy reached? What does success mean? Is there more that needs to be done, and how can this be achieved?

Activities for advocacy

There are a number of ways that NGOs, human rights defenders, advocates, and others operate to promote actions for human rights advocacy. In addition to working with UN, regional,
national, and grass roots, organisations, as discussed previously, individuals can advocate for
human rights through a variety of other platforms, including through digital channels, such as
social media and personal blogs, by working with journalists, and by engaging with governments through submissions and formal lobbying.

Using digital platforms

Human rights advocates and defenders have been using digital means to progress their work
and amplify their message for decades. In 1992, WITNESS began partnering with on the
ground human rights organisations to document through video and photography human
rights violations and their consequences (Gregory 2010). WITNESS was created with the
idea that if all human rights defenders had a camera in their hands, it would be easier to
get the public's attention when human rights were being violated. WITNESS has partnered
with hundreds of human rights organisations all over the world documenting human rights
abuses including the use of child soldiers in the Democratic Republic of Congo, violence
against women in Mexico, modern day slavery in Brazil, and elder abuse in the United States
(Gregory 2010).

Thanks to advances in technology, the idea behind the creation of WITNESS, that every
human rights defender has a camera in their hand, is now a reality. Two-thirds of the world's
population has a smartphone, allowing users to access the internet at almost all times. This
immediate internet access has made it increasingly easy to receive, share, and be involved in
individualised acts of political expression and to participate in digital advocacy (McKay and
Dunn 2017). Advocacy in the form of letter writing and donating money or goods, as well as
petition signing, boycotts, and blogging, have become easier thanks to their integration into
the online space. Digital advocacy now includes the use of websites, blogs, newsletters, online
petitions, and social media including Twitter, Facebook, Instagram, and Snapchat, and can
employ video and photography.

There are many examples of good digital human rights advocacy. For example, social
media has often been used to champion human rights. In Uganda, with a recent campaign
to promote democratic governance, protect civic spaces, demand government accountability,
safeguard freedom of expression, and champion social justice, Connecting Voices, promoted
through blogging and social media. In the United States, digital media were used to protest
the death and campaign for justice for Trayvon Martin, who at the age of seventeen was shot
and killed by a neighbourhood watchman (Hon 2015). Social media included a Facebook
page, a Twitter hashtag, an online petition on change.org, and national and international news
stories as a result of the social media activity. Social media in Fiji is increasingly being used to
demand accountability and transparency from the government. Recently, the Fiji Women's
Rights Movement have begun to use social media to advocate for women's rights in Fiji,
and as a way to garner further national and international media attention (Brimacombe et al.
2018).

There are also examples where the use of digital media can have a negative impact on
human rights, particularly with growing nationalistic sentiments and the phenomena of 'fake

news'. In Myanmar, social media, particularly Facebook, has been used by ultranationalist groups to spread hate speech and violence against the minority Muslim Rohingya (Fink 2018). Facebook is widely used in Myanmar, with many assuming that Facebook, thanks to the widespread use of Facebook Basic, is the internet (Lee 2019). In 2018, a number of Facebook posts, authored by Myanmar's military, falsely accused Rohingya Muslims of raping Buddhist women, and claiming that Islam was a threat to Buddhism. These posts turned Facebook into a tool for ethnic cleansing, with devastating outcomes for many thousands of Rohingya.

Journalism and human rights

Journalists have long played a role in reporting on and exposing human rights abuses. Human rights journalism is a type of reporting that can offer a critical reflection of the experiences of both the victims and perpetrators of physical, cultural, and/or structural human rights violations (Shaw 2011). Common among human rights journalism is an attempt to understand the reasons for the violations, while at the same time, seeking to challenge, rather than reinforce, the status quo of the dominant voices.

Some journalism with the greatest impact is that which is dangerous for the journalist, as the journalist seeks to expose human rights abuses that perpetrators would rather keep hidden. Many journalists have been arrested or detained arbitrarily, tortured, or disappeared because of their reporting, forcing journalists to work from increased distances, while also putting their sources in danger. Reporting from China provides an example of reporting that places the journalist in danger but provides the broader public with a greater understanding of the human rights issues of the one party, authoritarian state. China has a poor human rights record, with regular extrajudicial killings, censorship, and arbitrary detention of human rights defenders, activists, and lawyers. Recently there has been an increase in reporting from the autonomous western region of Xinjiang, where at least 120,000 (but possibly up to one million) members of the of Muslim Uyghur minority have been detained in re-education camps, aimed at changing the political thinking of detainees, their identities, and their religious beliefs via indoctrination and torture (HRW 2019a). Some official reporting has been facilitated by the government of China, who, while providing 'official' camp tours for diplomats and media outlets, are preventing independent journalism. A number of Chinese journalists have been arrested as a result of their reports on the camps at Xinjiang, while foreign journalists have been deported from China for reporting on the situation (HRW 2019a).

Working with governments

Lobbying is one method of advocacy and can be used to influence legislation. Lobbying, often referred to as interest representation, is typically considered to be the act of seeking to influence the actions, policies, or decisions of officials, usually legislators.

Lobbying can work when legislative reform needs to happen for human rights to be realised. Legislative reform relating to access to emergency contraception in Honduras is one example. According to the WHO, emergency contraception, which includes any method of contraception used to prevent pregnancy by delaying ovulation or preventing fertilisation taken after sexual intercourse, is a human right and should be included in all national family planning programs (WHO 2019a). Honduras has some of the strictest abortion laws; abortion illegal in all circumstances and women who seek an abortion are sentenced for up to six years in prison (HRW 2019b). Emergency contraception has been banned since a coup backed by powerful religions leaders in 2009 in Honduras, forcing women to find illegal ways to prevent unwanted pregnancies, with Honduras having one of the highest rates of teen pregnancy in the region (HRW 2019b). A coalition of both small and large human rights organisations are now working in Honduras to have these laws changed, and at the same time are employing a broad community education process to dispel some of the myths surrounding emergency contraception.

Many governments also accept submissions through formal inquiries on issues and prior to the passage of new legislation. For example, the Parliament of New Zealand allows for community feedback on new laws after they has been drafted and read in Parliament. The public are asked to provide feedback in writing, presenting any views or expertise they have on the issue. These submissions are then taken into consideration when preparing the final Bill for Parliament (New Zealand Parliament 2019).

The future of human rights advocacy

Human rights advocacy has a variety of activities, objectives, and methods, however, all advocacy works to address infringement of human rights, whether these are of an individual, community, or people. Human rights advocates work all around the world to promote and protect human rights through a variety of means that at times can be dangerous to themselves, and to those they are seeking to protect. The future of advocacy is likely to include an increased reliance on social media and the internet more generally. While these methods of communication come with increased connectivity, they also come with risks. Finding ways to ameliorate and to protect from these risks will play an essential role in future advocacy as breaches in human rights dealt with through advocacy start to impact on more people.

References

The Advocates for Human Rights 2019. *10 Steps to Becoming a Human Rights Advocate* [Online], Minneapolis. Available: www.theadvocatesforhumanrights.org/10_steps_to_becoming_a_human_rights_advocate

AFHRD 2019. *Human Rights Defenders at Risk in Asia* [Online], Geneva. Available: www.forum-asia.org/?p=28897 [Accessed 19/09/2019].

Allen, H 2006. Village savings and loans associations: Sustainable and cost-effective rural finance, *Small Enterprise Development*, 17(1): 61–68. doi.org/10.3362/0957-1329.2006.009

Amnesty International 2019a. *Amnesty International* [Online]. Available: www.amnesty.org/en/ [Accessed 29/06/2019].

Amnesty International 2019b. *Death Sentences and Executions 2018*, London: Amnesty International Ltd.

Amnesty International 2019c. *Saving Lives Is Not a Crime: Politically Motivated Legal Harassment against Migrant Human Rights Defenders by the USA*, London: Amnesty International.

Brimacombe, T, Kant, R, Finau, G, Tarai, J, & Titifanue, J 2018. A new frontier in digital activism: An exploration of digital feminism in Fiji, *Asia & the Pacific Policy Studies*, 5(3): 508–521. doi.org/10.1002/app5.253

Buchanan, T 2002. The truth will set you free: The making of Amnesty International, *Journal of Contemporary History*, 37(4): 575–597. doi.org/10.1177/00220094020370040501

CARE 2019. *CARE International* [Online], Atlanta. Available: www.care.org/

CARE International 2019a. *CARE International* [Online]. Available: www.care.org [Accessed 30/06/2019].

CARE International 2019b. *Gender Equality and Women's Empowerment Programme (GEWEP) II Result Highlights 2016–2019*, Norway: CARE International.

Druba, V 2002. The problem of child soldiers, *International Review of Education*, 48(3): 271–278. doi. org/10.1023/A:1020309527289

ESCR-Net 2019. *International Network for Economic, Social and Cultural Rights* [Online], New York. Available: www.escr-net.org/ILOendGBV [Accessed 30/06/2019].

Fink, C 2018. Dangerous speech, anti-muslim violence, and facebook in Myanmar, *Journal of International Affairs*, 71(1.5): 43–52.

Global Witness 2018. *At What Cost? Irresponsible Business and the Murder of Land and Environmental Defenders in 2017* [Online], London: Global Witness. Available: www.globalwitness.org/en-gb/campaigns/environmental-activists/at-what-cost [Accessed 02/07/2019].

Gregory, S 2010. Cameras everywhere: Ubiquitous video documentation of human rights, new forms of video advocacy, and considerations of safety, security, dignity and consent, *Journal of Human Rights Practice*, 2(2): 191–207. doi.org/10.1093/jhuman/huq002

Hankey, S, & Ó Clunaigh, D 2013. Rethinking risk and security of human rights defenders in the digital age, *Journal of Human Rights Practice*, 5(3): 535–547. doi.org/10.1093/jhuman/hut023

Henry, KM 1999. CARE International: Evolving to meet the challenges of the 21st century, *Nonprofit and Voluntary Sector Quarterly*, 28(Suppl. 1): 109–120. doi.org/10.1177/089976499773746465

Hon, L 2015. Digital social advocacy in the justice for Trayvon campaign, *Journal of Public Relations Research*, 27(4): 299–321. doi.org/10.1080/1062726X.2015.1027771

HRW 2019a. *China and Tibet* [Online]. Available: www.hrw.org/asia/china-and-tibet [Accessed 09/07/2019].

HRW 2019b. *Honduras* [Online]. Available: www.hrw.org/americas/honduras [Accessed 09/07/2019].

HRW 2019c. *Human Rights Watch* [Online], New York. Available: www.hrw.org [Accessed 29/06/2019].

ILO 2019. *New International Labour Standard to Combat Violence, Harassment, at Work Agreed* [Online], New York: ILO. Available: www.ilo.org/ilc/ILCSessions/108/media-centre/news/WCMS_711321/lang-en/index.htm [Accessed 30/06/2019].

JASS 2019. *Just Associates* [Online]. Available: https://justassociates.org [Accessed 04/07/2019].

Lake, DA, & Wong, W 2007. The politics of networks: Interests, power, and human rights norms, *Power, and Human Rights Norms*, May 12. doi.org/10.2139/ssrn.1004199

Landman, T 2006. Holding the line: Human rights defenders in the age of terror, *The British Journal of Politics and International Relations*, 8(2): 123–147. doi.org/10.1111/j.1467-856x.2006.00216.x

Lee, R 2019. Extreme speech| extreme speech in Myanmar: The role of state media in the Rohingya forced migration crisis, *International Journal of Communication*, 13(22).

McKay, FH, & Dunn, M 2017. Can online participation on issues of asylum seeking lead to action? Understanding the intent to act, *Australian Journal of Psychology*. doi.org/10.1111/ajpy.12147

MSF 2018. *International Activity Report 2017*, Geneva: MSF.

MSF 2019a. *Campaign for Access to Essential Medicines* [Online], Geneva. Available: https://msfaccess.org/about-us [Accessed 29/06/2019].

MSF 2019b. *Médecins Sans Frontières* [Online], Geneva. Available: www.msf.org [Accessed 29/06/2019].

Nah, AM, Bennett, K, Ingleton, D, & Savage, J 2013. A research agenda for the protection of human rights defenders, *Journal of Human Rights Practice*, 5(3): 401–420. doi.org/10.1093/jhuman/hut026

Nelson, PJ, & Dorsey, E 2008. *New Rights Advocacy: Changing Strategies of Development and Human Rights NGOs*, Washington: Georgetown University Press.

New Zealand Parliament 2019. *Make a Submission* [Online]. Available: www.parliament.nz/en/pb/sc/make-a-submission/ [Accessed 09/07/2019].

O'Keefe, LK, Drew, JS, & Bailey, L 1991. Guide to the records of CARE, *New York Public Library*.

OHCHR 1998. *Declaration on Human Rights Defenders* [Online], Geneva. Available: www.ohchr.org/en/issues/srhrdefenders/pages/declaration.aspx [Accessed 30/06/2019].

OHCHR 2016. They spoke truth to power and were murdered in cold blood, in M Forst & G Tognoni (eds.) *Assistenza infermieristica e ricerca: AIR*, Geneva: United Nations Special Rapporteur on the Situation of Human Rights Defenders.

OHCHR 2019a. *Human Rights Defenders* [Online], Geneva. Available: www.ohchr.org/EN/Issues/SRHRDefenders/Pages/SRHRDefendersIndex.aspx [Accessed 04/07/2019].

OHCHR 2019b. Situation of women human rights defenders, in *Human Rights Council*, Geneva: Report of the Special Rapporteur on the Situation of Human Rights defenders.

OHCHR 2019c. *Special Procedures of the Human Rights Council* [Online], Geneva: United Nations. Available: www.ohchr.org/EN/HRBodies/SP/Pages/Welcomepage.aspx [Accessed 17/07/2019].

PHM 2019. *People's Health Movement* [Online]. Available: https://phmovement.org/ [Accessed 04/07/2019].

Picard, M 2005. Principles into practice: Learning from innovative rights-based programmes, *CARE International*, September.

Power, J 1981. *Amnesty International: The Human Rights Story*, New York: Elsevier.

Save the Children 2019. *US Border Crisis* [Online], Connecticut. Available: www.savethechildren.org/us/what-we-do/emergency-response/historical-emergencies/us-border-crisis

Shaw, IS 2011. 'Human rights journalism': A critical conceptual framework of a complementary strand of peace journalism, *Expanding Peace Journalism: Comparative and Critical Approaches*: 96–121. doi.org/10.1057/9780230358874_2

Tucker, D 2017. Making a killing: A special index investigation looking at why Mexico is an increasingly deadly place to be a journalist as reporters face threats from corrupt police to deadly drug gangs, *Index on Censorship*, 46(3): 81–86. doi.org/10.1177/0306422017730967

United Nations 2019. *Treaty Collection* [Online], Geneva. Available: https://treaties.un.org/ [Accessed 08/04/2019].

WGNRR 2019. *Women's Global Network for Reproductive Rights* [Online]. Available: http://wgnrr.org [Accessed 04/07/2019].

WHO 2019a. *Emergency Contraception* [Online], Geneva. Available: www.who.int/news-room/fact-sheets/detail/emergency-contraception [Accessed 06/07/2019].

WHO 2019b. *Preventing Unsafe Abortion* [Online]. Available: www.who.int/en/news-room/fact-sheets/detail/preventing-unsafe-abortion [Accessed 04/07/2019].

Zambrano, R, & Seward, RK 2012. *Mobile Technologies and Empowerment: Enhancing Human Development Through Participation and Innovation*, New York, NY: UNDP.

13

CONCLUSION

Ann Taket and Fiona H. McKay

Introduction

The World Health Organisation, WHO, (2002) makes a strong statement about the value of human rights work in health, highlighting that human rights approaches can provide lever actions for the protection and promotion of public health, and provide important tools to tackle health inequity. The final chapter of the first edition of this book (Taket 2012), offered a detailed analysis of the evidence for the value of human rights approaches for each of WHO's eleven different types of 'value-added' by human rights. This is not repeated this here but note that in the seven years that have elapsed since the first edition, there are many more example of the instrumental value of human rights in public health. There is now a much larger evidence base for the successful use of such approaches, and earlier chapters have already introduced some of these. In this concluding chapter we look at a number of important areas: the value of rights-based approaches, whether the multi-layered human rights system represents a strength or a weakness, the challenges of transnational corporations, the question of rights for non-human agents, and future opportunities and challenges.

The value of rights-based approaches

This book has presented a wealth of examples of the positive effects of the use of rights-based approaches at the international, regional, national, and local levels in terms of policy formulation and in the design, implementation, and evaluation of specific programs and activities. The examples considered cover the whole range of countries at different stages of development, and in particular have focused attention on the most disadvantaged or marginalised groups. One reason for the underlying success of the rights-based approach in health has been identified by Jonsson (2003, p. 20), who compares needs-based approaches to human rights-based approaches in the context of development planning, noting that:

> *Although human rights are need-based claims, a human rights approach to programming differs sharply from the basic needs approach. Most importantly, the basic needs approach does not imply*

the existence of a duty-bearer. When demands for meeting needs have no 'object', nobody has a clear-cut duty to meet needs, and rights are vulnerable to ongoing violation.

It is important to acknowledge however, that rights-based approaches are not a 'magic wand' that can be waved to solve all problems. As illustrated throughout this book, rights-based approaches do not provide solutions in terms of difficult resource allocation decisions between competing health problems and target groups, although they do help define appropriate processes by which such decisions can be reached (Rumbold et al. 2007).

Necessary complexity or needless bureaucracy?

This book has also examined the various human rights systems that exist, at the global, regional, and national levels; a complex system of systems with multiple points of interaction and leverage. At first sight, this can be confusing to navigate as an individual or group with a human rights concern. However, this complexity allows for multiple points of influence and leverage that do, in particular circumstances, assist in addressing human rights issues. One example of the complexity and interrelatedness of the system is Japan, which does not connect directly into any regional human rights system, and has no national human rights institution; nonetheless, Japan has been influenced and is influential within the international system (see Chapter 4).

When considering regional and global systems, it has been suggested that in some cases, particularly in newly emerged democracies, countries have agreed to participate in such systems as a way to consolidate, or 'lock-in', recent domestic democratic reforms. International human rights bodies can operate in a range of ways to prevent reversion into authoritarian practices and are therefore a useful tool for newly democratic governments who face internal challenges (both actual and anticipated) to their democratic gains (Munro 2009). This theory was first suggested by Moravcsik (2000), and his examination of the European Convention of Human Rights showed evidence for this, particularly when individual citizens bring cases of human rights breaches to national level courts and institutions. Conversely, Simmons (2002), in her study of six UN human rights treaties (CAT, CEDAW, CRC, ICCPR, ICESCR, and ICERD) finds that most evidence of socialisation is through persuasion, and occurs from actors external to the country which she calls 'external socialisation', rather than pressure by powerful state actors or democratic lock-in. Similarly, Munro (2009) concludes that regional groupings may find it 'appropriate' or 'necessary' to construct human rights regimes to remain active participants in the international community. They may fear a 'pariah status' and even sanctions if they do not participate in the established international discourse on human rights.

Charged with promoting and protecting human rights, including the right to health, the UN is challenged by the difficulty of doing this in the face of the current neoliberal global finance and trade mechanisms, adhered to by its own agencies. The actions of, for example, the World Bank, the International Monetary Fund, and the World Trade Organization have been found to directly sustain many human rights violations (see Macdonald (2008) and Stiglitz (2006)). A major challenge for the UN is to address the tensions this causes, hopefully with the result of reaffirming human rights as the central principle for the operation of all the UN agencies. The UN however, is not without its critics.

While documenting considerable criticism of the UN, Macdonald (2008) rejects the conclusion that the UN should be abandoned. Instead he argues for its reform, in both organisational and philosophical terms, placing human rights at the centre of all its operations. Fox and Meier (2009) argue that focusing on the collective human right to development would prove a more powerful legal framework to create a just and equitable international economic order for the improvement of health in developing countries, and that this would support improvements in the whole array of social determinants of health. These arguments are taken further in the book edited by Meier and Gostin (2018), which explores in detail the mainstreaming of human rights in institutions of global health governance.

The most recent annual report of the High Commissioner for Human Rights (OHCHR 2018: 4) discusses the need to 'build a broad global constituency for human rights; the need to protect and expand civic space; prevention of conflict, violence and insecurity; and human rights aspects of climate change, corruption, digital space, inequality and migration'. An important part of this challenge is ensuring helpful collaboration between the global, regional, and national human rights frameworks and monitoring systems, so that they are mutually reinforcing.

The challenges of transnational corporations and philanthrocapitalism

In terms of the right to health in particular, Macdonald (2007) argues that under present global economic models, global equity in health is impossible, and achieving the right to health requires the adoption of an alternative economic paradigm; he identifies promising avenues in the use of international health impact assessments and regional fair-trade zones. In this context ongoing debates about global health governance are particularly important (Ng and Ruger 2011, Meier and Gostin 2018). Ongoing concern is being expressed about the impact of trade agreements on health. For example, Hirono and colleagues (2015) present a health impact assessment of the Trans-Pacific Partnership Agreement, demonstrating potential negative health impacts on the health of Australians in a number of different areas, likely to result in increasing health inequalities. President Trump withdrew the United States from this agreement in 2017, leaving the remaining countries to negotiate a new trade deal, largely identical to the previous deal, but without the twenty-two items specifically relating to the United States.

The main beneficiaries of neoliberal globalisation have been the transnational corporations, which saw their share of profits as a part of global GDP increase by 30% between 1980 and 2013 (Flues and van Schaik 2018). This has had widespread effects on health, increasing inequality and environmental degradation. As ENCO (2018: 40) puts it:

> European transnational corporations are involved in human rights and environmental violations across the planet and largely succeed in escaping accountability. The emphasis put on the old continent's "respectability" leads to a disturbing pattern of outsourcing the worse environmental and social impacts of European multinationals and European consumption of resources in the Global South. A pattern that is facilitated if not encouraged by key EU policies such as the pursuit of trade and investment agreements or the focus on carbon permit trading.

The human rights community has not yet developed an effective strategy to deal with globalisation (Chapman 2016). As yet, there are few ways to hold corporations responsible for negatively impacting human rights. While there is some movement toward a UN treaty, discussed in Chapter 5, as the analyses offered in Flues and van Schaik (2018) and ENCO (2018) demonstrate, these negotiations have not proceeded with public health goals in mind, but rather seek to protect the interests of corporations. Transnational corporations benefit the richest members of our societies and exploit workers, both paid and unpaid, denying them basic human rights and compromising their right to health (Freudenberg 2014; Pimentel et al. 2018). There is some movement toward corporations becoming more socially responsible, particularly those with a larger amount of public scrutiny. For example, pharmaceutical companies are being increasingly pressured to act responsibly, however, there appears still to be some way to go toward achieving this goal.

Changing governance of the global health agenda has also played its part. As Horton (2018) identifies, the private sector seeks to exploit the calls for partnerships in global health for their own ends, and he calls for their activities to be more accountable to scrutiny by the scientific community and subject to rules for participation in global health events.

Philanthrocapitalism refers to infusing philanthropy with the principles and practices of for-profit enterprise and to demonstrating capitalism's so-called benevolent potential through innovations that allegedly 'benefit everyone, sooner or later, through new products, higher quality and lower prices' (Bishop and Green 2009). Underlying this is the assumption that the market solves rather than creates problems. Birn and Richter (2018) contrast the workings of the Rockefeller and Bill and Melinda Gates Foundations, demonstrating how the first supports public health as a public responsibility, while the second has 'challenged the leadership and purview of public, intergovernmental agencies, fragmenting health coordination and allotting a massive global role for corporate and philanthropic "partners"' (Birn and Richter 2018: p 156). They argue that action is urgently needed to overturn philanthrocapitalism's influence and reclaim a global health agenda based on social justice and human rights. Latham (2018) discusses how the Gates foundation's Ceres2030 Plan supports the agenda of agribusiness. In this context, struggles over global health governance are extremely important.

Non-human agents: rights for artificial intelligence and nature?

Rights for non-human entities have been created in law for a variety of different organisational types: businesses, corporations, trade unions, associations, and so forth. More recently there have been increasing calls for rights for animals or nature. Chapron and colleagues (2019) summarises the arguments why the introduction of legal rights for nature could protect natural systems from destruction and the grounds on which such rights are based. Arguments include those based on the moral assertion that nature has an intrinsic value, those based on spiritual or religious connections to nature, as well as rights created under the law, in an analogous fashion to the rights (and duties) accorded to business enterprises and other non-human entities. Pelizzon and Gagliano (2015) consider the sentience of plants, exploring the intersections of animal rights and rights of nature. Stephens et al. (2019) explore recent developments in plant science that have led to consideration of the importance of considering rights for non-human agents.

There are a number of examples where rights have been accorded to nature. Ecuador recognises the rights of nature (or Pacha Mama) in its constitution (Political Database of the Americas, Republic of Ecuador 2008) and New Zealand has recognised the legal person Te Awa Tupua as an indivisible and living whole, comprising the Whanganui River from the mountains to the sea (Chapron et al. 2019). In the Indian state of Uttarakhand, in July 2018, the high court accorded the entire animal kingdom, including avian and aquatic animals the status of living people, further charging human citizens with standing in loco parentis for the welfare and protection of animals (The Hindu 2018).

GARN, the Global Alliance for the Rights of Nature was created in 2010. Their position is that rather than treating nature as property under the law, nature in all its life forms has the right to exist, persist, maintain, and regenerate its vital cycles. Its website provides a resource hub and it has instituted an International Rights of Nature Tribunal to hear cases as part of activities running parallel to the conferences associated with the United Nations Framework Convention on Climate Change. A number of cases have been heard since its creation, including that of the Great Barrier Reef in Australia (Maloney 2015) and the case of Bolivia who are in the process of implementing a set of laws that also recognize certain rights for nature (Humphreys 2017).

Debates concerning the rights of non–humans take a different direction when scholars ask at what point rights might be demanded or considered for entities that have artificial intelligence (for example: Robertson 2014; Ashrafian 2015a, 2015b). Schwitzgebel and Garza (2015) identify four different grounds for ascribing rights to such entities: no relevant difference; a psychosocial view of moral status and liberalism about embodiment and architecture; subjecting the binary opposition of artificial/non–artificial to critical scrutiny; and the impossibility of establishing psychological difference in consciousness, free will, or insight. As advances in artificial intelligence proceed, this will obviously require further consideration. At the moment within the global human rights system, debate is centred on the risks to human rights posed by artificial intelligence and machine learning (Raso et al 2018).

Looking to the future: opportunities and challenges

Many challenges remain, first and foremost perhaps is that of ensuring that rights-based approaches are used to their full effect for public health purposes, especially in the demanding socio-political context, increased forced migration, and the health threats posed by climate change (Watts et al. 2018a, 2018b). Even when considering HIV/AIDS, the field in which rights-based approaches started to be developed and honed, considerable work needs still to be done to tackle rights violations for specific population groups. UNAIDS (2019) identifies 48 that countries impose some form of restriction on entry, stay or residence based on people's HIV status alone. The latest report by the UN Secretary General (2018) on HIV/AIDS acknowledges the stigma, discrimination, and gender inequality that continue to undermine efforts to achieve universal access to HIV prevention, treatment, care, and support, and calls for a continued focus on human rights as a part of the solution. Perl and Hamill (2017) demonstrate how multinational food, soda, and alcohol giants are employing the same tactics that tobacco companies used to rely on, and require, the same careful rights-based contestation. Calls for the use of rights-based approaches are becoming more widespread. A review by Mann et al (2016) has investigated the role of rights-based approaches in care and treatment for mental health finding that human rights based approaches can be cost effective and lead to positive health outcomes. Other work investigating the role of rights-based approaches in health care for women and children has found that rights-based approaches are best understood across a spectrum of change that includes the individual, group, and society level (Thomas et al 2015).

Felner (2009) argues that a further challenge remains in terms of monitoring progressive realisation of economic, social, and cultural rights. Progressive realisation in the terms of the ICESCR is qualified by 'to the maximum of the state's available resources', which brings into play questions of resource prioritisation. Monitoring methods that focus on this area could provide powerful tools for social change, with Felner (2009) setting out a framework within which such monitoring could be located. It remains to be seen whether such an approach, and the more sophisticated methods he overviews briefly, including the use of econometric tools and economic models, are taken up by human rights activists and/or NHRIs.

Trends in increasing development of NHRIs have been mentioned as well as their increased integration into UN system; the full implications of this remain to be explored. There is also an increased emphasis on citizen education about human rights and on the further potential of human rights defenders. This is supported by the growing sections on the OHCHR website dedicated to human rights education, and the production of guides and resource books for use by concerned individuals, human rights defenders, or activists. For example, at global level, AHRC (2011) is a guide to using the Optional Protocol to CEDAW and other international complaint mechanisms; OHCHR (2008) is a handbook for civil society on working with the United Nations Human Rights Programme; Asher (2004) is a resource manual for NGOs on the right to health; and Asher and colleagues (2007) is a tool kit for health professionals on the right to health and their day-to-day work. There are also regional and national guides, for example, Kagoiya (2009) on women's rights in Africa, MacNeil (2011) on rights work with local government in South Africa and Tiwana et al. (2006) on Human Rights Commissions in India. Alongside this, an increasing discussion of human rights fieldwork as a profession can be identified, see for example, O'Flaherty and Ulrich (2010). WHO (2016) have produced the Innov8 framework to assist in identifying actions needed in the health system to achieve the SDGs, and Friedmann (2019) has described a rights-based approach for use in all health programs. The Danish Institute for Human Rights has developed two important websites to assist in operationalising a human rights-based approach to the implementation of sustainable development, in a manner that leaves no one behind: the Human Rights Guide to the SDGs (The Danish Institute for Human Rights 2019a), and the SDG-Human Rights Data Explorer (The Danish Institute for Human Rights 2019b).

The links between human rights and the social determinants of health are becoming increasingly recognised; Blas et al. (2011) examine social determinants approaches to public health and provide many examples of where programs and initiatives have justified their activities in terms of achievements of particular rights, and in some cases (Hargreaves et al. 2011) have used explicitly rights-based approaches. ILO (2011: 6) takes up the question of the "pivotal role of freedom of association in fostering and maintaining sustainable development" and illustrating this through examples taken from areas such as inclusive economic growth and poverty reduction, positive business environments, crisis response, and finally democracy and governance. Rasanathan and colleagues (2010) provide thoughtful discussions of some of the challenges and opportunities in taking this work further in the future.

Rights-based approaches have a potentially highly significant role to play in global health governance. Ooms (2011) analyses the global response to HIV/AIDS and argues that there is scope for developing a global social contract for health with its basis in the right to health. The WHO European Regional Office sees human rights as providing the 'value frame' within which its new regional health policy, Health 2020, will sit (EURO 2011). A coalition of civil society organisations and academics has initiated a program of work aimed at securing a global health agreement and supporting social mobilisation around the right to health (Gostin et al. 2011). In 2017, WHO signed a memorandum of understanding with the OHCHR.

Ng and Ruger (2011) argue that the state of global health governance evidenced in the literature was one beset by the continuance of problems such as insufficient coordination, dominance of narrow national and or organisational self-interest, insufficient participation, and resource shortage. This landscape has changed considerably as the different chapters in Meier and Gostin (2018) demonstrate, so that "the rights based approach is now seen as a principal normative framework for health-related policies, programs, and practices" (p. 569).

At the end of this book, it should be clear that rights-based approaches do not represent an easy solution to ensure universal achievement of human rights and the removal of health inequity under all circumstances. However, different examples of useful rights-based approaches have been identified, as have other examples of more qualified success. As the work of CARE International discussed at some length in Chapter 12 explicitly demonstrated, there may well be situations where it is not considered appropriate to use the language of rights.

Although human rights-based approaches do not provide the response to every challenge, they may represent one of the most useful frameworks we have in meeting the challenge of health inequities globally, nationally, and at local levels. The challenge for the future is to continue to develop these, and to disseminate them widely, both amongst health and social care or welfare professionals and amongst the general population. It remains to be seen exactly how far the potential provided by rights-based approaches can assist public health practitioners in working for health and social justice. Alston (2017: 14) summarises the challenges that we face today in achieving this goal and as he concludes: 'These are extraordinarily dangerous times, unprecedentedly so in my lifetime. Even during most of the Cold War there was a degree of certainty, but today we have lost much of that and almost anything seems possible. The response is really up to us.'

References

Ashrafian, H 2015a. AIonAI: A humanitarian law of artificial intelligence and robotics, *Science and Engineering Ethics*, 21(1): 29–40. doi.org/10.1007/s11948-013-9513-9

Ashrafian, H 2015b. Artificial intelligence and robot responsibilities: Innovating beyond rights, *Science and Engineering Ethics*, 21(2): 317–326. doi.org/10.1007/s11948-014-9541-0

AHRC 2011. *Mechanisms for Advancing Women's Human Rights: A Guide to Using the Optional Protocol to CEDAW and Other International Complaint Mechanisms*, Sydney: AHRC.

Alston, P 2017. The populist challenge to human rights, *Journal of Human Rights Practice*, 9: 1–15. doi.org/10.1093/jhuman/hux007

Asher, J 2004. *The Right to Health: A Resource Manual for NGOs*, London: Commonwealth Medical Trust.

Asher, J, Hamm, D, & Sheather, J 2007. *The Right to Health: A Toolkit for Health Professionals*, London: British Medical Association.

Birn, A-E, & Richter, J 2018. U.S. philanthrocapitalism and the global health agenda: The Rockefeller and Gates Foundations, past and present, in H Waitzkin & the Working Group for Health Beyond Capitalism (eds.) *Health Care Under the Knife: Moving Beyond Capitalism for Our Health*, New York: Monthly Review Press.

Bishop M, & Green, M 2009. *Philanthrocapitalism: How Giving Can Save the World*. New York: Bloomsbury Press. Available: http://philanthrocapitalism.net/about/faq/

Blas, E, Sommerfeld, J, & Kurup, AS (eds.) 2011. *Social Determinants Approaches to Public Health: From Concept to Practice*, Geneva: WHO.

Chapman, A 2016. Health and human rights in the neoliberal era, in *Global Health, Human Rights, and the Challenge of Neoliberal Policies*, Cambridge: Cambridge University Press. doi.org/10.1017/CBO9781316104576

Chapron, G, Epstein, Y, & López-Bao, JV 2019. A rights revolution for nature, *Science*, 363(6434): 1392–1393. doi.org/10.1126/science.aav5601

The Danish Institute for Human Rights 2019a. *The Human Rights Guide to the Sustainable Development Goals* [Online], Denmark. Available: sdg.humanrights.dk [Accessed 09/08/2019].

The Danish Institute for Human Rights 2019b. *SDG: Human Rights Data Explorer* [Online], Denmark. Available: https://sdgdata.humanrights.dk/en [Accessed 09/08/2019].

ENCO 2018. *The EU and the Corporate Impunity Nexus: Building the UN Binding Treaty on Transnational Corporations and Human Rights*, Amis de la Terre France, CETIM, Observatoire des multinationales, OMAL and the Transnational Institute (TNI). Available: www.tni.org/files/publication-downloads/the_eu_and_corporate_impunity_nexus.pdf [Accessed 25/04/2019].

EURO 2011. *Governance for Health in the 21st Century*, Copenhagen: WHO Regional Office for Europe, EUR/RC61/Inf.Doc./6.

Felner, E 2009. Closing the 'escape hatch': A toolkit to monitor the progressive realization of economic, social and cultural rights, *Journal of Human Rights Practice*, 1(3): 402–435. doi.org/10.1093/jhuman/hup023

Flues, F, & van Schaik, A 2018. *The EU's Double Agenda on Globalisation: Corporate Rights vs People's Rights*. Available: www.foeeurope.org/sites/default/files/corporate_accountability/2018/un_treaty_report_v5_screen.pdf [Accessed 25/04/2019].

Fox, AM, & Meier, BM 2009. Health as freedom: Addressing social determinants of global health inequities through the human right to development, *Bioethics*, 23(2): 112–122. doi.org/10.1111/j.1467-8519.2008.00718.x

Friedmann, EA 2019. *Health Equity Programs of Action: An Implementation Framework*, Georgetown: O'Neill Institute.

Freudenberg, N 2014. *Lethal but Legal: Corporations, Consumption, and Protecting Public Health*, New York, NY: Oxford University Press.

Gostin, LO, Friedman, EA, Ooms, G, Gebauer, T, Gupta, N, Sridhar, D, Chenguang, W, Rttingen, J, & Sanders, D 2011. The joint action and learning initiative: Towards a global agreement on national and global responsibilities for health, *PLOS Medicine*, 8(5): e1001031. doi.org/10.1371/journal.pmed.1001031

Hargreaves, J, Hatcher, A, Busza, J, Strange, V, Phetla, G, Kim, J, Watts, C, Morison, L, Porter, J, Pronyk, P, & Bonell, C 2011. What happens after a trial? Replicating a cross-sectoral intervention addressing the social determinants of health: The case of the Intervention with Microfinance for AIDS and Gender Equity (IMAGE) in South Africa, in E Blas, J Sommerfeld, & AS Kurup (eds.) *Social Determinants Approaches to Public Health: From Concept to Practice*, Geneva: WHO.

Hirono, K, Haigh, F, Gleeson, D, Harris, P, & Thow, AM 2015. *Negotiating Healthy Trade in Australia: Health Impact Assessment of the Proposed Trans-Pacific Partnership Agreement*, Liverpool, NSW: Centre for Health Equity Training Research and Evaluation, UNSW. Available: http://hiaconnect.edu.au/wp-content/uploads/2015/03/TPP_HIA.pdf [Accessed 26/04/2019].

Horton, R 2018. Offline: Global health and the private sector, *The Lancet*, 391: 2196. doi.org/10.1016/S0140-6736(18)31253-4

Humphreys, D 2017. Rights of Pachamama: The emergence of an earth jurisprudence in the Americas, *Journal of International Relations and Development*, 20(3): 459–484. doi.org/10.1057/s41268-016-0001-0

ILO 2011. *Freedom of Association and Development*, Geneva: ILO.

Jonsson, U 2003. *Human Rights Approach to Development Programming*, Nairobi: UNICEF.

Kagoiya, R (ed.) 2009. *Freedom of Information and Women's Rights in Africa*, Nairobi: African Women's Development and Communication Network.

Latham, J 2018. *The Gates Foundation's Ceres2030 Plan Pushes Agenda of Agribusiness*. Available: www.independentsciencenews.org/environment/the-gates-foundations-ceres2030-plan-pushes-agenda-of-agribusiness/ [Accessed 26/04/2019].

Macdonald, TH 2007. *The Global Human Right to Health: Dream or Possibility?*, Oxford: Radcliffe Publishing.

Macdonald, TH 2008. *Health, Human Rights and the United Nations: Inconsistent Aims and Inherent Contradictions?*, Oxford: Radcliffe Publishing.

MacNeil, C 2011. *Making Local Government Work: An Activist's Guide*, South Africa: Section27, Treatment Action Campaign and Read Hope Phillips. Available: www.localgovernmentaction.org [Accessed 01/09/2011].

Maloney, M 2015. Finally being heard: The great barrier reef and the international rights of nature tribunal, *Griffith Journal of Law & Human Dignity*, 3(1).

Mann, SP, Bradley, VJ, & Sahakian, BJ 2016. Human rights-based approaches to mental health: A review of programs, *Health and Human Rights*, 18(1): 263.

Meier, BM, & Gostin, LO (eds.) 2018. *Human Rights in Global Health: Rights-Based Governance for a Globalizing World*, Oxford: Oxford University Press. doi.org/10.1093/oso/9780190672676.003.0004

Moravcsik, A 2000. The origins of human rights regimes, *International Organization*, 54(2): 217–252. doi.org/10.1162/002081800551163

Munro, J 2009. Why states create international human rights mechanisms: The ASEAN intergovernmental commission on human rights and democratic lock-in theory, *Asia Pacific Journal on Human Rights and the Law*, 10(1): 1–26. doi.org/10.1163/138819009X12589762582493

Ng, NY, & Ruger, JP 2011. Global health governance at a crossroads, *Global Health Governance*, 4(2): 1–37. doi.org/10.1057/9780230299474_1

O'Flaherty, M, & Ulrich, G 2010. The professionalization of human rights field work, *Journal of Human Rights Practice*, 2(1): 1–27. doi.org/10.1093/jhuman/hup014

OHCHR 2008. *Working with the United Nations Human Rights Programme: A Handbook for Civil Society*, Geneva: OHCHR.

OHCHR 2018. *UN Human Rights Report 2017*, Geneva: OHCHR.

Ooms, G 2011. *Global Health: What Is Has Been so Far, What It Should be, and What It Could Become*, Studies in Health Services Organisation and Policy, Working paper no. 2, Antwerp: Institute of Tropical Medicine.

Pelizzon, A, & Gagliano, M 2015. The sentience of plants: Animal rights and the rights of plants intersecting?, *Australian Animal Protection Law Journal*, 11: 5–13.

Perl, R, & Hamill, S 2017. *NCD Advocacy Report: Fool me Twice*. Vital Strategies. Available: www.vitalstrategies.org/publications/fool-twice-ncd-advocacy-report/ [Accessed 11/12/2017].

Pimentel, DAV, Aymar, IM, & Lawson, M 2018. *Reward Work, Not Wealth*, Oxfam. Available: www.oxfam.org/en/research/reward-work-not-wealth [Accessed 16/04/2019].

Political Database of the Americas 2008. *Republic of Ecuador: Constitution of 2008*. [Online] Available: http://www.pdba.georgetown.edu/.Constitutions/Ecuador/ecu ador08.html [Accessed 08/02/2020].

Rasanathan, K, Norenhag, J, & Valentine, N 2010. Realizing human rights-based approaches for action on the social determinants of health, *Health and Human Rights*, 12(2): 49–59.

Raso, FA, Hilligoss, H, Krishnamurthy, V, Bavitz, C, & Kim, L 2018. *Artificial Intelligence & Human Rights: Opportunities & Risks*. Berkman Klein Center Research Publication, (2018–6). doi.org/10.2139/ssrn.3259344

Robertson, J 2014. Human rights vs. robot rights: Forecasts from Japan, *Critical Asian Studies*, 46(4): 571–598. doi.org/10.1080/14672715.2014.960707

Rumbold, B, Baker, R, Ferraz, O, Hawkes, S, Krubiner, C, Littlejohns, P, Norheim, OF, Pegram, T, Rid, A, Venkatapuram, S, Voorhoeve, A, Wang, D, Weale, A, Wilson, J, & Sarelin, AL 2007. Human rights-based approaches to development cooperation, HIV/ AIDS, and food security, *Human Rights Quarterly*, 29(2): 460–488. doi.org/10.1353/hrq.2007.0022

Schwitzgebel, E, & Garza, M 2015. A defense of the rights of artificial intelligences, *Midwest Studies in Philosophy*, 39(1): 98–119. doi.org/10.1111/misp.12032

Simmons, B 2002. *Why Commit? Explaining State Acceptance of International Human Rights Obligations*, Cambridge, MA: Weatherhead Center for International Affairs, Harvard University. doi.org/10.1002/sres.2532

Stephens, A, Taket, A, & Gagliano, M 2019. Ecological justice for nature in critical systems thinking, *Systems Research and Behavioral Science*, 36(1): 3–19.

Stiglitz, J 2006. *Making Globalisation Work*, Harmondsworth: Penguin.

Taket, AR 2012. *Health Equity, Social Justice and Human Rights*, Routledge. London.

The Hindu 2018. Uttarakhand HC Declares Animals to be 'Legal Persons', *The Hindu*. Available: www.thehindu.com/news/national/uttarakhand-hc-declares-animals-to-be-legal-persons/article24335973.ece [Accessed 03/05/2019].

Thomas, R, Kuruvilla, S, Hinton, R, Jensen, SL, Magar, V, & Bustreo, F 2015. Assessing the impact of a human rights-based approach across a spectrum of change for women's, children's, and adolescents' health, *Health & Human Rights: An International Journal*, 17(2).

Tiwana, M, Aurora, S, & Punj, A 2006. *Human Rights Commissions: A Citizen's Handbook*, New Delhi: Commonwealth Human Rights Initiative.

UN Secretary-General 2018. *Leveraging the AIDS Response for United Nations Reform and Global Health, Report of the Secretary-General*, A/72/815, New York: UN.

UNAIDS 2019. *No End to AIDS Without Respecting Human Rights*. Available: www.unaids.org/en/keywords/travel-restrictions [Accessed 09/08/2019].

Watts, N et al 2018a. The Lancet Countdown on health and climate change: From 25 years of inaction to a global transformation for public health, *The Lancet*, 392: 2479–2514. doi.org/10.1016/S0140-6736(17)32464-9

Watts, N et al 2018b. The 2018 report of the Lancet Countdown on health and climate change: Shaping the health of nations for centuries to come, *The Lancet*, 391: 581–586.

WHO 2002. *25 Questions and Answers on Health and Human Rights*, Geneva: World Health Organization.

WHO 2016. *Innov8 Approach for Reviewing National Health Programmes*, Geneva: WHO.

NOTES ON SOURCES

Throughout a number of chapters in this book, in discussing the basic history and structures of human rights systems use has been made of websites and a few key references. Rather than compromise the readability of the text by attempting to reference each point explicitly, basic notes on these sources are provided here. Sources specific to chapters are listed in those chapters.

References

Alfreðsson, GS, & Tomaševski, K (eds.) 1998. *A Thematic Guide to Documents on Health and Human Rights: Global and Regional Standards Adopted by Intergovernmental Organizations, International Non-Governmental Organizations and Professional Associations*, Vol. 2, Leiden, Netherlands: Martinus Nijhoff Publishers.

Flynn, MM, Garkawe, S, & Holt, YJ 2011. *Human Rights: Treaties, Statutes, and Cases*, New York: LexisNexis Butterworths.

Levinson, D (ed.) 2003. *The Wilson chronology of Human Rights*. New York: H.W. Wilson Company.

Marks, S 2006. *Health and Human Rights: Basic International Documents*, 2nd edn, Cambridge: François-Xavier Bagnoud Center for Health and Human Rights, Harvard School of Public Health.

Office of the United Nations High Commissioner for Human Rights 2002. *Human Rights: A Compilation of International Instruments: Universal Instruments*, 2 Vols, New York: United Nations.

APPENDIX

The UDHR

Preamble

Whereas recognition of the inherent dignity and of the equal and inalienable rights of all members of the human family is the foundation of freedom, justice and peace in the world,

Whereas disregard and contempt for human rights have resulted in barbarous acts which have outraged the conscience of mankind, and the advent of a world in which human beings shall enjoy freedom of speech and belief and freedom from fear and want has been proclaimed as the highest aspiration of the common people,

Whereas it is essential, if man is not to be compelled to have recourse, as a last resort, to rebellion against tyranny and oppression, that human rights should be protected by the rule of law,

Whereas it is essential to promote the development of friendly relations between nations,

Whereas the peoples of the United Nations have in the Charter reaffirmed their faith in fundamental human rights, in the dignity and worth of the human person and in the equal rights of men and women and have determined to promote social progress and better standards of life in larger freedom,

Whereas Member States have pledged themselves to achieve, in cooperation with the United Nations, the promotion of universal respect for and observance of human rights and fundamental freedoms,

Whereas a common understanding of these rights and freedoms is of the greatest importance for the full realization of this pledge,

Now, Therefore THE GENERAL ASSEMBLY proclaims THIS UNIVERSAL DECLARATION OF HUMAN RIGHTS as a common standard of achievement for all peoples and all nations, to the end that every individual and every organ of society, keeping this Declaration constantly in mind, shall strive by teaching and education to promote respect for these rights and freedoms and by progressive measures, national and international, to secure their universal and effective recognition and observance, both among the peoples of Member States themselves and among the peoples of territories under their jurisdiction.

Article I All human beings are born free and equal in dignity and rights. They are endowed with reason and conscience and should act towards one another in a spirit of brotherhood.

Article 2 Everyone is entitled to all the rights and freedoms set forth in this Declaration, without distinction of any kind, such as race, colour, sex, language, religion, political or other opinion, national or social origin, property, birth or other status. Furthermore, no distinction shall be made on the basis of the political, jurisdictional or international status of the country or territory to which a person belongs, whether it be independent, trust, non-self-governing or under any other limitation of sovereignty.

Article 3 Everyone has the right to life, liberty and security of person.

Article 4 No one shall be held in slavery or servitude; slavery and the slave trade shall be prohibited in all their forms.

Article 5 No one shall be subjected to torture or to cruel, inhuman or degrading treatment or punishment.

Article 6 Everyone has the right to recognition everywhere as a person before the law.

Article 7 All are equal before the law and are entitled without any discrimination to equal protection of the law. All are entitled to equal protection against any discrimination in violation of this Declaration and against any incitement to such discrimination.

Article 8 Everyone has the right to an effective remedy by the competent national tribunals for acts violating the fundamental rights granted him by the constitution or by law.

Article 9 No one shall be subjected to arbitrary arrest, detention or exile.

Article 10 Everyone is entitled in full equality to a fair and public hearing by an independent and impartial tribunal, in the determination of his rights and obligations and of any criminal charge against him.

Article 11

1   Everyone charged with a penal offence has the right to be presumed innocent until proved guilty according to law in a public trial at which he has had all the guarantees necessary for his defence.

2   No one shall be held guilty of any penal offence on account of any act or omission which did not constitute a penal offence, under national or international law, at the time when it was committed. Nor shall a heavier penalty be imposed than the one that was applicable at the time the penal offence was committed.

Article 12 No one shall be subjected to arbitrary interference with his privacy, family, home or correspondence, nor to attacks upon his honour and reputation. Everyone has the right to the protection of the law against such interference or attacks.

Article 13

1   Everyone has the right to freedom of movement and residence within the borders of each State.

2   Everyone has the right to leave any country, including his own, and to return to his country.

Article 14

1   Everyone has the right to seek and to enjoy in other countries asylum from persecution.

2   This right may not be invoked in the case of prosecutions genuinely arising from non-political crimes or from acts contrary to the purposes and principles of the United Nations.

Article 15

1   Everyone has the right to a nationality.

2   No one shall be arbitrarily deprived of his nationality nor denied the right to change his nationality.

Article 16

1   Men and women of full age, without any limitation due to race, nationality or religion, have the right to marry and to found a family. They are entitled to equal rights as to marriage, during marriage and at its dissolution.

2   Marriage shall be entered into only with the free and full consent of the intending spouses.

3   The family is the natural and fundamental group unit of society and is entitled to protection by society and the State.

Article 17

1   Everyone has the right to own property alone as well as in association with others.

2   No one shall be arbitrarily deprived of his property.

Article 18 Everyone has the right to freedom of thought, conscience and religion; this right includes freedom to change his religion or belief, and freedom, either alone or in community with others and in public or private, to manifest his religion or belief in teaching, practice, worship and observance.

Article 19 Everyone has the right to freedom of opinion and expression; this right includes freedom to hold opinions without interference and to seek, receive and impart information and ideas through any media and regardless of frontiers.

Article 20

1   Everyone has the right to freedom of peaceful assembly and association.

2   No one may be compelled to belong to an association.

Article 21

1   Everyone has the right to take part in the government of his country, directly or through freely chosen representatives.

2   Everyone has the right to equal access to public service in his country.

3   The will of the people shall be the basis of the authority of government; this will shall be expressed in periodic and genuine elections which shall be by universal and equal suffrage and shall be held by secret vote or by equivalent free voting procedures.

Article 22 Everyone, as a member of society, has the right to social security and is entitled to realization, through national effort and international cooperation and in accordance with the organization and resources of each State, of the economic, social and cultural rights indispensable for his dignity and the free development of his personality.

Article 23

1   Everyone has the right to work, to free choice of employment, to just and favourable conditions of work and to protection against unemployment.

2   Everyone, without any discrimination, has the right to equal pay for equal work.

3   Everyone who works has the right to just and favourable remuneration ensuring for himself and his family an existence worthy of human dignity, and supplemented, if necessary, by other means of social protection.

4   Everyone has the right to form and to join trade unions for the protection of his interests.

Article 24 Everyone has the right to rest and leisure, including reasonable limitation of working hours and periodic holidays with pay.

Article 25

1   Everyone has the right to a standard of living adequate for the health and well-being of himself and of his family, including food, clothing, housing and medical care and necessary social services, and the right to security in the event of unemployment, sickness, disability, widowhood, old age or other lack of livelihood in circumstances beyond his control.

2   Motherhood and childhood are entitled to special care and assistance. All children, whether born in or out of wedlock, shall enjoy the same social protection.

Article 26

1   Everyone has the right to education. Education shall be free, at least in the elementary and fundamental stages. Elementary education shall be compulsory. Technical and professional education shall be made generally available and higher education shall be equally accessible to all on the basis of merit.

2   Education shall be directed to the full development of the human personality and to the strengthening of respect for human rights and fundamental

freedoms. It shall promote understanding, tolerance and friendship among all nations, racial or religious groups, and shall further the activities of the United Nations for the maintenance of peace.

3 Parents have a prior right to choose the kind of education that shall be given to their children.

Article 27

1 Everyone has the right freely to participate in the cultural life of the community, to enjoy the arts and to share in scientific advancement and its benefits.

2 Everyone has the right to the protection of the moral and material interests resulting from any scientific, literary or artistic production of which he is the author.

Article 28 Everyone is entitled to a social and international order in which the rights and freedoms set forth in this Declaration can be fully realized.

Article 29

1 Everyone has duties to the community in which alone the free and full development of his personality is possible.

2 In the exercise of his rights and freedoms, everyone shall be subject only to such limitations as are determined by law solely for the purpose of securing due recognition and respect for the rights and freedoms of others and of meeting the just requirements of morality, public order and the general welfare in a democratic society.

3 These rights and freedoms may in no case be exercised contrary to the purposes and principles of the United Nations.

Article 30 Nothing in this Declaration may be interpreted as implying for any State, group or person any right to engage in any activity or to perform any act aimed at the destruction of any of the rights and freedoms set forth herein.

From the Universal Declaration of Human Rights, by The United Nations General Assembly, ©1948 United Nations. Reprinted with the permission of the United Nations.

INDEX